Springer Texts in Statistics

Series editors

R. DeVeaux
S. Fienberg
I. Olkin

More information about this series at http://www.springer.com/series/417

Richard A. Berk

Statistical Learning from a Regression Perspective

Second Edition

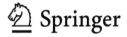 Springer

Richard A. Berk
Department of Statistics
The Wharton School
University of Pennsylvania
Philadelphia, PA
USA

and

Department of Criminology
Schools of Arts and Sciences
University of Pennsylvania
Philadelphia, PA
USA

ISSN 1431-875X   ISSN 2197-4136   (electronic)
Springer Texts in Statistics
ISBN 978-3-319-44047-7   ISBN 978-3-319-44048-4   (eBook)
DOI 10.1007/978-3-319-44048-4

Library of Congress Control Number: 2016948105

This Springer imprint is published by Springer Nature
The registered company is Springer International Publishing AG Switzerland

*In God we trust. All others
must have data.*

W. Edwards Deming

In memory of Peter H. Rossi,
a mentor, colleague, and friend

Preface to the Second Edition

Over the past 8 years, the topics associated with statistical learning have been expanded and consolidated. They have been expanded because new problems have been tackled, new tools have been developed, and older tools have been refined. They have been consolidated because many unifying concepts and themes have been identified. It has also become more clear from practice which statistical learning tools will be widely applied and which are likely to see limited service. In short, it seems this is the time to revisit the material and make it more current.

There are currently several excellent textbook treatments of statistical learning and its very close cousin, machine learning. The second edition of *Elements of Statistical Learning* by Hastie, Tibshirani, and Friedman (2009) is in my view still the gold standard, but there are other treatments that in their own way can be excellent. Examples include *Machine Learning: A Probabilistic Perspective* by Kevin Murphy (2012), *Principles and Theory for Data Mining and Machine Learning* by Clarke, Fokoué, and Zhang (2009), and *Applied Predictive Modeling* by Kuhn and Johnson (2013).

Yet, it is sometimes difficult to appreciate from these treatments that a proper application of statistical learning is comprised of (1) data collection, (2) data management, (3) data analysis, and (4) interpretation of results. The first entails finding and acquiring the data to be analyzed. The second requires putting the data into an accessible form. The third depends on extracting instructive patterns from the data. The fourth calls for making sense of those patterns. For example, a statistical learning data analysis might begin by collecting information from "rap sheets" and other kinds of official records about prison inmates who have been released on parole. The information obtained might be organized so that arrests were nested within individuals. At that point, support vector machines could be used to classify offenders into those who re-offend after release on parole and those who do not. Finally, the classes obtained might be employed to forecast subsequent re-offending when the actual outcome is not known. Although there is a chronological sequence to these activities, one must anticipate later steps as earlier steps are undertaken. Will the offender classes, for instance, include or exclude juvenile offenses or vehicular offenses? How this is decided will affect the choice of statistical learning tools, how they are implemented, and how they are interpreted. Moreover, the preferred statistical learning procedures anticipated place constraints on how the offenses are coded, while the ways in which the results are likely to be used affect how the procedures are tuned. In short, no single activity should be considered in isolation from the other three.

Nevertheless, textbook treatments of statistical learning (and statistics textbooks more generally) focus on the third step: the statistical procedures. This can make good sense if the treatments are to be of manageable length and within the authors' expertise, but risks the misleading impression that once the key statistical theory is understood, one is ready to proceed with data. The result can be a fancy statistical analysis as a bridge to nowhere. To reprise an aphorism attributed to Albert Einstein: "In theory, theory and practice are the same. In practice they are not."

The commitment to practice as well as theory will sometimes engender considerable frustration. There are times when the theory is not readily translated into practice. And there are times when practice, even practice that seems intuitively sound, will have no formal justification. There are also important open questions leaving large holes in procedures one would like to apply. A particular problem is statistical inference, especially for procedures that proceed in an inductive manner. In effect, they capitalize on "data snooping," which can invalidate estimation, confidence intervals, and statistical tests.

In the first edition, statistical tools characterized as supervised learning were the main focus. But a serious effort was made to establish links to data collection, data management, and proper interpretation of results. That effort is redoubled in this edition. At the same time, there is a price. No claims are made for anything like an encyclopedic coverage of supervised learning, let alone of the underlying statistical theory. There are books available that take the encyclopedic approach, which can have the feel of a trip through Europe spending 24 hours in each of the major cities.

Here, the coverage is highly selective. Over the past decade, the wide range of real applications has begun to sort the enormous variety of statistical learning tools into those primarily of theoretical interest or in early stages of development, the niche players, and procedures that have been successfully and widely applied (Jordan and Mitchell, 2015). Here, the third group is emphasized.

Even among the third group, choices need to be made. The statistical learning material addressed reflects the subject-matter fields with which I am more familiar. As a result, applications in the social and policy sciences are emphasized. This is a pity because there are truly fascinating applications in the natural sciences and engineering. But in the words of Dirty Harry: "A man's got to know his limitations" (from the movie *Magnum Force*, 1973).[1] My several forays into natural science applications do not qualify as real expertise.

---

[1]"Dirty" Harry Callahan was a police detective played by Clint Eastwood in five movies filmed during the 1970s and 1980s. Dirty Harry was known for his strong-armed methods and blunt catch-phrases, many of which are now ingrained in American popular culture.

The second edition retains it commitment to the statistical programming language R. If anything the commitment is stronger. R provides access to state-of-the-art statistics, including those needed for statistical learning. It is also now a standard training component in top departments of statistics so for many readers, applications of the statistical procedures discussed will come quite naturally. Where it could be useful, I now include the R-code needed when the usual R documentation may be insufficient. That code is written to be accessible. Often there will be more elegant, or at least more efficient, ways to proceed. When practical, I develop examples using data that can be downloaded from one of the R libraries. But, R is a moving target. Code that runs now may not run in the future. In the year it took to complete this edition, many key procedures were updated several times, and there were three updates of R itself. *Caveat emptor.* Readers will also notice that the graphical output from the many procedures used do not have common format or color scheme. In some cases, it would have been very difficult to force a common set of graphing conventions, and it is probably important to show a good approximation of the default output in any case. Aesthetics and common formats can be a casualty.

In summary, the second edition retains its emphasis on supervised learning that can be treated as a form of regression analysis. Social science and policy applications are prominent. Where practical, substantial links are made to data collection, data management, and proper interpretation of results, some of which can raise ethical concerns (Dwork et al., 2011; Zemel et al., 2013). I hope it works.

The first chapter has been rewritten almost from scratch in part from experience I have had trying to teach the material. It much better reflects new views about unifying concepts and themes. I think the chapter also gets to punch lines more quickly and coherently. But readers who are looking for simple recipes will be disappointed. The exposition is by design not "point-and-click." There is as well some time spent on what some statisticians call "meta-issues." A good data analyst must know what to compute and what to make of the computed results. How to compute is important, but by itself is nearly purposeless.

All of the other chapters have also been revised and updated with an eye toward far greater clarity. In many places greater clarity was sorely needed. I now appreciate much better how difficult it can be to translate statistical concepts and notation into plain English. Where I have still failed, please accept my apology.

I have also tried to take into account that often a particular chapter is downloaded and read in isolation. Because much of the material is cumulative, working through a single chapter can on occasion create special challenges. I have tried to include text to help, but for readers working cover to cover, there are necessarily some redundancies, and annoying pointers to material in other chapters. I hope such readers will be patient with me.

I continue to be favored with remarkable colleagues and graduate students. My professional life is one ongoing tutorial in statistics, thanks to Larry Brown, Andreas Buja, Linda Zhao, and Ed George. All four are as collegial as they are smart. I have learned a great deal as well from former students Adam Kapelner, Justin Bleich, Emil Pitkin, Kai Zhang, Dan McCarthy, and Kory Johnson. Arjun

Gupta checked the exercises at the end of each chapter. Finally, there are the many students who took my statistics classes and whose questions got me to think a lot harder about the material. Thanks to them as well.

But I would probably not have benefited nearly so much from all the talent around me were it not for my earlier relationship with David Freedman. He was my bridge from routine calculations within standard statistical packages to a far better appreciation of the underlying foundations of modern statistics. He also reinforced my skepticism about many statistical applications in the social and biomedical sciences. Shortly before he died, David asked his friends to "keep after the rascals." I certainly have tried.

Philadelphia, PA, USA   Richard A. Berk

example, the interaction patterns among children at school: who plays with whom. These too are not discussed.

Other topics can be considered regression analysis only as a formality. For example, a common data mining application in marketing is to extract from the purchasing behavior of individual shoppers patterns that can be used to forecast future purchases. But there are no predictors in the usual regression sense. The conditioning is on each individual shopper. The question is not what features of shoppers predict what they will purchase, but what a given shopper is likely to purchase.

Finally, there are a large number of procedures that focus on the conditional distribution of the response, much as with any regression analysis, but with little attention to how the predictors are related to the response (Horváth and Yamamoto, 2006; Camacho et al., 2006). Such procedures neglect a key feature of regression analysis, at least as discussed in this book, and are not considered. That said, there is no principled reason in many cases why the role of each predictor could not be better represented, and perhaps in the near future that shortcoming will be remedied.

In short, although using a regression framework implies a big-tent approach to the topics included, it is not an exhaustive tent. Many interesting and powerful tools are not discussed. Where appropriate, however, references to that material are provided.

I may have gone a bit overboard with the number of citations I provide. The relevant literatures are changing and growing rapidly. Today's breakthrough can be tomorrow's bust, and work that by current thinking is uninteresting can be the spark for dramatic advances in the future. At any given moment, it can be difficult to determine which is which. In response, I have attempted to provide a rich mix of background material, even at the risk of not being sufficiently selective. (And I have probably missed some useful papers nevertheless.)

In the material that follows, I have tried to use consistent notation. This has proved to be very difficult because of important differences in the conceptual traditions represented and the complexity of statistical tools discussed. For example, it is common to see the use of the expected value operator even when the data cannot be characterized as a collection of random variables and when the sole goal is description.

I draw where I can from the notation used in *The Elements of Statistical Learning* (Hastie et al., 2001). Thus, the symbol X is used for an input variable, or predictor in statistical parlance. When X is a set of inputs to be treated as a vector, each component is indexed by a subscript (e.g., X_j). Quantitative outputs, also called response variables, are represented by Y, and categorical outputs, another kind of response variable, are represented by G with K categories. Upper case letters are used to refer to variables in a general way, with details to follow as needed. Sometimes these variables are treated as random variables, and sometimes not. I try to make that clear in context.

Observed values are shown in lower case, usually with a subscript. Thus x_i is the ith observed value for the variable X. Sometimes these observed values are nothing more than the data on hand. Sometimes they are realizations of random variables. Again, I try to make this clear in context.

Matrices are represented in bold uppercase. For example, in matrix form the usual set of p predictors, each with N observations, is an $N \times p$ matrix $\mathbf{X}$. The subscript i is generally used for observations and the subscript j for variables. Bold lowercase letters are used for vectors with N elements, commonly columns of X. Other vectors are generally not represented in boldface fonts, but again, I try to make this clear in context.

If one treats Y as a random variable, its observed values y are either a random sample from a population or a realization of a stochastic process. The conditional means of the random variable Y for various configurations of X-values are commonly referred to as "expected values," and are either the conditional means of Y for different configurations of $\mathbf{X}$-values in the population or for the stochastic process by which the data were generated. A common notation is $E(Y|X)$. The $E(Y|X)$ is also often called a "parameter." The conditional means computed from the data are often called "sample statistics," or in this case, "sample means." In the regression context, the sample means are commonly referred to as the fitted values, often written as $\hat{y}|X$. Subscripting can follow as already described.

Unfortunately, after that it gets messier. First, I often have to decipher the intent in the notation used by others. No doubt I sometimes get it wrong. For example, it is often unclear if a computer algorithm is formally meant to be an estimator or a descriptor.

Second, there are some complications in representing nested realizations of the same variable (as in the bootstrap), or model output that is subject to several different chance processes. There is a practical limit to the number and types of bars, asterisks, hats, and tildes one can effectively use. I try to provide warnings (and apologies) when things get cluttered.

There are also some labeling issues. When I am referring to the general linear model (i.e., linear regression, analysis of variance, and analysis of covariance), I use the terms classical linear regression, or conventional linear regression. All regressions in which the functional forms are determined before the fitting process begins, I call parametric. All regressions in which the functional forms are determined as part of the fitting process, I call nonparametric. When there is some of both, I call the regressions semiparametric. Sometimes the lines among parametric, nonparametric, and semiparametric are fuzzy, but I try to make clear what I mean in context. Although these naming conventions are roughly consistent with much common practice, they are not universal.

All of the computing done for this book was undertaken in R. R is a programming language designed for statistical computing and graphics. It has become a major vehicle for developmental work in statistics and is increasingly being used by practitioners. A key reason for relying on R for this book is that most of the newest developments in statistical learning and related fields can be found in R. Another reason is that it is free.

Readers familiar with S or S-plus will immediately feel at home; R is basically a "dialect" of S. For others, there are several excellent books providing a good introduction to data analysis using R. Dalgaard (2002), Crawley (2007), and Maindonald and Braun (2007) are all very accessible. Readers who are especially interested in graphics should consult Murrell (2006). The most useful R website can be found at http://www.r-project.org/.

The use of R raises the question of how much R-code to include. The R-code used to construct all of the applications in the book could be made available. However, detailed code is largely not shown. Many of the procedures used are somewhat in flux. Code that works one day may need some tweaking the next. As an alternative, the procedures discussed are identified as needed so that detailed information about how to proceed in R can be easily obtained from R help commands or supporting documentation. When the data used in this book are proprietary or otherwise not publicly available, similar data and appropriate R-code are substituted.

There are exercises at the end of each chapter. They are meant to be hands-on data analyses built around R. As such, they require some facility with R. However, the goals of each problem are reasonably clear so that other software and datasets can be used. Often the exercises can be usefully repeated with different datasets.

The book has been written so that later chapters depend substantially on earlier chapters. For example, because classification and regression trees (CART) can be an important component of boosting, it may be difficult to follow the discussion of boosting without having read the earlier chapter on CART. However, readers who already have a solid background in material covered earlier should have little trouble skipping ahead. The notation and terms used are reasonably standard or can be easily figured out. In addition, the final chapter can be read at almost any time. One reviewer suggested that much of the material could be usefully brought forward to Chap. 1.

Finally, there is the matter of tone. The past several decades have seen the development of a dizzying array of new statistical procedures, sometimes introduced with the hype of a big-budget movie. Advertising from major statistical software providers has typically made things worse. Although there have been genuine and useful advances, none of the techniques have ever lived up to their most optimistic billing. Widespread misuse has further increased the gap between promised performance and actual performance. In this book, therefore, the tone will be cautious, some might even say dark. I hope this will not discourage readers from engaging seriously with the material. The intent is to provide a balanced discussion of the limitations as well as the strengths of the statistical learning procedures.

While working on this book, I was able to rely on support from several sources. Much of the work was funded by a grant from the National Science Foundation: SES-0437169, "Ensemble Methods for Data Analysis in the Behavioral, Social and Economic Sciences." The first draft was completed while I was on sabbatical at the Department of Earth, Atmosphere, and Oceans, at the Ecole Normale Supérieur in Paris. The second draft was completed after I moved from UCLA to the University of Pennsylvania. All three locations provided congenial working environments. Most important, I benefited enormously from discussions about statistical learning with colleagues at UCLA, Penn and elsewhere: Larry Brown, Andreas Buja, Jan de

Leeuw, David Freedman, Mark Hansen, Andy Liaw, Greg Ridgeway, Bob Stine, Mikhail Traskin and Adi Wyner. Each is knowledgeable, smart and constructive. I also learned a great deal from several very helpful, anonymous reviews. Dick Koch was enormously helpful and patient when I had problems making TeXShop perform properly. Finally, I have benefited over the past several years from interacting with talented graduate students: Yan He, Weihua Huang, Brian Kriegler, and Jie Shen. Brian Kriegler deserves a special thanks for working through the exercises at the end of each chapter.

Certain datasets and analyses were funded as part of research projects undertaken for the California Policy Research Center, The Inter-America Tropical Tuna Commission, the National Institute of Justice, the County of Los Angeles, the California Department of Correction and Rehabilitation, the Los Angeles Sheriff's Department, and the Philadelphia Department of Adult Probation and Parole. Support from all of these sources is gratefully acknowledged.

Philadelphia, PA   Richard A. Berk
2006

The original version of the book was revised:
Belated corrections have been incorporated.
The erratum to the book is available at https://
doi.org/10.1007/978-3-319-44048-4_10

Contents

Chapter 1
Statistical Learning as a Regression Problem

Before getting into the material, it may be important to reprise and expand a bit on three points made in the first and second prefaces — most people do not read prefaces. First, any credible statistical analysis combines sound data collection, intelligent data management, an appropriate application of statistical procedures, and an accessible interpretation of results. This is sometimes what is meant by "analytics." More is involved than applied statistics. Most statistical textbooks focus on the statistical procedures alone, which can lead some readers to assume that if the technical background for a particular set of statistical tools is well understood, a sensible data analysis automatically follows. But as some would say, "That dog won't hunt."

Second, the coverage is highly selective. There are many excellent encyclopedic, textbook treatments of machine/statistical learning. Topics that some of them cover in several pages, are covered here in an entire chapter. Data collection, data management, formal statistics, and interpretation are woven into the discussion where feasible. But there is a price. The range of statistical procedures covered is limited. Space constraints alone dictate hard choices. The procedures emphasized are those that can be framed as a form of regression analysis, have already proved to be popular, and have been throughly battle tested. Some readers may disagree with the choices made. For those readers, there are ample references in which other materials are well addressed.

Third, the ocean liner is slowly starting to turn. Over the past decade, the 50 years of largely unrebutted criticisms of conventional regression models and extensions have started to take. One reason is that statisticians have been providing useful alternatives. Another reason is the growing impact of computer science on how data are analyzed. Models are less salient in computer science than in statistics, and

---

The original version of this chapter was revised: See the "Chapter Note" section at the end of this chapter for details. The erratum to this chapter is available at https://doi.org/10.1007/978-3-319-44048-4_10.

© Springer International Publishing Switzerland 2016
R.A. Berk, *Statistical Learning from a Regression Perspective*,
Springer Texts in Statistics, DOI 10.1007/978-3-319-44048-4_1

far less salient than in popular forms of data analysis. Yet another reason is the
growing and successful use of randomized controlled trials, which is implicitly an
admission that far too much was expected from causal modeling. Finally, many of the
most active and visible econometricians have been turning to various forms of quasi-
experimental designs and methods of analysis in part because conventional modeling
often has been unsatisfactory. The pages ahead will draw heavily on these important
trends.

1.1 Getting Started

As a first approximation, one can think of statistical learning as the "muscle car" version of Exploratory Data Analysis (EDA). Just as in EDA, the data can be approached
with relatively little prior information and examined in a highly inductive manner.
Knowledge discovery can be a key goal. But thanks to the enormous developments
in computing power and computer algorithms over the past two decades, it is possible to extract information that would have previously been inaccessible. In addition,
because statistical learning has evolved in a number of different disciplines, its goals
and approaches are far more varied than conventional EDA.

In this book, the focus is on statistical learning procedures that can be understood
within a regression framework. For a wide variety of applications, this will not pose
a significant constraint and will greatly facilitate the exposition. The researchers in
statistics, applied mathematics and computer science responsible for most statistical
learning techniques often employ their own distinct jargon and have a penchant for
attaching cute, but somewhat obscure, labels to their products: bagging, boosting,
bundling, random forests, and others. There is also widespread use of acronyms:
CART, LOESS, MARS, MART, LARS, LASSO, and many more. A regression
framework provides a convenient and instructive structure in which these procedures
can be more easily understood.

After a discussion of how statisticians think about regression analysis, this chapter
introduces a number of key concepts and raises broader issues that reappear in later
chapters. It may be a little difficult for some readers to follow parts of the discussion,
or its motivation, the first time around. However, later chapters will flow far better
with some of this preliminary material on the table, and readers are encouraged to
return to the chapter as needed.

1.2 Setting the Regression Context

We begin by defining regression analysis. A common conception in many academic
disciplines and policy applications equates regression analysis with some special case
of the generalized Linear model: normal (linear) regression, binomial regression,
Poisson regression, or other less common forms. Sometimes, there is more than
one such equation, as in hierarchical models when the regression coefficients in one
equation can be expressed as responses within other equations, or when a set of

Fig. 1.1 Birthweight by
mother's weight (*Open
circles* are the data, *filled
circles* are the conditional
means, the *solid line* is a
linear regression fit, the
dashed line is a fit by a
smoother. $N = 189$.)

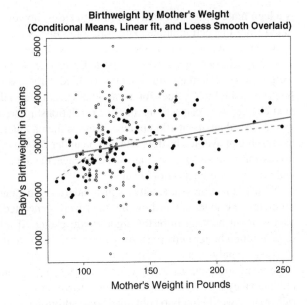

equations is linked though their response variables. For any of these formulations, inferences are often made beyond the data to some larger finite population or a data generation process. Commonly these inferences are combined with statistical tests and confidence intervals. It is also popular to overlay causal interpretations meant to convey how the response distribution would change if one or more of the predictors were independently manipulated.

But statisticians and computer scientists typically start farther back. Regression is "just" about conditional distributions. The goal is to understand "as far as possible with the available data how the conditional distribution of some response y varies across subpopulations determined by the possible values of the predictor or predictors" (Cook and Weisberg 1999: 27). That is, interest centers on the distribution of the response variable Y conditioning on one or more predictors X. Regression analysis fundamentally is the about conditional distributions: $Y|X$.

For example, Fig. 1.1 is a conventional scatter plot for an infant's birth weight in grams and the mother's weight in pounds.[1] Birthweight can be an important indicator of a newborn's viability, and there is reason to believe that birthweight depends in part on the health of the mother. A mother's weight can be an indicator of her health.

In Fig. 1.1, the open circles are the observations. The filled circles are the conditional means and the likely summary statistics of interest. An inspection of the pattern of observations is by itself a legitimate regression analysis. Does the conditional distribution of birthweight vary depending on the mother's weight? If the conditional mean is chosen as the key summary statistic, one can consider whether the conditional means for infant birthweight vary with the mother's weight. This too

---

[1] The data, *birthwt*, are from the MASS package in R.

is a legitimate regression analysis. In both cases, however, it is difficult to conclude much from inspection alone. The solid blue line is a linear least squares fit of the data. On the average, birthweight increases with the mother's weight, but the slope is modest (about 44 g for every 10 pounds), especially given the spread of the birth-weight values. For many, this is a familiar kind of regression analysis. The dashed red line shows the fitted values for a smoother (i.e., lowess) that will be discussed in the next chapter. One can see that the linear relationship breaks down when the mother weighs less than about 100 pounds. There is then a much stronger relationship with the result that average birthweight can be under 2000 g (i.e., around 4 pounds). This regression analysis suggests that on the average, the relationship between birthweight and mother's weights is nonlinear.

None of the regression analyses just undertaken depend on a "generative" model; no claims are made about how the data were generated. There are also no causal claims about how mean birthweight would change if a mother's weight is altered (e.g., through better nutrition). And, there is no statistical inference whatsoever. The regression analyses apply solely to the data on hand and are not generalized to some large set of observations. A regression analysis may be enhanced by such extensions, although they do not go to the core of how regression analysis is defined. In practice, a richer story would likely be obtained were additional predictors introduced, perhaps as "controls," but that too is not a formal requirement of regression analysis. Finally, visualizations of various kinds can be instructive and by themselves can constitute a regression analysis.

The same reasoning applies should the response be categorical. Figure 1.2 is a spine plot that dichotomizes birth weight into two categories: low and not low. For each decile of mothers' weights, the conditional proportions are plotted. For example, if a mother's weight is between 150 and 170 pounds, a little under 20 % of the

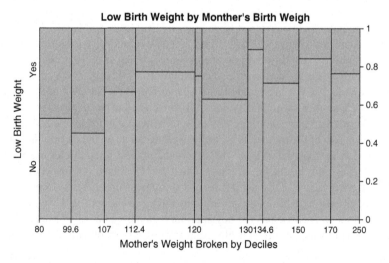

Fig. 1.2 Low birth weight by mother's weight with birth weight dichotomized (Mother's weight is binned by deciles. $N = 189$.)

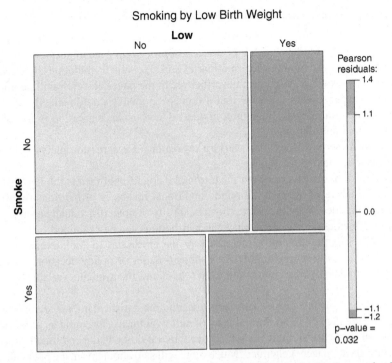

Fig. 1.3 Whether the mother smokes by low birth weight with Pearson residuals assuming independence (*Red* indicates fewer cases than expected under independence. *Blue* indicates more cases than expected under independence. $N = 189$.)

newborns have low birth weights. But if a mother's weight is less than 107 pounds, around 40 % of the newborns have low birth weights.

The reasoning applies as well if both the response and the predictor are categorical. Figure 1.3 shows a mosaic plot for whether or not a newborn is underweight and whether or not the newborn's mother smoked. The area of each rectangle is proportional to the number of cases in the respective cell of the corresponding 2×2 table. One can see that the majority of mothers do not smoke and a majority of the newborns are not underweight. The red cell contains fewer observations than would be expected under independence, and the blue cell contains more observations than would be expected under independence. The metric is the Pearson residual for that cell (i.e., the contribution to the χ^2 statistic). Mothers who smoke are more likely to have low birth weight babies. If one is prepared to articulate a credible generative model consistent with a conventional test of independence, independence is rejected at the .03 level. But even without such a test, the mosaic represents a legitimate regression analysis.[2]

[2]The spine plot and the mosaic plot were produced using the R package *vcd*, which stands for "visualizing categorical data." Its authors are D. Meyer et al. (2007).

There are several lessons highlighted by these brief illustrations.

- As discussed in more depth shortly, the regression analyses just conducted made no direct use of models. Each is best seen as a *procedure*. One might well have preferred greater use of numerical summaries and algebraic formulations, but regression analyses were undertaken nevertheless. In the pages ahead, it will be important to dispense with the view that a regression analysis automatically requires arithmetic summaries or algebraic models. Once again, regression is just about conditional distributions.
- Visualizations of various kinds can be a key feature of a regression analysis. Indeed, they can be the defining feature.
- A regression analysis does not have to make conditional means the key distributional feature of interest, although conditional means or proportions dominate current practice. With the increasing availability of powerful visualization procedures, for example, entire conditional distributions can be examined.
- Whether it is the predictors of interest or the covariates to "hold constant," the choice of conditioning variables is a subject-matter or policy decision. There is nothing in data by itself indicating what role, if any, the available variables should play.[3]
- There is nothing in regression analysis that requires statistical inference: inferences beyond the data on hand, formal tests of null hypotheses, or confidence intervals. And when statistical inference is employed, its validity will depend fundamentally on how the data were generated. Much more will said about this in the pages ahead.
- If there is to be cause-and-effect overlay, that too is a subject-matter or policy call unless one has conducted an experiment. When the data result from an experiment, the causal variables are determined by the research design.
- A regression analysis can serve a variety of purposes.

1. For a "level I" regression analysis, the goal is solely description of the data on hand. Level I regression is effectively assumption-free and should always be on the table. Too often, description is undervalued as a data analysis tool perhaps because it does not employ much of the apparatus of conventional statistics. How can a data analysis without statistical inference be good? The view taken here is that p-values and all other products of statistical inference can certainly be useful, but are worse than useless when a credible rationale cannot be provided (Berk and Freedman 2003). Assume-and-proceed statistics is not likely to advance science or policy. Yet, important progress frequently can be made from statistically informed description alone.

2. For a "level II" regression analysis, statistical inference is the defining activity. Estimation is undertaken using the results from a level I regression, often in

---

[3]Although there are certainly no universal naming conventions, "predictors" can be seen as variables that are of subject-matter interest, and "covariates" can be seen as variables that improve the performance of the statistical procedure being applied. Then, covariates are not of subject-matter interest. Whatever the naming conventions, the distinction between variables that matter substantively and variables that matter procedurally is important. An example of the latter is a covariate included in an analysis of randomized experiments to improve statistical precision.

concert with statistical tests and confidence intervals. Statistical inference forms the core of conventional statistics, but proper use with real data can be very challenging; real data may not correspond well to what the inferential tools require. For the statistical procedures emphasized here, statistical inference will often be overmatched. There can be a substantial disconnect between the requirements of proper statistical inference and adaptive statistical procedures such as those central to statistical learning. Forecasting, which will play an important role in the pages ahead, is also a level II activity because projections are made from data on hand to the values of certain variables that are unobserved.

3. For a "level III" regression analysis, causal inference is overlaid on the results of a level I regression analysis, sometimes coupled with level II results. There can be demanding conceptual issues such as specifying a sensible "counterfactual." For example, one might consider the impact of the death penalty on crime; states that have the death penalty are compared to states that do not. But what is the counterfactual to which the death penalty is being compared? Is it life imprisonment without any chance of parole, a long prison term of, say, 20 years, or probation? In many states the counterfactual is life in prison with no chance of parole. Also, great care is needed to adjust for the possible impact of confounders. In the death penalty example, one might want to control for average clearance rate in each of the state's police departments. Clearance rates for some kinds of homicides are very low, which means that it is pretty easy to get away with murder, and the death penalty is largely irrelevant.[4] Level III regression analysis will not figure significantly in the pages ahead because of a reliance on algorithmic methods rather than model-based methods (Breimen 2001b).

In summary, a focus on conditional distributions will be a central feature in all that follows. One does not require generative models, statistical inference, or causal inference. On the one hand, a concentration on conditional distribution may seem limiting. On the other hand, a concentration on conditional distributions may seem liberating. In practice, both can be true and be driven substantially by the limitations of conventional modeling to which we now briefly turn.

Of necessity, the next several sections are more technical and more conceptually demanding. Readers with a substantial statistical background should have no problems, although some conventional ways of thinking will need to be revised. There may also need to be an attitude adjustment. Readers without a substantial statistical background may be best served by skimming the material primarily to see the topics addressed, and then returning to the material as needed when in subsequent chapters those topics arise.

---

[4]A crime is "cleared" when the perpetrator is arrested. In some jurisdictions, a crime is cleared when the perpetrator has been identified, even if there has been no arrest.

1.3   Revisiting the Ubiquitous Linear Regression Model

Although conditional distributions are the foundation for all that follows, linear regression is its most common manifestation in practice and needs to be explicitly addressed. For many, linear regression is the canonical procedure for examining conditional relationship, or at least the default. Therefore, a brief review of its features and requirements can be a useful didactic device to highlight similarities to and differences from statistical learning.

When a linear regression analysis is formulated, conventional practice combines a level I and level II perspective. Important features of the data are conceptually embedded in how the data were generated. Y is an $N \times 1$ numerical response variable, where N is the number of observations. There is an $N \times (p + 1)$ "design matrix" $\mathbf{X}$, where p is the number of predictors (sometimes called regressors). A leading column of 1s is usually included in $\mathbf{X}$ for reasons that will clear momentarily. Y is treated as a random variable. The p predictors in $\mathbf{X}$ are taken to be fixed. Whether predictors are fixed or random is not a technical detail, but figures centrally in subsequent material.

The process by which the values of Y are realized then takes the form

$$y_i = \beta_0 + \beta_1 x_{1i} + \beta_2 x_{2i} + \cdots + \beta_p x_{pi} + \varepsilon_i, \qquad (1.1)$$

where

$$\varepsilon_i \sim \text{NIID}(0, \sigma^2). \qquad (1.2)$$

β_0 is the y-intercept associated with the leading column 1s. There are p regression coefficients, and a random perturbation ε_i. One might say that for each case i, nature sets the values of the predictors, multiplies each predictor value by its corresponding regression coefficient, sums these products, adds the value of the constant, and then adds a random perturbation. Each perturbation, ε_i, is a random variable realized as if drawn at random and independently from a single distribution, often assumed to be normal, with a mean of 0.0. In short, nature behaves as if she adopts a linear model.

There are several important implications. To begin, the values of Y can be realized repeatedly for a given case because its values will vary solely because of ε. The predictor values do not change. Thus, for a given high school student, one imagines that there could be a limitless number of scores on the mathematics SAT, solely because of the "noise" represented by ε_i. All else in nature's linear combination is fixed: the number of hours spent in an SAT preparation course, motivation to perform well, the amount of sleep the night before, the presence of distractions while the test is being taken, and so on. This is more than an academic formality. It is a substantive theory about how SAT scores come to be. For a given student, nature requires that an observed SAT score could have been different by chance alone, but not because any of variation in the predictors.[5]

---

[5]If on substantive grounds one allows for nature to set more than one value for any given predictor and student, a temporal process is implied, and there is systematic temporal variation to build into the regression formulation. This can certainly be done, but the formulation is more complicated,

From Eqs. 1.1 and 1.2, it can be conceptually helpful to distinguish between the mean function and the disturbance function (also called the variance function). The mean function is the expectation of Eq. 1.1. When in practice a data analyst specifies a conventional linear regression model, it will be "first-order correct" when the data analyst (a) knows what nature is using as predictors, (b) knows what transformations, if any, nature applies to those predictors, (c) knows that the predictors are combined in a linear fashion, and (d) has those predictors in the dataset to be analyzed. For conventional linear regression, these are the first-order conditions. The only unknowns in the mean function are the values of the y-intercept and the regression coefficients. Clearly, these are daunting hurdles.

The disturbance function is Eq. 1.2. When in practice the data analyst specifies a conventional linear regression model, it will be "second-order correct" when the data analyst knows that each perturbation is realized independently of all other perturbations and that each is realized from a single distribution that has an expectation of 0.0. Because there is a single disturbance distribution, one can say that the variance of that distribution is "constant." These are the usual second-order conditions. Sometimes the data analyst also knows the functional form of the distribution. If that distribution is the normal, the only distribution unknown whose value needs to be estimated is its variance σ^2.

When the first-order conditions are met and ordinary least squares is applied to the data, estimates of the slope and y-intercept are unbiased estimates of the corresponding values that nature uses. When in addition to the first-order conditions, the second-order conditions are met, and ordinary least squares is applied to the data, the disturbance variance can be estimated in an unbiased fashion using the residuals from the realized data. Also, conventional confidence intervals and statistical tests are valid, and by the Gauss–Markov theorem, each estimated β has the smallest possible sampling variation of any other linear estimator of nature's regression parameters. In short, one has the ideal textbook results for a level II regression analysis. Similar reasoning properly can be applied to the entire generalized linear model and its multi-equation extensions, although usually that reasoning depends on asymptotics.

Finally, even for a conventional regression analysis, there is no need to move to level III. Causal interpretations are surely important when they can be justified, but they are an add-on, not an essential element. With observational data, moreover, causal inference can be in principle very controversial (Freedman 1987, 2004).

1.3.1 Problems in Practice

There are a wide variety of practical problems with the conventional linear model, many recognized well over a generation ago (e.g., Leamer 1978; Rubin 1986, 2008; Freedman 1987, 2004; Berk 2003). This is not the venue for an extensive review, and

---

(Footnote 5 continued)
requires that nature be even more cooperative, and for the points to be made here, adds unnecessary complexity.

David Freedman's excellent text on statistical models (2009a) can be consulted for an unusually cogent discussion. Nevertheless, it will prove useful later to mention now a few of the most common and vexing difficulties.

There is effectively no way to know whether the model specified by the analyst is the means by which nature actually generated the data. And there is also no way to know how close to the "truth" a specified model really is. One would need to know that truth to quantify a model's disparities from the truth, and if the truth were known, there would be no need to analyze any data to begin with. Consequently, all concerns about model specification are translated into whether the model is good enough.

There are two popular strategies addressing the "good enough" requirement. First, there exist a large number of regression diagnostics taking a variety of forms and using a variety of techniques including graphical procedures, statistical tests, and the comparative performance of alternative model specifications (Weisberg 2014). These tools can be useful in identifying problems with the linear model, but they can miss serious problems as well. Most are designed to detect single difficulties in isolation when in practice, there can be many difficulties at once. Is evidence of nonconstant variance a result of mean function misspecification, disturbances generated from different distributions, or both? In addition, diagnostic tools derived from formal statistical tests typically have weak statistical power (Freedman 2009b), and when the null hypothesis is not rejected, analysts commonly "accept" the null hypothesis that all is well. In fact, there are effectively a limitless number of other null hypotheses that would also not be rejected.[6] Finally, even if some error in the model is properly identified, there may be little or no guidance on how to fix it, especially within the limitation of the data available.

Second, claims are made on subject-matter grounds that the results make sense and are consistent with – or at least not contradicted by – existing theory and past research. This line of reasoning can be a source of good science and good policy, but also misses the point. One might learn useful things from a data analysis even if the model specified is dramatically different from how nature generated the data. Indeed, this perspective is emphasized many times in the pages ahead. But advancing a scientific or policy discourse does not imply that the model used is right, or even close.

If a model's results are sufficiently useful, why should this matter? It matters because one cannot use the correctness of the model to justify the subject-matter claims made. For example, interesting findings said to be the direct product of an elaborate model specification might have surfaced just as powerfully from several scatter plots. The findings rest on a very few strong associations easily revealed by simple statistical tools. The rest is pretense.

It matters because certain features of the analysis used to bolster substantive claims may be fundamentally wrong and misleading. For example, if a model is not first-order correct, the probabilities associated with statistical tests are almost certainly incorrect. Even if asymptotically valid standard errors are obtained with such tools as the sandwich estimator (White 1980a, b), the relevant estimate from the data will

---

[6]This is sometimes called "the fallacy of accepting the null" (Rozeboom 1960).

on the average be offset by its bias. If the bias moves the estimate away from the null hypothesis, the estimated p-values will be on the average too small. If the bias moves the estimate toward the null hypothesis, the estimated p-values will on the average be too large. In a similar fashion, confidence intervals will be offset in one of the two directions.

It matters because efforts to diagnose and fix model specification problems can lead to new and sometime worse difficulties. For example, one response to a model that does not pass muster is to re-specify the model and re-estimate the model's parameters. But it is now well known that model selection and model estimation undertaken on the same data (e.g., statistical tests for a set of nested models) lead to biased estimates even if by some good fortune the correct model happens to be found (Leeb and Pötscher 2005; 2006; 2008; Berk et al. 2010; 2014).[7] The model specification itself is a product of the realized data and a source of additional uncertainty — with a different realized dataset, one may arrive at a different model. As a formal matter, statistical tests assume that the model has been specified *before* the data are examined.[8] This is no longer true. The result is not just more uncertainty overall, but a particular form of uncertainty that can result in badly biased estimates of the regression coefficients and pathological sampling distributions.

And finally, it matters because it undermines the credibility of statistical procedures. There will be times when an elaborate statistical procedure is really needed that performs as advertised. But why should the results be believed when word on the street is that data analysts routinely make claims that are not justified by the statistical tools employed?

1.4 Working with Statistical Models that Are Wrong

Is there an alternative way to proceed that can be more satisfactory? The answer requires a little deeper look at conventional practice. Emphasis properly is placed on the word "practice." There are no fundamental quarrels with the mathematical statistics on which conventional practice rests.

Model misspecification is hardly a new topic, and some very smart statisticians and econometricians have been working on it for decades. One tradition concentrates on patching up models that are misspecified. The other tradition tries to work constructively with misspecified models. We will work within the second tradition. For many statisticians and practitioners, this can require a major attitude adjustment.

Figure 1.4 is a stylized representation of the sort of practical problems that can follow for a level II analysis when for a linear model one assumes that the first-

---

[7]Model selection in some disciplines is called variable selection, feature selection, or dimension reduction.

[8] Actually, it can be more complicated. For example, if the predictors are taken to be fixed, one is free to examine the predictors. Model selection problems surface when the response variable is examined as well. If the predictors are taken to be random, the issues are even more subtle.

Fig. 1.4 Estimation of a
nonlinear response surface
under the true linear model
perspective (The *broken line*
is an estimate from a given
dataset, *solid line* is the
expectation of such
estimates, the *vertical dotted
lines* represent conditional
distributions of Y with the
red bars as each
distribution's mean.)

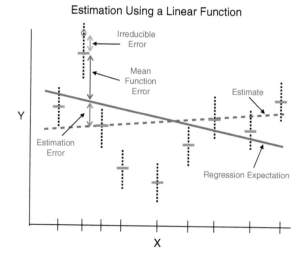

and second-order conditions are met. The Figure is not a scatterplot but an effort
to illustrate some key ideas from the relevant statistical theory. For simplicity, but
with no important loss of generality for the issues to be addressed, there is a single
predictor on the horizontal axis. For now, that predictor is assumed to be fixed.[9] The
response variable is on the vertical axis.

The red, horizontal lines in Fig. 1.4 are the true conditional means that constitute
nature's response surface. The vertical, black, dotted lines are meant to show the
distribution of y-values around each conditional mean. Those distributions are also
nature's work. No assumptions are made about what form the distributions take, but
for didactic convenience each conditional distribution is assumed to have the same
variance.

An eyeball interpolation of the true conditional means reveals an approximate U-
shaped relationship but with substantial departures from that simple pattern. Nature
provides a data analyst with realized values of Y by making independent draws from
the distribution associated with each conditional mean. The red circle is one such
y-value; the red circle is one output from nature's data generation process.

A data analyst assumes the usual linear model $y_i = \beta_0 + \beta_1 x_i + \varepsilon_i$. With a set
of realized y values and their corresponding x values (not shown), estimates $\hat{\beta}_0$, $\hat{\beta}_1$
and $\hat{\sigma}^2$ are obtained. The broken blue line shows the estimated mean function. One
can imagine nature generating many (formally, a limitless number) such datasets
so that there are many mean function estimates that will naturally vary because the
realized values y will change from dataset to dataset. The solid blue line represents
the expectation of those many estimates.

---

[9]If one prefers to think about the issues in a multiple regression context, the single predictor can be
replaced by the predictor adjusted, as usual, for its linear relationships with the other predictors.

Clearly, the assumed linear mean function is incorrect because the true conditional means do not fall on a straight line. The blue, two-headed arrow shows the bias at one value of x. The size and direction of the biases differ over the values of x because the disparities between regression expectation and the true conditional means differ.

The data analyst does not get to work with the expectation of the estimated regression lines. Usually, the data analyst gets to work with one such line. The random variation captured by one such line is shown with the magenta, double-headed error. Even if the broken blue line fell right on top of the solid blue line, and if both went exactly through the true conditional mean being used as an illustration, there would still be a gap between the observed value of Y (the red circle) and that conditional mean (the short red horizontal line). In Fig. 1.4, that gap is represented by the green, double-headed arrow. It is sometimes called "irreducible error" because it exists even if nature's response surface is known.

Summarizing the implications for the conventional linear regression formulation, the blue double-headed arrow shows the bias in the estimated regression line, the magenta double-headed arrow shows the impact of the variability of that estimate, and the green double-headed arrow shows the irreducible error. For any given estimated mean function, the distance between the estimated regression line and a realized y-value is a combination of mean function error (also called mean function misspecification), random variation in the estimated regression line caused by ε_i, and the variability in ε_i itself. Sometimes these can cancel each other out, at least in part, but all three will always be in play.

Some might claim that instrumental variables provide a way out. It is true that instrumental variable procedures can correct for some forms of bias if (a) a valid instrument can be found and if (b) the sample size is large enough to capitalize on asymptotics. But the issues are tricky (Bound et al. 1995). A successful instrument does not address all mean function problems. For example, it cannot correct for wrong functional forms. Also, it can be very difficult to find a credible instrumental variable. Even if one succeeds, an instrumental variable may remove most of the regression coefficient bias and simultaneously cause a very large increase in the variance of the regression coefficient estimate. On the average, the regression line is actually farther away from the true conditional means even through the bias is largely eliminated. One is arguably worse off.

It is a simple matter to alter the mean function. Perhaps something other than a straight line can be used to accurately represent nature's true conditional means. However, one is still required to get the first-order conditions right. That is, the mean function must be correct. Figure 1.5 presents the same kinds of difficulties as Fig. 1.4. All three sources of error remain: model misspecification, sampling variability in the function estimated, and the irreducible error. Comparing the two figures, the second seems to have on the average a less biased regression expectation, but in practice it is difficult know whether that is true or not. Perhaps more important, it is impossible to know how much bias remains.[10]

---

[10]We will see later that by increasing the complexity of the mean function estimated, one has the potential to reduce bias. But an improved fit in the data on hand is no guarantee that one is

Fig. 1.5 Estimation of a nonlinear response surface under the true nonlinear model perspective (The *broken line* is an estimate from a given dataset, *solid line* is the expectation of such estimates, the *vertical dotted lines* represent conditional distributions of Y with the *red bars* as each distribution's mean.)

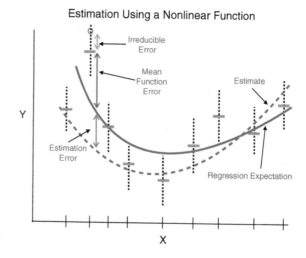

One important implication of both Figs. 1.4 and 1.5 is that the variation in the realized observations around the fitted values will not be constant. The bias, which varies across x-values, is captured by the least squares residuals. To the data analyst, this will look like heteroscedasticity even if the variation in ε_i is actually constant. Conventional estimates of σ^2 will likely be incorrect. Incorrect standard errors for the intercept and slope follow, which jeopardize statistical tests and confidence intervals.

When faced with non-constant variance, the "sandwich" estimator (White 1980b) can provide asymptotically valid standard errors. But the mean function must be correctly specified. The requirement of proper mean function specification too commonly is overlooked.

It seems that we are at a dead end. But we are not. All of the estimation difficulties are level II regression problems. If one can be satisfied with a level I regression analysis, these difficulties disappear. Another option is to reformulate conventional linear regression so that the estimation task is more modest. We turn to that next. Yet another option considered in later chapters requires living with, and even reveling in, at least some bias. Unbiased estimates of the nature's response surface are not a prerequisite if one can be satisfied with estimates that are as close as possible on the average to nature's response surface over realizations of the data. There can be bias if in trade, there is a substantial reduction in the variance; on the average, the regression line is then closer to nature's response surface. We will see that in practice, it is difficult to decrease both the bias and the variance, but often there will be ways which arrive at a beneficial balance in what is called the "bias–variance tradeoff." Still, as long as any bias remains, statistical tests and confidence intervals need to be reconsidered. As for the irreducible variance, it is still irreducible.

(Footnote 10 continued)
more accurately representing the mean function. One complication is that greater mean function complexity can foster overfitting.

1.4.1 An Alternative Approach to Regression

The material in this section can be conceptually demanding and has layers. There are also lots of details. It may be helpful, therefore, to make two introductory observations. First, in the words of George Box, "All models are wrong..." (Box 1976). It follows that one must learn to work with wrong models and not proceed as if they are right. This is a large component of what follows. Second, if one is to work with wrong models, the estimation target is also a wrong model. Standard practice has the "true" model as the estimation target. In other words, one should be making correct inferences to an incorrect model and not be making incorrect inferences to a correct model. Let's see how these two observations play out.

If a data analyst wants to employ a level II regression analysis, inferences from the data must be made to something. Within conventional conceptions, that something is the parameter of a linear model used by nature to generate the data. The parameters are the estimation targets. Given the values of those parameters and the fixed-x values, each y_i is realized by the linear model shown in Eqs. 1.1 and 1.2.[11]

Consider as an alternative what one might call the "joint probability distribution model." It has much the same look and feel as the "correlation model" formulated by Freedman (1981), and is very similar to a "linear approximation" perspective proposed by White (1980a). Both have important roots in the work of Huber (1967) and Eicker (1963, 1967). Angrist and Pischke (2008: Sect. 3.1.2) provide a very accessible introduction.

For the substantive or policy issues at hand, one imagines that there exists a materially relevant, joint probability distribution composed of variables represented by $\mathbf{Z}$. The joint probability distribution has familiar parameters such the mean (i.e., the expected value) and variance for each variable and the covariances between variables. No distinctions are made between predictors and responses. Nature can "realize" independently any number of observations from the joint probability distribution. This is how the data are generated. One might call the process by which observations are realized from the joint probability distribution the "true generative model." This is the "what" to which inferences are to be made in a level II analysis.

A conceptually equivalent "what" is to consider a population of limitless size that represents all possible realizations from the joint probability distribution. Inferences are made from the realized data to this "infinite population." In some circles, this is called a "superpopulation." Closely related ideas can work for finite populations (Cochran 1977: Chap. 7). For example, the data are a simple random sample from a well-defined population that is in principle observable. This is the way one usually thinks about sample surveys, such as well-done political polls. The population is all registered voters and a probability sample is drawn for analysis. In finite populations, the population variables are fixed. There is a joint distribution of all the variables in the population that is just a multivariate histogram.

---

[11] The next several pages draw heavily on Berk et al. (2014) and Buja et al. (2016).

Switching to matrix notation for clarity, from $\mathbf{Z}$, data analysts will typically distinguish between predictors $\mathbf{X}$ and the response $\mathbf{y}$. Some of $\mathbf{Z}$ may be substantively irrelevant and ignored. These distinctions have nothing to do with how the data are generated. They derive from the preferences of the individuals who will be analyzing the data.

For any particular regression analysis, attention then turns to a conditional distribution of $\mathbf{y}$ given some $\mathbf{X} = \mathbf{x}$. For example, $\mathbf{X}$ could be predictors of longevity, and $\mathbf{x}$ is the predictor values for a given individual. The distribution of $\mathbf{y}$ is thought to vary from one $\mathbf{x}$ to another $\mathbf{x}$. Variation in the mean of $\mathbf{y}$, $\mu(\mathbf{x})$, is usually the primary concern. But now, because the number of observations in the population is limitless, one must work with the $\mathrm{E}[\mu(\mathbf{x})]$.

The values for $\mathrm{E}[\mu(\mathbf{x})]$ constitute the "true response surface." The true response surface is the way the expected values of Y are actually related to $\mathbf{X}$ within the joint probability distribution. It is unknown. Disparities between the $\mathrm{E}[\mu(\mathbf{x})]$ and the potential values of Y are the "true disturbances" and necessarily have an expectation of 0.0 (because they are deviations around a mean – or more properly, an expected value)

The data analyst specifies a working regression model using a conventional, linear mean function meant to characterize *another* response surface within the same joint probability distribution. Its conditional expectations are equal to $\mathbf{X}\boldsymbol{\beta}$. The response $\mathbf{y}$ is then taken to be $\mathbf{X}\boldsymbol{\beta} + \boldsymbol{\varepsilon}$, where $\boldsymbol{\beta}$ is an array of least squares coefficients. Because $\boldsymbol{\varepsilon}$ also is a product of least squares, it has by construction an expectation of 0.0 and is uncorrelated with $\mathbf{X}$. For reasons that will be clear later, there is no requirement that $\boldsymbol{\varepsilon}$ have constant variance. Nevertheless, thanks to least squares, one can view the conditional expectations from the working model as the *best linear approximation* of the true response surface. We will see below that it is the best linear approximation of the true response surface that we seek to estimate, not the true response surface itself.

This is a major reformulation of conventional, fixed-x linear regression. For the working model, there is no a priori determination of how the response is related to the predictors and no commitment to linearity as the truth. In addition, the chosen predictors share no special cachet. Among the random variables $\mathbf{Z}$, a data analyst determines which random variables are predictors and which random variables are responses. Hence, there can be no such thing as an omitted variable that can turn a correct model into an incorrect model. If important predictors are overlooked, the regression results are just incomplete; the results are substantively insufficient but still potentially very informative. Finally, causality need not be overlaid on the analysis. Although causal thinking may well have a role in an analyst's determination of the response and the predictors, a serious consideration of cause and effect is not required at this point. For example, one need not ponder whether any given predictor is actually manipulable holding all other predictors constant.

Still to come is a discussion of estimation, statistical tests and confidence intervals. But it may be important to pause and give potential critics some air time. They might well object that we have just traded one fictional account for another.

From an epistemological point of view, there is real merit in such concerns. However, in science and policy settings, it can be essential to make empirically based claims that go beyond the data on hand. For example, when a college admissions office uses data from past applicants to examine how performance in college is related to the information available when admission decisions need to be made, whatever is learned will presumably be used to help inform future admission decisions. Data from past applicants are taken to be realizations from the social processes responsible for academic success in college. Insofar as those social processes are reasonably consistent over several years, the strategy can have merit. A science fiction story? Perhaps. But if better admissions decisions are made as a result, there are meaningful and demonstrable benefits. To rephrase George Box's famous aphorism, all models are fiction, but some stories are better than others. And there is much more to this story.

1.4.1.1   Statistical Inference with Wrong Models

Figure 1.6 can be used to help understand estimation within the "wrong model" framework. It is a stylized rendering of the joint probability distribution. There is a single predictor treated as a random variable. There is a single response, also treated as a random variable. Some realized values of Y are shown as red circles. The solid back line represents nature's unknown, true response surface, the "path" of the conditional means, or more accurately, the path of the conditional expectations.

The true response surface is allowed to be nonlinear, although for ease of exposition, the nonlinearity in Fig. 1.6 is rather well behaved. For each location along the response surface, there is a conditional distribution represented in Fig. 1.6 by the dotted, vertical lines. Were one working with a conventional regression perspective, the curved black line would be the estimation target.

Under the wrong model perspective, the straight blue line in Fig. 1.6 represents the mean function implied by the data analyst's working linear model. Clearly, the linear mean function is misspecified. It is as if one had fitted a linear least squares regression within the joint probability distribution. The blue line is the new estimation target that can be interpreted as the best linear approximation of the true response surface. It can be called "best" because it is conceptualized as a product of ordinary least squares; it is best by the least square criterion. Although the best linear approximation is the estimation target, one also gets estimates of the regression coefficients responsible. These may be of interest for least squares regression applications and procedures that are a lot like them. By the middle of the next chapter, however, most of the connections to least squares regression will be gone.

Consider the shaded vertical slice of the conditional distribution toward the center of Fig. 1.6. The disparity between the true response surface and the red circle near the top of the conditional distribution results solely from the irreducible error. But when the best linear approximation is used as a reference, the apparent irreducible error is much smaller. Likewise, the disparity between the true response surface and the red circle near the bottom of the conditional distribution results solely from the

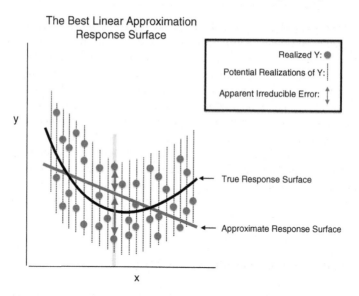

Fig. 1.6 Within the joint probability distribution, mean function error as a cause of nonconstant variance (The *black curved line* is the true response surface, and the *straight blue line* is the best linear approximation of that response surface.)

irreducible error. But when the best linear approximation is used as a reference, the apparent irreducible error is much larger. Both distortions result from the gap between the true response surface and the best linear approximation response surface. Because X is a random variable, mean function misspecification is a random variable captured as a component of the *apparent* irreducible error. Similar issues arise for the full range of x-values in the figure.

Suppose a data analyst wanted to estimate from data the best linear approximation of nature's true response surface. The estimation task can be usefully partitioned into five steps. The first requires making the case that each observation in the dataset was independently realized from a relevant joint probability distribution. Much more is required than hand waving. Required is usually subject-matter expertise and knowledge about how the data were collected. There will be examples in the pages ahead. Often a credible case cannot be made, which takes estimation off the table. Then, there will probably be no need to worry about step two.

The second step is to define the target of estimation. For linear regression of the sort just discussed, an estimation target is easy to specify. Should the estimation target be the true response surface, estimates will likely be of poor statistical quality. Should the estimation target be the best linear approximation of the true response surface, the estimates can be of good statistical quality, at least asymptotically. We will see in later chapters that defining the estimation target often will be far more difficult because there will commonly be no model in the conventional regression sense. One cannot sensibly proceed to step three unless there is clarity about what is to be estimated.

The third step is to select an estimator. Sometimes the best estimator will be apparent. The least squares estimator used in conventional regression is a good example. There are other relatively straightforward examples when the mean function is determined without any formal model selection or data snooping. But most of the procedures considered in later chapters capitalize on model selection, even if not quite in plain sight, and informal data snooping is a common practice. Getting the estimator right can then be challenging. The risk is that an inappropriate estimator is used by default, justified by performance claims that are incorrect.

Fourth, the estimator needs to be applied to the data. This is usually the easiest step because the requisite software is often easily found and easily deployed. But there are exceptions when the data have unusual properties or the questions being asked of the data are unusual. One hopes that appropriate software can be easily written, but sometimes the underlying statistical problems are unsolved.

In the final step, the estimates and any associated confidence intervals and tests are interpreted. The major risk is that the results of earlier steps are not properly taken into account. A common example is asserting asymptotic properties with far too few observations in the data.

Let us play this through for estimates of the best linear approximation. In the absence of real data not much can be said here about the first step. It will figure large

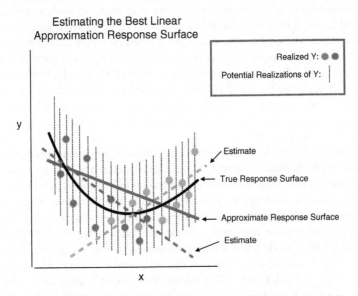

Fig. 1.7 Bias in the estimates of the best linear approximation (The *black curved line* is the true response surface, and the *straight blue line* is the best linear approximation of that response surface, and estimates are shown as *broken lines*.)

in real applications later. The second step has already been addressed. The estimation target is the best linear approximation of the true response surface.

Important technical complications materialize for steps three, four, and five. Consider Fig. 1.7. Suppose that in the data, the realized values of X tend to be concentrated at the smaller values. This is illustrated by the red filled circles in Fig. 1.7. Because the nonlinear true response surface is sloping downward where the red observations are more likely to be concentrated, estimated least squares lines tend to have a negative slope. In contrast, suppose that the realized values of X tend to be concentrated at the larger values. This is illustrated by the green filled circles in Fig. 1.7. Because the nonlinear true response surface is sloping upward where the green observations are more likely to be concentrated, estimated least squares lines will tend to have a positive slope. For a conventional fixed X regression, this leads to based estimates of the best linear approximation.

However, under the joint probability distribution approach, all observations are realized by the equivalent of random sampling, and all the predictors are random variables. One can show, therefore, that conventional estimates of the best linear approximation are asymptotically unbiased (Buja et al. 2016). And there is more good news. Despite the nonconstant variance described earlier, asymptotically valid standard errors may be obtained using a sandwich procedure or a nonparametric bootstrap. Asymptotically valid statistical tests and confidence intervals follow (Buja et al. 2016).

These conclusions apply to nonlinear parametric approximations as well. For example, one might choose to approximate the true response surface with a cubic polynomial function of X. One would have the best cubic approximation of the true response surface. The conclusions also apply to the entire generalized linear model (White 1980a). For example, the response might be binary and a form of binomial regression might be the estimation procedure. In short, the standard estimators can work well in large samples, and in those large samples, the sandwich or a bootstrap estimator of the regression coefficient standard errors can work well too. And there is readily available software for both. Asymptotically, valid statistical tests and confidence intervals follow.

It may seem that in the second step, the selection of the best linear approximation as the estimation target comes perilously close to a resurrection of conventional model-based procedures. But there is absolutely no reason to be limited to a linear model, and subject-matter knowledge may suggest a better mean function. There remains a very important role for subject-matter theory and the results from past research. One is still trying to learn about the true response surface, but that knowledge will come from working models that are, in conventional terms, misspecified. The way one learns from models that are wrong is not to pretend they are right. The way one learns from wrong models is to acknowledge their imperfections and exploit their instructive features nevertheless. There can be important complications to be sure, but they will be constructively addressed in the chapters ahead.

Given the goal of learning about the true response surface with a misspecified model, one can imagine using that model to forecast the response. That is, for a *new* vector of x-values realized from the same joint probability distribution, the misspecified model is used to produce a good guess about the response when the response value is not known. Ideally, that forecast will fall right on the true response surface, but in practice this will not happen very often. (And how would you know?) One hopes, therefore, to be close most of the time. But, if the forecasting target is the true response surface, one has reintroduced all of the estimation problems faced when working with wrong models assumed to be specified correctly. We seem to be back where we started.

Actually, we are not. In principle, one can obtain estimates of the best linear approximation that have good asymptotic properties. The approximation can provide useful information about how the response is related to the predictors, informed by asymptotically valid statistical tests and confidence intervals. None of this is available within the conventional approach to linear regression when the model's mean function is misspecified. Then, as an *additional* step, one can try to forecast accurately values of true response surface. This step necessarily reintroduces the problems just discussed. But, we will see that there are ways to make good progress here too. In the spirit of the approximation approach to estimation, one gives up the goal of unbiased forecasts and settles for trying to get forecasts that are close. How this can be done depends on the fitting procedure used and will be discussed in some detail in the pages ahead.

For many readers, the wrong model formulation addressed in the past few pages may seem odd and perhaps even heretical. But from a sampling perspective, our wrong model formulation was anticipated in the work of Willian Cochran over 50 years ago (1977: Chap. 7). One has a finite population, such as all students at a university. A simple random sample is drawn, and a conventional linear regression applied. The predictors are random variables because in new random samples, the students and their x-values will change. The estimation target is the response surface of the same regression specification were it applied in the population. It does not matter whether the mean function for population regression is specified properly; wrong models are fine. Estimates of the wrong model's response surface are biased. When the number of observations in the sample approaches the number of observations in the finite population, the bias disappears. Valid statistical inference can follow (Thompson 2002: Sect. 8.1).

1.4.1.2 Wrong Regression Models with Binary Response Variables

Up to this point, analyses with quantitative response variables have dominated the discussion, in part because of a desire to make connections to conventional linear regression. The majority of subsequent chapters will introduce procedures for the analysis of categorical response variables in part because that is where some of the most interesting and useful work on statistical learning can be found.

To help set the stage, in Fig. 1.8, there is a binary response coded as 1 or 0, and as before, a single numerical X. Dropping out of high school might be coded as 1, and graduating might be coded as 0. The fuzzy lines at y-values of 1 and 0 are the potential realized values of Y. There is, as before, a true response surface and an approximation. The latter is the estimation target although there can be interest in the regression coefficients responsible. Fitted values can range from 0 to 1. For a level I analysis, the fitted values often can be interpreted as proportions. For a level II analysis, the fitted values often can be interpreted as probabilities.

Typically, the fitted values are used to determine class membership. In Fig. 1.8, there are two classes: A and B. A might be dropping out of high school and B might be graduating. There is also a threshold shown at an illustrative value of .30. Fitted values at or above the threshold imply membership in class A. Fitted values below that threshold imply membership in class B. Notice that the true response surface and its approximation classify many cases differently. For the value of X at the gray vertical rectangle, the true response surface would classify a case as an A, and the approximation would classify a case as a B. The use of .30 as a threshold might seem strange, but we will see later that there can principled reasons for choosing threshold values other than .50.

Within a parametric perspective, one might apply logistic regression to the data. Typically, fitted values of .50 or larger imply membership in one class ("50–50 or better"). Fitted values smaller than .50 imply membership in the other class ("less than 50–50"). Hence, the threshold is .50. Within statistical learning traditions, there are several effective ways to estimate the nonlinear approximation in a nonparametric fashion. These will be discussed in later chapters.

1.4.1.3 Wrong Models in Practice

We are adopting a perspective for level II regression in which the data are generated as independent realizations from a joint probability distribution. All the realized

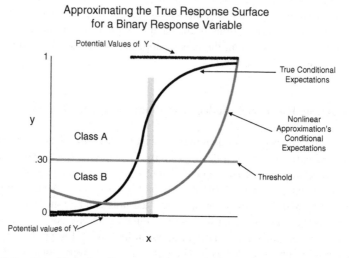

Fig. 1.8 Estimation with the best linear approximation for a binary response Class A or B

variables are random variables. Responses and predictors are determined by the data analyst, not by nature. There is a true response surface of conditional expectations of a response that is unknown. The true response surface is not the estimation target. The estimation target is an approximation of that response surface whose relation to the true response surface is undetermined. No restrictions are placed on the approximation's functional form, and it can be specified before looking at the data or, as we will see later, arrived at inductively. When specified in advance, the approximation can be estimated in an asymptotically unbiased fashion with valid standard errors, confidence intervals, and statistical tests. When the specification is determined as part of the data analysis, the issues are more complicated, and we will address them subsequently. With an estimate of the approximation in hand, one can compute fitted values that may be used as estimates of the true response surface. One should proceed assuming that these estimates are biased, even asymptotically. The goal is to get close to the true response surface on the average. Getting the response surface right on the average usually is too hard.

A superficial reading of the last several pages might suggest that in practice one could proceed with linear or logistic regression as usual by simply providing a more cautious interpretations of the results. This typically will not be a good idea. Because the estimation target is still the true response surface, estimates of the regression coefficients and fitted values will be biased, even asymptotically. It follows that even if valid asymptotic standard errors could be computed, statistical tests and confidence intervals will not be correct. There is also the likely prospect of substantial additional work trying to diagnose model misspecifications and their consequences. And in the end, justification of results will often look like just so much hand waving.

So, what should be done in practice? For each of the special cases of the generalized linear model, one computes as one ordinarily would, but uses either sandwich or nonparametric bootstrap standard error estimates. Then, proper asymptotic statistical tests and confidence intervals can be constructed. The regression coefficients can be interpreted as usual with one critical caveat: they are the product of *an incorrect model*. That is, they are covariance adjusted measures of association as usual, but the adjustments differ from those of a correct model. For example, one can obtain an estimate of the how the probability of a fatal car accident differs for 18 year olds compared to 25 year olds, which could be useful for insurance companies to know. But that estimate might well differ if covariance adjustments were made for average miles driven per month, the kind of vehicle driven, and use of alcohol. A more formal and complete discussion can be found in the paper by Buja and his colleagues (2016), but moving to a level III analysis will likely be ill advised.

1.5 The Transition to Statistical Learning

As a first approximation, statistical learning can be seen as a form of nonparametric regression in which the search for an effective mean function is especially data intensive. For example, one might want to capture how longevity is related to genetic and lifestyle factors. A statistical learning algorithm could be turned loose on a large dataset with no preconceptions about what the nature of the relationships might be. Fitted values from the exercise could then be used to anticipate which kinds of patients are more likely to face life-threatening chronic diseases. Such information would be of interest to physicians or actuaries. Likewise, a statistical learning algorithm could be applied to credit card data to determine which features of transactions are associated with fraudulent use. Again, there would be no need for any preconceptions about the relationships involved. With the key relationships determined, banks that issue credit cards would be able to alert their customers when their cards were likely being misused.

So far, this sounds little different from conventional regression analyses. And in fact, there has been considerable confusion in the applications literature about the nature of statistical learning and which procedures qualify (Baca-García et al. 2006; Kessler et al. 2015). In truth, the boundaries are fuzzy. The difference between models and algorithms is a good place to start clarifying the issues.

1.5.1 Models Versus Algorithms

Consider again the pair of equations for the conventional linear model.

$$y_i = \beta_0 + \beta_1 x_{1i} + \beta_2 x_{2i} + \cdots + \beta_p x_{p_i} + \varepsilon_i, \tag{1.3}$$

where

$$\varepsilon_i \sim \text{NIID}(0, \sigma^2). \tag{1.4}$$

Equations 1.3 and 1.4 are a theory of how each case i came to be. They are generative models because they represent the data generation mechanisms. When a data analyst works with these equations, a substantial amount of thought goes into model specification. What predictors should be used? What, if any, transformations are needed? What might be done about possible dependence among the disturbances or about nonconstant disturbance variances? But once these decisions are made, the necessary computing follows almost automatically. Usually, the intent is to minimize the sum of the squared residuals, and there is a convenient closed-form solution routinely implemented. On occasion, a more robust fitting criterion is used, such as minimizing the sum of the absolute value of the residuals, and although there is no closed form solution, the estimation problem is easily solved with linear programming.

Statistical learning allocates a data analysts' effort differently. Equations 1.3 and 1.4 often can be replaced by

$$y_i = f(\mathbf{X}_i) + \varepsilon_i, \tag{1.5}$$

where $f(\mathbf{X}_i)$ is some unknown function of one or more predictors, and ε_i is a residual if the analysis is level I. In a level II analysis, ε_i is a random disturbance whose assumed properties can depend on the data and statistical procedure used.

There can be two level II interpretations of Eq. 1.5. Consistent with conventional practice in regression, Eq. 1.5 may be interpreted as how nature generated the data, and then ε_i has its usual properties. It is just that the form of the mean function is not specified. However, that interpretation is inconsistent with the joint probability distribution framework used in statistical learning and raises again all of the problems with conventional linear regression.

The second interpretation builds on the mean function approximation approach used above for working with incorrect models. The $f(\mathbf{X}_i)$ is the estimation target taken to be some approximation of the true response surface, and ε_i is an additive disturbance whose properties we will consider shortly. But Eq. 1.5 is not a model of the data generation process.

Very little is asked of the data analyst because no commitment to any particular mean function is required. Indeed, the only decision may be to introduce ε_i additively. There is effectively no concern about whether the mean function is right or wrong because for all practical purposes there is no model responsible for the data. In practice, the objective is to arrive at fitted values from a computed $\hat{f}(\mathbf{X}_i)$ that make subject-matter sense and that correspond as closely as possible to realized values of Y. What form the $\hat{f}(\mathbf{X}_i)$ takes to get the job done can be of little concern.

In contrast, there needs to be serious thought given to the algorithm through which the fitted values are computed. Hence, the methods often are called "algorithmic." A simple and somewhat stylized outline of one kind of algorithmic method proceeds as follows.

1. Specify a linear mean function of the form of Eq. 1.3 and apply least squares as usual.
2. Compute the fitted values.
3. Compute the residuals.
4. Compute a measure of fit.
5. Apply least squares again, but weight the data so that observations with larger residuals are given more weight.
6. Update the fitted values obtained from the immediately preceding regression with the new fitted values weighted by their measure of fit.
7. Repeat steps 2–6 until the quality of the fit does not improve (e.g., 1000 times).
8. Output the fitted values.

In a process that has some of the same look and feel as boosting, a regression analysis is repeated over and over, each time with altered data so that hard-to-fit values of the Y are given more weight. In that sense, the hard-to-fit observations are counted more heavily when the sum of squared residuals is computed. The final result is a single set of fitted values that is a weighted sum of the many sets of fitted values. Hard thought must be given to whether this algorithm is an effective way to link predictors to a response and whether other algorithms might do the job better.

Fig. 1.9 Inputs W, X, and Z linked to the output Y through a black box algorithm

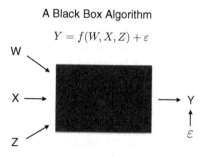

A Black Box Algorithm

$$Y = f(W, X, Z) + \varepsilon$$

There are also interpretative issues. In this algorithm, there can be a very large number of regressions and an even larger number of regression coefficients. For example, if there are 1000 regressions and 10 predictors, there are 10,000 regression coefficients. It is effectively impossible to make subject matter sense of 10,000 regression coefficients. Moreover, each set is computed for data with different weights so that the fitting task is continually changing.

In the end, one has a "black box" algorithm of the form shown in Fig. 1.9. There are in Fig. 1.9 three inputs $\{W, X, Z\}$, and a single output Y, connected by complicated computations that provide no information of substantive importance.[12] One can get from the inputs to the final set of fitted values. But, there is no model. The many regressions are just a computational device. In other terms, one has a procedure not a model.

Thinking back to the college admissions example, one can use the results of the algorithm to forecast a college applicant's freshman GPA *even though one does not know exactly how the predictors are being used to make that forecast.* In a similar fashion, one can use such methods to determine the dollar value of insurance claims a given driver is likely to make over the course of a year or the total precipitation a city will receive in a particular month. When Y is binary, one can project which parolees are likely to be rearrested or which high school students are likely to drop out of school.

There can be more interpretative information when one is able to change what inputs are used and re-run the algorithm. One could determine, for example, how the fitted values for college GPA change whether or not gender is included as an input. One could determine how much any measures of fit change as well. We will see later that there are special algorithms operating in much the same spirit that allow one to at least peep into the black box.

But one must be clear about exactly what might be learned. Suppose the association between gender and GPA operates in concert with age. The association between gender and college GPA is stronger for younger students perhaps because male stu-

---

[12]Some academic disciplines like to call the columns of **X** "inputs," and Y an "output" or a "target." Statisticians typically prefer to call the columns of **X** "predictors" and Y a "response." By and large, the terms predictor (or occasionally, regressor) and response will be used here except when there are links to computer science to be made. In context, there should be no confusion.

dents do not mature as rapidly as female students. As a result, should the quality of the fit improve when gender is included, the improvement results from a main effect and an interaction effect. Moreover, the algorithm might have transformed age in a manner that is unknown to the data analyst. A claim that on the average gender improves the quality of the fit is technically correct, but how gender is related to college GPA remains obscure.

A metaphor may help fix these ideas. Suppose one wants to bake some bread. The recipe calls for the following:

1. 2 packages of yeast
2. 2 cups of warm water
3. 2 tablespoons of melted butter
4. 2 tablespoons of sugar
5. 1 tablespoon of salt
6. 4 cups of all-purpose flour.

These ingredients are mixed and stirred until the batter is stiff, adding more flour if needed. The stiff batter is then kneaded until it is smooth and elastic, put into a greased bowl and allowed to rise for about an hour. The dough is then punched down and divided in half, placed into two greased loaf pans and again allowed to rise for about 30 min. Finally, the two loaves are baked at $400°$ for about 25 min.

The bread baking begins with known ingredients in specified amounts. From that point onward — the knead and baking — complicated physical and chemical processes begin that change the molecular structure of the ingredients as they are combined so that a bland watery batter can be turned into a delicious solid punctuated by air holes. The baker knows little about such details, and there is no way for the baker to document exactly how the ingredients are turned into bread. But if bread is tasty, the recipe will be repeated in the future. Looking again at Fig. 1.9, the ingredients are $\{W, X, Z\}$. The bread is Y. The black box is all of the physics and chemistry in-between.

It is possible to alter the bread recipe. For example, one might use 1 teaspoon of sugar rather than 2. That would likely lead to changes in the bread that comes out of the oven. It might be more preferable or less. Or one might choose to substitute whole wheat flour for the all-purpose flour. It is possible therefore, to see how changing the ingredients and/or their proportions affects the quality of the bread. But the baker does not learn much about the processes by which those ingredients are transformed into bread.[13]

Why might one prefer black box algorithmic methods rather than a traditional parametric regression? If the primary goal of the data analysis is to understand how the predictors are related to the response, one would not. But if the primary goal of the data analysis is to make decisions based at least in part on information provided by fitted values, statistical learning really has no downside. It should perform at least as well as model-based methods, and often substantially better. The reasons will

---

[13]In later chapters, several procedures will be discussed that can help one consider the "importance" of each input and how inputs are related to outputs.

be considered in later chapters when particular statistical learning procedures are discussed.

What roles do estimation, statistical tests and confidence intervals play? As before, they are effectively irrelevant for a level I analysis. For a level II analysis, the broader issues are the same as those already discussed. Inferences are being made to an approximation of the unknown response surface using the fitted values constructed from the data. However, that approximation is not model-based and is derived directly from the data. In the algorithm just summarized, for instance, each new weighted regression is altered because of the results of the earlier regressions. The algorithm is engaged in a very extensive form of data snooping. The resulting problems are similar to those produced by model selection, but with additional complications. One important complication is that there are tuning parameters whose values need to be determined by the data, and the number of observations can make an important difference. For example, if the sample size is 1000, the algorithm might well be tuned differently from when the sample size is 10,000, and the joint probability distribution to which inferences are being made has a limitless number of observations. What does tuning mean in that setting? In later chapters, when particular statistical learning procedure is discussed, the conceptual issues will be revisited and potential solutions provided.

Forecasting remains a level II activity. The approximation is used to compute forecasts and consequently, the forecasts will contain bias. One hopes that the forecasts are close to the truth, but there is no way to know for sure. As before, we will see that real progress can be made nevertheless.

Finally, we need to briefly address what to call an algorithmic approach for linking inputs to outputs. Suppose again that we have a set of fitted values constructed from 1000 linear, residual-weighted regressions. Do we call the computed relationships between the inputs and the outputs a model? In statistics, the term "model" is often reserved for the "generative model." The model conveys how the data were generated. But we are proceeding, at least for level II applications, assuming the data are generated as realizations from a joint probability distribution. That is not what is represented by each of the 1000 regressions. So, calling those 1000 regressions a model can be confusing.

Unfortunately, there seems to be no commonly accepted alternative term. We will proceed from here on with one of four terms: "algorithmic model," "algorithmic procedure," "statistical learning procedure," or most simply, "procedure." There should be no confusion in context.

1.6 Some Initial Concepts

Within a regression analysis framework, a wide variety of statistical learning procedures are examined in subsequent chapters. But, before going much farther down that road, a few key concepts need to be briefly introduced. They play central roles in the chapters ahead and, at this point, would benefit from some initial exposure. We return to these ideas many times, so nothing like mastery is required now. And that is a good thing. Important details can only be addressed later in the context of particular statistical learning procedures. For now, we consider what statistical learning looks like from 30,000 ft up.

1.6.1 Overall Goals of Statistical Learning

The range of procedures we examine have been described in several different ways (Christianini and Shawe-Taylor 2000; Witten and Frank 2000; Hand et al. 2001; Breiman 2001b; Dasu and Johnson, 2003; Bishop 2006; Hastie et al. 2009; Barber 2012; Marsland 2014; Sutton and Barto 2016), and associated with them are a variety of names: statistical learning, machine learning, supervised learning, reinforcement learning, algorithmic modeling, and others. The term "Statistical learning" as emphasized in the pages that follow, is based on the following notions.

The definition of regression analysis still applies, but as already noted, some statisticians like a function estimation framework. Thus,

$$Y = f(X) + \varepsilon \qquad (1.6)$$

or

$$G = f(X) + \varepsilon. \qquad (1.7)$$

For a quantitative response variable, the goal is to examine $Y|X$ for a response Y and one or more predictors X. If the response variable is categorical, the goal is to examine $G|X$ for a response G and a set of predictors X. X may be categorical, quantitative, or a mix of the two. Consistent with a data generated from a joint probability distribution, X is a random variable, although it is sometimes convenient to condition on the values of X that happen to be realized in the sample.

In conventional level II regression models, ε is assumed to be IID, with a mean of 0 and a constant variance. Drawing on the best linear approximation perspective, ε now conflates, as before, irreducible error, estimation (sampling) error, and bias. The new wrinkle is that at this point, no structure is imposed on the mean function. For a level I analysis, ε is just a residual.

Many different features of $Y|X$ and $G|X$ can be examined with statistical learning procedures. Usually conditional means or proportions, respectively, are of primary interest. For a level I analysis, fitted values suffice with no additional conceptual scaffolding. For a level II analysis, the fitted values are taken to be estimates of the conditional expectations of the response surface approximation discussed earlier. But there are several different flavors of this undertaking depending on the statistical procedure and the nature of the data.

When the response is categorical, the conditional expectations are usually interpreted as probabilities. The categories of G are often called "classes," and the data analysis exercise is often called "classification." There are also some issues that are unique to classification.

As anticipated in our earlier discussion of linear regression, it is very important to distinguish between fitted values computed when the response values are known and fitted values computed when the response values are unknown. Suppose for the moment that the response values are known. One then hopes that a statistical learning procedure succeeds in finding substantial associations between a set of predictors and a response. But, what is the task when a new set of predictor values is provided without known response values? This motivates a very different, but related, enterprise. The goals differ, but one cannot undertake the second unless the first has been reasonably well accomplished.[14]

When the response is known, the usual intent is to characterize how well the procedure is performing and for some statistical learning approaches, to describe how the inputs are related to the outputs. The aims may be substantive, but how the procedure performs will often lead to tuning. In our illustrative algorithm shown earlier, one might decide to slow down the speed at which the fitted values are updated even if that means re-running the regressions many more times.[15] There can sometimes be additional analysis steps making the statistical learning results more understandable.

When the response is unknown, there are two different analysis activities that depend on why the response is not known. The first kind of analysis is imputation. The response values exist but are not in the data. For example, can the carbon emissions from a coal-powered energy plant be approximated from information about the kind of technology the plant uses and amount of coal burned over a day? Can a student's true score in a standardized test be inferred from a pattern of answers that suggests cheating? Can the fish biomass of a tropical reef be estimated from information about the kinds of coral of which the reef is composed, the size of the reef, water temperature, and the amount of fishing allowed?

The second kind of analysis is forecasting: an outcome of interest is not just unknown, it has not occurred yet. What is the likely return from a given investment? What will be the top wind speed when a particular hurricane makes shore? For a certain county in Iowa, how many bushels of corn per acre can be expected in September from information available in June?

For categorical responses, one might try to impute an unknown class. For example, does a pattern of expenditures indicate that a credit card is being used fraudulently? Does a DNA test place a given suspect at the crime scene? Do the injuries from a car crash indicate that the driver was not wearing a seat belt? But just as with quantitative responses, forecasts are commonly undertaken as well. Will a particular

---

[14] When there is no interest whatsoever in a response Y, and attention is limited exclusively to X, supervised learning is no longer on the table, but unsupervised learning can be. Some kinds of cluster analysis can be seen as examples of unsupervised learning. Supervised learning becomes unsupervised learning when there is no response variable. In computer science terms, there is no "labeled" response.

[15] For instance, one might divide the updating set of fitted values by 10 making their updating impact 10 times weaker.

prison inmate be rearrested within two years when later released on parole? Will a certain earthquake fault rupture in the next decade? Will a given presidential candidate win the overall popular vote when a year later the election is held?

Why does the difference between imputation and forecasting matter? There are usually operational matters such as for imputation trying to understand why the data are missing? The answers help determine what remedies might be appropriate. The deeper difference is that in contrast to imputation, forecasting involves the realization of new cases from a joint probability distribution. One has to consider whether the same joint probability distribution is the source and whether the new cases are random realizations.

In short, statistical learning focuses on fitted values as the primary algorithmic product. They may be used for description, especially when associations with predictors can be calculated or displayed. As important in practice, associations between predictors and a response are used to compute fitted values when the response values are unknown. The enterprise can be imputation or forecasting.

1.6.2 Data Requirements: Training Data, Evaluation Data and Test Data

It is well known that all statistical procedures are vulnerable to overfitting. The fitting procedure capitalizes on the noise in the dataset as well as the signal. This is an especially important problem for statistical learning because there can be many ways to conflate noise with signal.

For a statistical learning level I analysis, the result can be an unnecessarily complicated summary of relationships and the risk of misleading interpretations. For a level II analysis, the problems are more complex and troubling. An important consequence of overfitting is that when performance of the procedure is examined with new data, even if realized from the same joint probability distribution, predictive accuracy will often degrade substantially. If out-of-sample performance is meaningfully worse than in-sample performance, generalizing the results from original data is compromised.

Overfitting can be exacerbated when the statistical learning procedure is allowed to seek a complex $f(X)$. Recall that in conventional linear regression, the greater the number of non-redundant regression coefficients whose values are to be estimated, the better the in-sample fit, other things equal. There have been, therefore, many attempts to develop measures of fit that adjust for this source of overfitting, typically by taking the degrees of freedom used by the procedure into account. Mallows' Cp is an example (Mallows 1973). Adjusting for the degrees of freedom used can counteract an important contributor to overfitting. Unfortunately, that does not solve the problem because the adjustments are all in-sample.

Probably the most important challenge to out-of-sample performance stems from various kinds of data snooping. It is common for data analysts to fit a regression model, look at the results and revise the regression model in response. This has become a widely promoted practice over the past several decades as various forms of regression diagnostic techniques have been developed. Thus, if evidence of non-constant variance is found in the residuals, a transformation of the response variable may be undertaken and the regression run again. Sometimes there is automated data snooping. Stepwise regression is a popular example. Many different models are compared in-sample, and the "best" one is chosen. Statistical learning procedures also data snoop because typically they are tuned. Sometimes the tuning is automated, and sometimes tuning is done by the data analyst. For example, tuning can be used to determine how complex the $\hat{f}(X)$ should be.

Data snooping can have especially pernicious effects because the problems caused go far beyond overly optimistic measure of performance. Data snooping introduces *model* uncertainty that is not included in standard formulations of statistical inference. That is, with different realizations of the data, there can be different models chosen. Canonical frequentist statistical inference assumes a known, fixed model before the data analysis begins. When data snooping leads to revising a mean function specification, the new mean function will typically lead to biased estimates, even asymptotically, and all statistical tests and confidence intervals can be invalid (Leeb and Pötscher 2005, 2006, 2008; Berk et al. 2010).[16] For level II analyses, these problems apply to statistical learning as well as conventional modeling.

Several in-sample solutions have been proposed (Berk et al. 2014; Lockhart et al. 2014), but they are not fully satisfactory, especially for statistical learning (Dwork et al. 2015). When a sufficient amount of data is available, the problems of overfitting and model selection sometimes can be effectively addressed with an out-of-sample approach. The realized data to which the statistical learning procedure is initially applied are usually called "training data." Training data provide the information through which the algorithm learns. There is then a second dataset, sometimes called "evaluation data," realized from the same joint probability distribution, used in the tuning process. The statistical learning procedure is tuned not by its performance in the training data, but by its performance in the evaluation data. One uses the results from the training data to predict the response in the evaluation data. How well the predicted values correspond to the actual evaluation data outcomes provides feedback on performance. Finally, there is a third dataset, commonly called "test data," also realized from the same joint probability distribution, used to obtain an "honest" assessment of the procedure's performance. Once a statistical learning procedure has been satisfactorily tuned, there can be a proper measure of out-of-sample performance. Much as was done with the evaluation data, a fitting and/or prediction

---

[16]Data snooping can also begin before an initial model is specified, and the implications are much the same. For example, all bivariate correlations between predictors and a response can be used to determine which predictors are selected for use in a regression analysis (Fan and Lv 2008).

exercise can be undertaken with the test data. The new set of fitted values can then be compared to the actual outcomes. In practice, there may be extensions of this process and interpretative complications, both of which will be addressed in subsequent chapters. For example, a lot depends on exactly what one is trying to estimate. Also, it can be useful to represent the uncertainty in the test sample results .

Arguably the most defensible approach is to have three datasets of sufficient size: a training dataset, an evaluation dataset, and a test dataset. "Sufficient" depends on the setting, but a minimum of about 500 cases each can be effective. All three should be realizations from the same joint probability distribution. If there is only one dataset on hand that is at least relatively large (e.g., 1500 cases), a training dataset, an evaluation dataset, and a test dataset can be constructed as three random, disjoint subsets. Then, there can important details to consider, such as the relative sizes of the three splits (Faraway 2014).

In addition, the split-sample approach is only justified asymptotically, and it is not clear how large a sample has to be before one is close enough. For example, if one or more of the key variables are highly skewed, no observations from the tails may have been included in the data overall, or in each of the data splits. Thus, in a study of sexually transmitted diseases (STDs), the very few individuals who have unprotected sex with a very large number of different individuals, may not be in the data. Yet these are the individuals who are most responsible for STD transmission. The chances that such a problem will materialize get smaller as the sample size gets bigger. But how big is big enough is not clear, at least in the abstract.

Finally, randomly splitting the data introduces a new source of uncertainty. Were the data split again, the fitted values would be at least somewhat different. In principle, this could be addressed with resampling. A large number of different splits could be used, and the fitted values in the test data across the different splits averaged. The main obstacle would be an additional computational burden.

When only training data are available, and the dataset on hand has too few observations for data splitting, there are several procedures one can use to try to approximate the out-of-sample ideal. Perhaps the most common is cross-validation. Consider a training data set with, say, 500 training observations and no evaluation or test data. Suppose the most pressing need is to document a procedure's performance conditional on the values of tuning parameters.

One can divide the data into five random, disjoint subsamples of 100 each, perhaps denoted by one of five letters A through E. The fitting procedure is applied to the 400 cases in subsets A–D and evaluated using remaining 100 "hold-out" cases in E. The fitting process is repeated for the 400 cases in subsets A, C, D, and E, and evaluated with the 100 hold-out cases in B. One proceeds in the same fashion until each of the five splits is used once as the holdout subset, and each split has four opportunities to be included with three other splits as training data. There are then five measures of performance that can be averaged to obtain an approximation of true evaluation data performance. For example, one might compute the average of five AICs (Akaike 1973). The tuning parameter values that lead to the best performance in the evaluation samples are selected. One has tuned using a fivefold cross-validation.

Cross-validation is no doubt a clever technique for level II analyses that might seem straightforward. It is not straightforward, and its use depends heavily on how the data were generated and the kind of statistical procedures undertaken. To begin, splitting the data five ways is somewhat arbitrary. Occasionally, there are as few as three splits and often as many as ten. Also, one can treat the jackknife as "leave-one-out" cross validation, in which case there are N splits. A larger number of splits means that the size of the training data relative to the test data is greater. This improves performance in the data training splits, but makes performance in the hold-out data less stable. The converse follows from a smaller number of splits. But, there is no formal justification for any particular number of splits which will typically depend on the setting. Common practice seems to favor either fivefold or tenfold cross-validation.

Much as with a split sample approach, there is a more fundamental issue: because there are no evaluations or test data, the results of cross-validation are conditional on the training data alone. Suppose one is trying to study the correlates of blindness for individuals under 50 years of age and has training data with 1000 observations. By the luck of the draw, 100 of those observations have macular degeneration whereas in the generative joint probability distribution, such cases are very rare. (Macular degeneration is usually found in substantially older people.) Moreover, that 10 % has a significant impact on any regression analyses. In all of those random splits of the data, about 10 % of the cases will be suffering from macular degeneration and the cross-validated regression results will be shaped accordingly. Again, defensible results depend on asymptotics.

In short, a lot can depend on having training data for which its distributional features are much like those of the generative joint probability distribution. And there is no way of knowing if this is true from the training data alone. Put another way, cross-validation is more likely to provide generalizable results from training data with a large number of observations. The empirical joint distribution in the data is more likely to correspond well to the joint probability distribution from which the data were realized. Formally, one needs to capitalize on asymptotics.

Finally, cross-validation is a popular procedure in part because single datasets that are too small to subdivide are common. But cross-validation shares with data splitting reductions in sample size. We will see later that many statistical learning procedures are sample size dependent. Smaller training datasets can increase bias in estimates of the true response surface. In addition, if the statistical learning results are sample size dependent, what does it mean to estimate features of a joint probably distribution for which the number of observations can be seen as limitless? We will address this matter in the next chapter.

In summary, for level II analyses one should try to avoid in-sample determination of tuning parameters and assessments of procedure performance. Having legitimate training data, evaluation data, and test data is probably the best option. Split samples are one fallback position, and cross-validation is another. They provide somewhat different challenges. Split samples provide separately for tuning and for honest performance assessments. Cross-validation forces a choice between proper tuning and honest performance assessments. Split samples do not immediately allow for representations of uncertainty, although there are extensions that can provide that information. Cross-validation can provide measures of uncertainty for many applications. There are also tradeoffs in how observations are allocated. Cross-validation uses most of the cases as training data. Split samples allow for a wide range of different data allocations. Sometimes, it effectively will not matter which one is used, and when it does matter, the choice will often be determined by the application. Later chapters have examples of both situations.

1.6.3 Loss Functions and Related Concepts

Loss functions can be used to quantify how well the output of a statistical procedure corresponds to certain features of the data. As the name implies, one should favor small loss function values. A very general expression for a loss function can be written as $L(Y, \hat{f}(X))$, where Y represents some feature of the data, and $\hat{f}(X)$ represents some empirical approximation of it. Often, Y is a response variable, and $\hat{f}(X)$ is the fitted values from some statistical procedure.[17]

In conventional treatments of estimation, there are loss functions that the estimators minimize with respect to the data on hand. Least squares regression, for example, minimizes the sum of the squared residuals. Least absolute residual regression, minimizes the sum of the absolute values of the residuals. For a level I analysis, these loss functions can be sensible ways to justify the summary statistics computed. Thus, least squares regression leads to fitted values for conditional means. Least absolute residual regression leads to fitted values for conditional medians. For a level II analysis, the resulting estimates have well-known and desirable formal properties as long as the requisite statistical assumptions are met. An absence of bias is a popular instance. But a key conceptual point is that when a loss function is minimized for the data on hand, performance is being addressed solely in-sample.

As already noted, there is a rich tradition of in-sample measures of fitting error that attempt to correct for the degrees of freedom used by the procedure. Recall that other things equal, a regression model that uses more degrees of freedom will automatically fit the data better. This is undesirable because a good fit should result from predictors that are strongly related to the response, not just because there are a lot of them. Measures that try to correct for the degrees of freedom used include the adjusted R^2, AIC, BIC, and Mallows Cp. The adjusted R^2 is popular because it seems easy to interpret, but it lacks a rigorous formal rationale. The other three measures each have good, but different, formal justifications (Hastie et al. 2009: Sect. 7.5).

---

[17]Loss functions are also called "objective functions" or "cost functions."

Unfortunately, they can still provide a falsely optimistic assessment of performance. The fitting is undertaken in-sample and capitalizes on idiosyncratic features of the data that undermine generalization. We need a better way.

For statistical learning, a better way can be especially important inasmuch as attention typically is directed to fitted values. A natural level II question, therefore, is how well the $\hat{f}(X)$ performs out-of-sample. One better way is to use *generalization error*, also called *test error*, as a performance metric (Hastie et al. 2009: 228). Suppose one has a test data observation denoted by (X^*, Y^*), where X^* can be a set of predictors. For the random variable Y, random variables X, and a statistical learning result constructed from the training data $\mathcal{T}$, generalization error is defined as

$$\text{Err}_{\mathcal{T}} = \text{E}_{(X^*, Y^*)}[L(Y^*, \hat{f}(X^*))|\mathcal{T})]. \tag{1.8}$$

The training data are treated as fixed once they are realized. A statistical procedure is applied to the training data in an effort minimize some loss function in-sample. The result is a set of parameter estimates. For example, in conventional regression, one obtains estimates of the regression coefficients and the intercept. At that point, the results of the minimization become fixed as well. Just as in many real forecasting settings, the training data and the parameters estimates are in the past and now do not change. Then, one may want to know how well the procedure performs with a test data observation. One can compare Y^* to $\hat{f}(X^*)$ within a loss function such as squared error.[18] But, $\text{E}_{(X^*, Y^*)}$ means that generalization error is the average loss over a limitless number of realized test observations, not a single observation. The result is an average loss in the test data. If one actually has test data, this is easy to operationalize. Cross-validation can be a fallback approach (Hastie et al. 2009: Sect. 7.12)

There can also be interest in the average generalization error, if in theory the training data $\mathcal{T}$ can also be realized over and over. With each realization of $\mathcal{T}$, the entire procedure represented in Eq. 1.8 is repeated. Then, *expected prediction error* (EPE) is defined as

$$\text{Err} = \text{E}_{\mathcal{T}} \text{E}_{(X^*, Y^*)}[L(Y^*, \hat{f}(X^*))|\mathcal{T})]. \tag{1.9}$$

If one has test data, the entire procedure can be wrapped in a resampling procedure such as a bootstrap. More will be said about the bootstrap in later chapters. Cross-validation once again can be a fallback position.

Whether one uses generalization error or expected prediction error depends on how much the X distribution matters. Because X and Y are treated as random variables and a response surface approximation is the estimation target, it can make sense to consider how the distribution of X can affect the results. Recall the earlier discussion of estimation with misspecified mean functions. But a lot depends on how the results of the estimation procedure will be used. With forecasting applications, for instance,

---

[18]In R, many estimation procedures have a *predict()* function that can easily be used with test data to arrive at test data fitted values.

generalization error may be more relevant than expected prediction error. Examples are provided in later chapters.

For categorical responses, generalization error can be written as

$$\text{Err}_\mathcal{T} = E_{(X^*, G^*)}[L(G^*, \hat{G}(X^*))|\mathcal{T})]. \tag{1.10}$$

As before, $E[\text{Err}_\mathcal{T}]$ is expected prediction error, and both $\text{Err}_\mathcal{T}$ and $E[\text{Err}_\mathcal{T}]$ can be of interest.

A look back at Fig. 1.8 will provide a sense of what generalization error and expected prediction error are trying to capture with $\hat{G}|X^*$. Suppose there are two actual response categories coded as 1 or 0. There are fitted values in the metric of proportions. A natural in-sample measure of fit is the deviance. There are also fitted classes depending on where a given proportion falls with respect to the classification threshold. A natural in-sample measure of fit is the proportion of cases for which the fitted value is the same as the actual class. Some very powerful statistical learning procedures classify without the intermediate step of computing proportions, but the correspondence between the actual class and the fitted class is still central.

The rationale for choosing generalization error or expected prediction error does not change for categorical response variables. The estimation options are also much the same. There will be examples later.

The loss functions considered so far are symmetric. For a numerical Y, a fitted value that is too large by some specific amount makes the same contribution to the loss function as a fitted value that is too small by that same amount. Consider, for example, the number of homeless in a census tract as the response variable, and predictors that are features of census tracts. Overestimating the number of homeless individuals in a census tract can have very different policy implications from underestimating the number of homeless individuals in a census tract (Berk et al. 2008). In the first instance, costly social services may be unnecessarily allocated to certain census tracts. In the second instance, those services may not be provided in census tracts that really need them. Yet, a symmetric loss function would assume that in the metric of costs, their consequences are exactly the same. One needs a loss function that properly takes the asymmetric costs into account so that the homeless estimates are responsive to how they will be used in practice.

Symmetric loss functions also dominate when the response variable is categorical. Suppose there are K exhaustive and mutually exclusive classes. Any misclassification — the fitted class is the wrong class — is given the same weight of 1.0. In a forecasting application, for instance, the error of predicting that a high school student will dropout when that student will not is given the same weight as predicting that a high school student will not dropout when that student will. (Correct classifications are given a value of 0.0.)

Once again, one must ask if symmetric costs are reasonable. Are the costs really the same, or even close? In the case of the potential high school dropout, are the

costs of interventions for a student who needs no interventions the same as failing
to provide interventions for a student who needs them? A lot depends on the content
of those interventions (e.g., academic tutoring, counseling). Especially in policy
settings where decision makers will be using the statistical learning results, symmetric
costs may not be reasonable. Some mistakes are much worse than others, and the
asymmetric costs must be allowed to affect how the statistical learning procedure
performs. In later chapters, this will be a central concern.

1.6.4 The Bias-Variance Tradeoff

Before we move into more of the nuts and bolts of estimation, we need to revisit a
bit more the bias–variance tradeoff. Recall that the bias–variance tradeoff is a level
II problem that arises when the true response surface is explicitly the estimation
target. The goal is to produce an estimate of the true response surface that is as close
as possible to the truth. In principle, this can be achieved by a judicious tradeoff
between the bias of the estimates and the variance in those estimates.

If the estimation target is the approximate response surface, there is no bias, at
least asymptotically, but a closely related tradeoff can be in play. When the focus is
on generalization error, for example, the goal is to impute or forecast as accurately
as possible even though one explicitly is using an approximation of the true response
surface. That is, the actual estimation target is the potential y-values in the joint
probability distribution responsible for the data.

To illustrate, using an asymptotically unbiased estimate of the mean function
approximation linking daily ozone concentrations in a city and emergency room visits for respiratory distress, one might want to forecast a day or two in advance how
many such visits there might be. Many factors affect emergency room visits, so one
is clearly working with a mean function approximation. Bias in the projected number
of emergency room visits might be reduced by using a different approximation; the
approximation could be made more complex. Thinking in parametric terms for the
moment, a 4th degree polynomial might be used instead of a second-degree polynomial. But with a more complex parametric approximation, the effective degrees of
freedom will be larger (more on that shortly). Other things equal, an increase in the
effective degrees of freedom will increase the variance in fitted values as estimates.
Hence, there is a potential tradeoff.

The tradeoff can be especially dicey with statistical learning because of the inductive nature of the procedures and the routine use of tuning. One problem is that the
meaning and calculation of the effective degrees of freedom can be a challenge
(Janson et al. 2015; Kauffman and Rosset 2014). Nevertheless, the split sample
approach can work satisfactorily, and there are fallback positions that can also lead
to useful results.

1.6 Some Initial Concepts

39

1.6.5 Linear Estimators

Level II statistical learning can capitalize on a wide variety of estimators. Linear
estimators are often preferred because they can be seen as variants of conventional
linear regression and are easily shown to have good statistical properties. Recall the
hat matrix from conventional, fixed-x linear regression:

$$\hat{\mathbf{y}} = \mathbf{X}\boldsymbol{\beta} = \mathbf{X}(\mathbf{X}^T\mathbf{X})^{-1}\mathbf{X}^T\mathbf{y} = \mathbf{H}\mathbf{y}. \tag{1.11}$$

The hat matrix $\mathbf{H}$ transforms the y_i in a linear fashion into $\hat{y}_i$.

A smoother matrix is a generalization of the hat matrix. Suppose there is a training
dataset with N observations, a single fixed predictor X, and a single value of X, x_0.
Generalizations to more than one predictor are provided in a later chapter. The fitted
value for $\hat{y}_0$ at x_0 can be written as

$$\hat{y}_0 = \sum_{j=1}^{N} \mathbf{S}_{0j} y_j. \tag{1.12}$$

$\mathbf{S}$ is an N by N matrix of fixed weights and is sometimes called a "smoother matrix."
$\mathbf{S}$ can be a product of a statistical learning procedure. The subscript 0 denotes the row
corresponding to the case whose fitted value of y is to be computed. The subscript j
denotes the column in which the weight is found. In other words, the fitted value $\hat{y}_0$ at
x_0 is a linear combination of all N values of y_i, with the weights determined by $\mathbf{S}_{0j}$.
In many applications, the weights decline with the distance from x_0. Sometimes the
declines are abrupt, as in a step function. In practice, therefore, a substantial number
of the values in $\mathbf{S}_{0j}$ can be zero.

Consider the following cartoon illustration in matrix format. There are five observations constituting a time series. The goal is to compute a moving average of three
observations going from the first observation to the last. In this case, the middle value
is given twice the weight of values on either side. Endpoints are often a complication
in such circumstances and here, the first and last observations are simply taken as is.

$$\begin{pmatrix} 1.0 & 0 & 0 & 0 & 0 \\ .25 & .50 & .25 & 0 & 0 \\ 0 & .25 & .50 & .25 & 0 \\ 0 & 0 & .25 & .50 & .25 \\ 0 & 0 & 0 & 0 & 1.0 \end{pmatrix} \begin{pmatrix} 3.0 \\ 5.0 \\ 6.0 \\ 9.0 \\ 10.0 \end{pmatrix} = \begin{pmatrix} 3.00 \\ 4.75 \\ 6.50 \\ 8.50 \\ 10.00 \end{pmatrix}. \tag{1.13}$$

The leftmost matrix is $\mathbf{S}$. It is post multiplied by the vector $\mathbf{y}$ to yield the fitted
values $\hat{\mathbf{y}}$. But from where do the values in $\mathbf{S}_{0j}$ come? If there are predictors, it only
makes sense to try to use them. Consequently, $\mathbf{S}_{0j}$ is usually constructed from X.

For a level II analysis, one has a linear estimator of the conditional means of Y. It
is a linear estimator because with $\mathbf{S}$ fixed, each value of y_i is multiplied by a constant
before the y_i are added together; $\hat{y}_0$ is a linear combination of the y_i. Linearity can

make it easier to determine the formal properties of an estimator, which are often highly desirable. Unbiasedness is a primary example.[19]

When one views the data as generated from a joint probability distribution, X is no longer fixed.[20] Linear estimators with fixed values of X become nonlinear estimators with random values of X. The use of turning parameters also can lead to nonlinear estimators. One has to rely on asymptotics to derive an estimator's formal statistical properties. Asymptotic unbiasedness can sometimes be demonstrated depending on precisely what features of the joint probability distribution are being estimated. One also will need to rely on asymptotics to arrive at, when appropriate, proper standard errors, statistical tests, and confidence intervals.

1.6.6 Degrees of Freedom

Woven through much of the discussion of level II analyses has been the term "degrees of freedom." It will prove useful to expand just a bit on the several related conceptual issues. Recall that, loosely speaking, the degrees of freedom associated with an estimate is the number of observations that are free to vary, given how the estimate is computed. In the case of the mean, if one knows the values of $N - 1$ of those observations, and one knows the value of the mean, the value of the remaining observation can be easily obtained. Given the mean, $N - 1$ observations are free to vary. The remaining observation is not. So, there are $N - 1$ degrees of freedom associated with the estimator of the mean.

This sort of reasoning carries over to many common statistics including those associated with linear regression analysis. The number of degrees of freedom used when the fitted values are computed is the number of regression parameters whose values need to be obtained (i.e., the intercept plus the regression coefficients). The degrees of freedom remaining, often called the "residual degrees of freedom," is the number of observations minus the number of these parameters to be estimated (Weisberg 2014: 26).

One of the interesting properties of the hat matrix is that the sum of its main diagonal elements (i.e., the trace) equals the number of regression parameters estimated. This is of little practical use with parametric regression because one can arrive at the same number by simply counting all of the regression coefficients and the intercept. However, the similarities between **H** and **S** (Hastie et al. 2009: Sect. 5.4.1) imply that for linear estimators, the trace of **S** can be interpreted as the degrees of freedom used. Its value is sometimes called the "effective degrees of freedom" and can

---

[19] "Linear" in regression can be used in two different ways. An estimator may or may not be linear. The relationship between Y and X may or may not be linear. For example, an estimator may be linear, and the relationship between Y and X may be highly nonlinear. In short, a linear estimator does not necessarily imply a linear relationship.

[20] Although as before, one can treat the random x-values as fixed once they are realized in the data, and as before, one is then limited to generalizing only to joint probability distributions with the exact same x-values.

roughly be interpreted as the "equivalent number of parameters" (Ruppert et al. 2003: Sect. 3.13). That is, the trace of **S** can be thought of as capturing how much less the data are free to vary given the calculations represented in **S**. One can also think of the trace as qualifying "*optimism* of the residual sum of squares as an estimate of the out-of-sample prediction error" (Janson et al. 2015: 3)[21] As already noted several times, when more degrees of freedom are used (other things equal), in-sample fit will provide an increasingly unjustified, optimistic impression of out-of-sample performance.[22]

There are other definitions of the degrees of freedom associated with a smoother matrix. In particular, Ruppert and his colleagues (2003: Sect. 3.14) favor

$$df_{\mathbf{S}} = 2\mathrm{tr}(\mathbf{S}) - \mathrm{tr}(\mathbf{S}\mathbf{S}^T). \tag{1.14}$$

In practice, the two definitions of the smoother degrees of freedom will not often vary by a great deal, but whether the two definitions lead to different conclusions depends in part on how they are used. If used to compute an estimate of the residual variance, their difference can sometimes matter. If used to characterize the complexity of the fitting function, their differences are usually less important because one smoother is compared to another applying the same yardstick. The latter application is far more salient in subsequent discussions. Beyond its relative simplicity, there seem to be interpretive reasons for favoring the first definition (Hastie et al. 2009: Sect. 5.4.1). Consequently, for linear estimators we use the trace of **S** as the smoother degrees of freedom.

Unfortunately, there are complications. When there is model selection, more degrees of freedom are being used than the number of non-redundant regression parameters in the final model chosen. This is no less true when tuning parameters are employed. It makes intuitive sense that tuning requires data snooping, even if automated, and degrees of freedom are spent in the process.

Efron's early work on prediction errors (1986) allows us to takes a step back to reformulate the issues. Effective degrees of freedom used boils down to how well the data are fit in training data compared to how well the data are fit in test data. Other things equal, the larger the gap, the larger the effective degrees of freedom used. Drawing from Efron (1986), Kaufman and Rosset (2014) and Janson and colleagues (2015), the effective degrees of freedom can be defined as

$$\mathrm{EDF} = \mathrm{E}\left[\sum_{i=1}^{N}(y_i^* - \hat{y}_i)^2\right], \tag{1.15}$$

where y_i^* is a realized y-value in test data, and $\hat{y}_i$ is a fitted value computed from the training data. The vector of x-values for case i does not change from realization to realization. Thus, one imagines two, fixed-x realizations of the response for each

---

[21]Emphasis in the original.

[22]The residual degrees of freedom can then be computed by subtraction (see also Green and Silverman 1994: Sect. 3.3.4).

case. One is included in the training data and used to construct a fitted value. The other is included in the test data. The effective degrees of freedom is the expectation of the summed (over N), squared disparities between the two. The greater the average squared disparities between the fitted values from the training data and the new, realized values of Y, the greater the EDF. The EDF captures how much the degrees of freedom used by the fitting procedure by itself inflates the quality of the fit.

When the fitted values are constructed from a procedure with IID finite variance disturbances, as discussed in Sect. 1.6.1, Eq. 1.15 becomes

$$\text{EDF} = \frac{1}{\sigma^2} \sum_{i=1}^{N} \text{Cov}(y_i, \hat{y}_i). \tag{1.16}$$

The covariance for each case i is defined over realizations of Y with the predictor values fixed, and σ^2 is the variance of the disturbances as usual. Equation 1.16 is a standardized representation of similarity between the realized values of Y and the fitted values of Y. The greater the standardized linear association between the two, the larger the effective degrees of freedom.

In practice, neither definition is operational. But there are important special cases for which estimates of the EDF can be obtained. One of the most useful is when the estimator for the fitted values is linear (e.g., for a smoother matrix $\mathbf{S}$). However, current thinking about the EDF appears to be limited to the fixed-x case, whereas statistical learning usually conceives both Y and X as random variables. How to formulate the EDF with random X is apparently unsolved. Indeed, the concept of EDF might usefully be abandoned and replaced by formulations for unjustified optimism. In a very wide set of circumstance, this could be addressed with training and test data, as suggested above.

1.6.7   Basis Functions

Another consideration in thinking about the effective degrees of freedom is that the procedures discussed in subsequent chapters commonly do not work directly with the given set of predictors. Rather, the design matrix in a level I or level II analysis can be comprised of linear basis expansions of X. Linear basis expansions allow for a more flexible fitting function, typically by increasing the dimensionality of the design matrix. A set of p predictors becomes a set of predictors much greater than p. This can make the fitted values more responsive to the data.

Consider first the case when there is but a single predictor. X contains two columns, one column with the values of that single predictor and one column solely of 1s for the intercept. The $N \times 2$ matrix is sometimes called the "basis" of a bivariate regression model. This basis can be expanded in a linear fashion as follows:

$$f(X) = \sum_{m=1}^{M} \beta_m h_m(X). \qquad (1.17)$$

There are M transformations of X, which can include the untransformed predictor, and typically a leading column of 1s is included (allowing for a y-intercept). β_m is the weight given to the mth transformation, and $h_m(X)$ is the mth transformation of X. Consequently, $f(X)$ is a linear combination of transformed values of X.

One common transformation employs polynomial terms such as $1, x, x^2, x^3$. Each term does not have to be a linear transformation of x, but the transformations are *combined* in a linear fashion. Then, Eq. 1.17 takes the form

$$f(X) = \beta_0 + \beta_1 x + \beta_2 x^2 + \beta_3 x^3. \qquad (1.18)$$

When least squares is applied, a conventional hat matrix follows, from which fitted values may be constructed.

Another popular option is to construct a set of indicator variables. For example, one might have predictor z, transformed in the following manner.

$$f(Z) = \beta_0 + \beta_1(I[z > 5]) + \beta_2(I[z > 8|z > 5]) + \beta_3(I[z < 2]). \qquad (1.19)$$

As before, fitting by least squares leads to a conventional hat matrix from which the fitted values may be constructed.[23]

Equation 1.17 can be generalized so that $p > 1$ predictors may be included:

$$f(X) = \sum_{j=1}^{p} \sum_{m=1}^{M_j} \beta_{jm} h_{jm}(X). \qquad (1.20)$$

There are p predictors, each denoted by j, and each with its own M_j transformations. All of the transformations for all predictors, each with its weight β_{jm}, are combined in a linear fashion. For example, one could combine Eqs. 1.18 and 1.19 with both X and Z as predictors. It is also possible, and even common in some forms of machine learning, to define *each* basis function as a complicated function of two or more predictors. For example, recall that the usual cross-product matrix so central to linear regression is $\mathbf{X}^T\mathbf{X}$. As we will see later, "kernels" broadly based on $\mathbf{X}\mathbf{X}^T$ can be constructed that serve is very effective linear basis expansions.

Linear basis expansions are no less central to many forms of classification. Figure 1.10 provides a visual sense of how. Decisions boundaries are essentially fitted values from some procedure that separate one class from another, and can then be used to decide in which class a new case belongs. In Fig. 1.10, there are two classes

---

[23] The symbol I denotes an indicator function. The result is equal to 1 if the argument in brackets is true and equal to 0 if the argument in brackets is false. The 1s and 0s constitute an indicator variable. Sometimes indicator variables are called a dummy variables.

represented by either a red circle or a blue circle. There are two predictors, X_1 and X_2. Figure 1.10 is a 3-dimensional scatterplot.

The upper plot shows in 2-D predictor space a linear decision boundary. All cases falling above the linear boundary are classified as red circles, because red circles are the majority. All cases falling below the linear boundary are classified as blue circles because blue circles are the majority. The linear decision boundary produces three classification errors. There is one blue circle above the decision boundary and two red circles below the decision boundary. Separation between the two classes is imperfect, and in this illustration, no linear decision boundary can separate the two classes perfectly. However, also shown is a nonlinear decision boundary that can. The trick would be to find transformations of the two predictors from which such a decision boundary could be constructed.

Sometimes there is an effective way to proceed. The lower plot in Fig. 1.10 shows the same binary outcomes in 3-D space. A third dimension has been added. The two curved arrows show how the locations for two illustrative points are moved. As just noted, new dimensions can result from transformations when there is a basis expansion. Here, the three transformation functions are shown as h_1, h_2 and h_3. Within this 3-D predictor space, all of the blue circles are toward the front of the figure, and all of the red circles are toward the back of the figure. The plane shown is a *linear* decision boundary that leads to perfect separation. By adding a dimension, perfect separation can be obtained, and one can work in a more congenial linear world. In 3-D, one has in principle an easier classification problem. Then if one wishes, the 3-D predictor space can be projected back to the 2-D predictor space to view the results as a function of the two original predictors. Back in 2-D predictor space, the decision boundary can then be nonlinear, often very nonlinear.

But if Eq. 1.20 is essentially multiple regression, where does statistical learning come in? The answer is that statistical learning procedures often "invent" their own linear basis expansions. That is, the linear basis expansions are inductively

Fig. 1.10 Reductions in classification errors under linear basis expansions (The *red filled circles* and the *blue filled circles* represent different classes. The *top figure* shows how classification errors can be reduced with a nonlinear decision boundary. The *bottom figure* shows how classification errors can be reduced by including a third predictor dimension.)

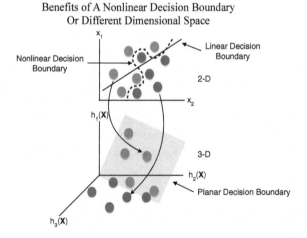

constructed as a product of how the algorithmic procedure "learns." Alternatively, a data analyst may provide the algorithm with far too many basis expansions terms, sometimes more terms than there are observations, and the algorithm decides inductively which are really needed.

Figure 1.11 provides an illustration. The observational units are all 50 states each year from 1978 to 1998, for a total of 1000 observations. For each state each year, the homicide rate and the number of executions for capital crimes were recorded. Data such as these have been central in debates about the deterrent value of the death penalty (Nagin and Pepper 2012).

Executions lagged by one year is on the horizontal axis. It is the only predictor and is included as a single vector of values. No position is taken by the data analyst about the nature of its relationship with the response; the values "as is" are input to the algorithm. The homicide rate per 1000 people is on the vertical axis. The blue, dashed line shows fitted values centered at zero. They are arrived at inductively though a linear basis expansion of the number of executions. The residuals around the fitted values are shown with small blue dots. Error bands around the fitted values are shown light blue. For reasons that will be discussed in the next chapter, the error bands only capture the variability in the fitted values; they are not confidence intervals. Still, if the error bands are used, one has a level II regression analysis.

Within a level I perspective, in most years, most states execute no one. Over 80 % of the observations have zero executions. A very few states in a very few years execute more than five individuals. Years in which more than five individuals in a state are executed represent about 1 % of the data (i.e., 11 observations out of 1000) and in this region of the figure, the data are very sparse.

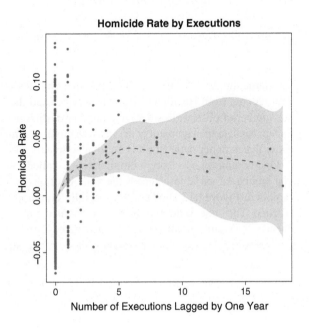

Fig. 1.11 The homicide rate per 1,000 as a function of the number of executions (The homicide rate is on vertical axis, and the number of executions one year earlier is on the horizontal axis. The *broken line* represents the fitted values, and the *light blue region* shows the error bands.)

When there are five executions or less, the relationship between the number of executions and the homicide rate one year later is positive. More executions are followed one year later by more homicides. Thus, there is a positive association for 99 % of the data. When a given state in a given year executes six or more individuals, the relationship appears to turn negative. With more executions, there are fewer homicides one year later. But there are almost no data supporting the change in sign, and from a level II perspective, the error bands around that portion of the curve show that the relationship could easily be flat and even positive.[24] In short, for 99 % of the data, the relationship is positive and for the atypical 1 %, one really cannot tell. (For more details, see Berk 2005.)

Figure 1.11 provides a visualization of how a response of great policy interest and a single predictor of great policy interest are related. There is no model in the conventional regression sense. The fitted values shown were arrived at inductively by a statistical learning algorithm. Had a linear mean function been imposed, the few influential points to the far right of the figure would have produced a negative regression coefficient. One might incorrectly conclude that on the average, there is evidence for the deterrent effect of executions. In practice, of course, the potential role of confounders would need to be considered.

In summary, linear basis expansions can be an important, and even essential, feature of statistical learning. Statistical learning algorithms can be seen as instruments in service of finding linear basis expansions that facilitate prediction. Where the algorithms differ is in exactly how they do that.

1.6.8   The Curse of Dimensionality

Linear basis expansions increase the dimensionality of a dataset. As just described, this is often a good thing. In this era of "Big Data" it is also increasingly common to have access to data not just with a very large number of observations, but with a very large number of variables. For example, the IRS might merge its own records with records from Health and Human Services and the Department of Labor. Both the number of observations (N) and number of dimensions (p) could be enormous. Except for data management concerns, one might assume that bigger data are always better than smaller data. But it is not that simple.

One common and vexing complication is called "the curse of dimensionality." The number of variables exceeds the number of observations that can be effectively exploited. Figure 1.12 shows two especially common difficulties that can arise in practice. The cube at the top illustrates that as the number of dimensions increases linearly, the volume of the resulting space increases as a power function of the number of dimensions. Hence, the 3 by 3 square has 9 units of space to fill with data, whereas

---

[24]To properly employ a level II framework, lots of hard thought would be necessary. For example, are the observations realized independently as the joint probability distribution approach requires? And if not, then what?

Fig. 1.12 Two consequences of the curse of dimensionality (The *top figure* shows how volume increases as a power function, the *bottom figure* shows how observations move farther away from the center.)

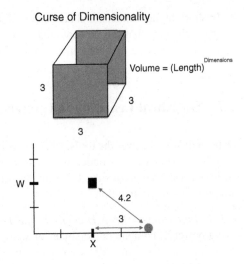

Curse of Dimensionality

Volume = (Length)^{Dimensions}

the 3 by 3 by 3 cube has 27 units of space to fill with data. The result for a dataset with a certain number of observations is that the distribution of the observations can become very sparse. The space is less adequately covered, so that the sample size per unit of space decreases. A data analysis one might like to do can become impractical. In particular, key regions of a nonlinear $f(\mathbf{X})$ may be very poorly estimated for lack of sufficient data.

Unless more observations can be obtained, some simplifications need to be imposed by the data analyst. A popular approach is to make the function some linear combination of the predictors. Sometimes that can improve the quality of the fitted values, and sometimes that can make the quality worse. This is another manifestation of the bias–variance tradeoff. Alternatively, one can try to reduce the dimensionality of the data using model selection procedures, shrinkage, an incomplete Cholesky decomposition, or principle components. But each of these comes with their own challenges. For example, if principle components analysis is used, one must determine how many of the principle components to include, which introduces a form of model selection.

The bottom figure illustrates a second complication. With an increase in the number of dimensions, the data move farther from the center of the space. For a very large p, the data can be concentrated toward the edges of the space. In the figure, a distance of 3 units in one dimension can become a distance of 4.2 in two dimensions. Thus, a hypercube with 5 sides of 3 units each has a maximum Euclidian distance of 6.7 units, whereas a hypercube with 10 sides of 3 units each has a maximum Euclidian distance of 22.3 units. The problem for a data analysis is that the region toward the center of the space becomes especially sparse. In that region, it will be very difficult to estimate effectively a response surface, especially if it is complicated. Once again, the data analyst has to simplify how the estimation is undertaken or reduce the number of dimensions.

In short, higher dimensional data can be very useful when there are more associations in the data that can be exploited. But at least ideally, a large p comes with a large N. If not, what may look like a blessing can actually be a curse.

1.7 Statistical Learning in Context

Data analysis, whatever the tools, takes place in a professional setting that can influence how the analysis is undertaken. Far more is involved than formal technique. Although we cannot consider these matters at any length, a few brief observations are probably worth mention.

- *It is Important to Keep Humans in the Loop* — With the increasing processing power of computers, petabytes of storage, efficient algorithms, and a rapidly expanding statistical toolbox, there are strong incentives to delegate data analyses to machines. At least in the medium term, this is a huge mistake. Humans introduce a host of critical value judgements, intuitions and context that computers cannot. Worse than a statistical bridge to nowhere is a statistical bridge to the wrong place. A better formulation is a structured computer–human partnership on which there is already interesting work in progress (Michelucci and Dickinson 2016).
- *Sometimes There is No Good Solution* — The moment one leaves textbook examples behind, there is a risk that problems with the data and/or the statistical procedures available will be insurmountable. That risk is to be expected in the real world of empirical research. There is no shame in answering an empirical question with "I can't tell." There is shame in manufacturing results for appearance's sake. Assume-and-proceed statistical practice can be a telling example. In later chapters, we will come upon unsolved problems in statistical learning where, in the words of Shakespeare's Falstaff, "The better part of valor is discretion" (Henry the Fourth, Part 1, Act 5, Scene 4).
- *The Audience Matters* — Results that are difficult to interpret in subject matter terms, no matter how good the statistical performance, are often of little use. This will sometimes lead to another kind of tradeoff. Algorithmic procedures that perform very well by various technical criteria may stumble when the time comes to convey what the results mean. Important features of the data analysis may be lost. It will sometimes be useful, therefore, to relax the technical performance criteria a bit in order to get results that effectively inform substantive or policy matters. One implication is that an effective data analysis is best done with an understanding of who will want to use the results and the technical background they bring. It can also be important to anticipate preconceptions that that might make it difficult to "hear" what the data analysis has to say. For example, it can be very difficult to get certain academic disciplines to accept the results from algorithmic procedures because those disciplines are so steeped in models.
- *Decisions That Can Be Affected* — Knowing your audience can also mean knowing what decisions might be influenced by the results of a data analysis. Simply put,

if one's goal is to bring information from a data analysis to bear on real decisions, the data analysis must be situated within the decision-making setting. This can mean making sure that the inputs and outputs are those that decision-makers deem relevant and that the details of the algorithmic procedures comport well with decision-maker needs. For example, if forecasting errors lead to asymmetric losses, asymmetric costs should be built into the algorithmic procedure.

- *Differences That Make No Difference* — In almost every issue of journals that publish work on statistical learning and related procedures, there will be articles offering some new wrinkle on existing techniques, or even new procedures, often with strong claims about superior performance compared to some number of other approaches. Such claims are often data-specific but even if broadly true, rarely translate into important implications for practice. Often the claims of improved performance are small by any standard. Some claims of improved performance are unimportant for the subject matter problem being tackled. But even when the improvements seem to be legitimately substantial, they often address secondary concerns. In short, although it is important to keep up with important developments, the newest are not necessarily important.

- *Software That Makes No Difference (or is actually worse)* — The hype can apply to software as well. While this edition is being written, the world is buzzing with talk of "data mining," "big data" and "analytics." Not surprisingly, there are in response a substantial number of software purveyors claiming to offer the very latest and very best tools, which perform substantially better than the competition. *Caveat Emptor.* Often, information on how the software runs is proprietary and no real competitive benchmarks are provided. Much like for the Wizard of Oz, there may be little behind a slick user interface. That is one reason why in this book we exclusively use the programming language R. It is free, so there are no sales incentives. The source code can be downloaded. If one wants to make the effort, it is possible to determine if anyone is hiding the ball. And with access to the source code, changes and enhancements in particular procedures can be written.

- *Data Quality Really Matters* — Just as in any form of regression analysis, good data are a necessary prerequisite. If there are no useful predictors, if the data are sparse, if key variables are highly skewed or unbalanced, or if the key variables are poorly measured, it is very unlikely that the choice of one among several statistical learning procedures will be very important. The problems are bigger than that. It is rare indeed when even the most sophisticated and powerful statistical learning procedures can overcome the liabilities of bad data. A closely related point is that a substantial fraction of the time invested in a given data analysis will be spent cleaning up the data and getting it into the requisite format. These tasks can require substantial skill only tangentially related to conventional statistical expertise.

- *The Role of Subject-Matter Expertise* — Subject-matter expertise can be very important in the following:

1. Framing the empirical questions to be addressed;
2. Defining a data generation mechanism;
3. Designing and implementing the data collection;

4. Determining which variables in the dataset are to be inputs and which are to be outputs;
5. Settling on the values of tuning parameters; and
6. Deciding which results make sense.

But none of these activities is necessarily formal or deductive, and they leave lots of room for interpretation. If the truth be told, subject-matter theory plays much the same role in statistical learning as it does in most conventional analyses. But in statistical learning, there is often far less posturing.

Demonstrations and Exercises

The demonstrations and exercises in the book emphasize data analysis, not the formalities of mathematical statistics. The goal is to provide practice in learning from data. The demonstrations and exercises for this chapter provide a bit of practice doing regression analyses by examining conditional distributions without the aid of conventional linear regression. It is an effort to get back to first principles unfiltered by least squares regression. Another goal is to show how data snooping can lead to misleading results. Commands in R are shown in italics. However, as already noted several times, R and the procedures in R are moving targets. What runs now may not run later, although there will almost certainly be procedures available that can serve as adequate substitutes. Often, examples of relevant code in R be found in the empirical applications provided in each chapter.

Set 1

Load the R dataset "airquality" using *data(airquality)*. Learn about the data set using *help(airquality)*. Attach the dataset "airquality" using *attach(airquality)*. If you do not have access to R, or choose to work with other software, exercises in the same spirit can be easily undertaken. Likewise, exercises in the same spirit can be easily undertaken with other data sets.

1. Using *summary()* take a look at some summary statistics for the data frame. Note that there are some missing data and that all of the variables are numeric.
2. Using *pairs()*, construct of a scatterplot matrix including all of the variables in the dataset. These will all be joint (bivarate) distributions. Describe the relationships between each pair of variables. Are there associations? Do they look linear? Are there outliers?
3. Using *boxplot()*, construct separate side-by-side boxplots for ozone concentrations conditioning on month and ozone concentrations conditioning on day. Does the ozone distribution vary by month of the year? In what way?
4. Construct a three-dimensional scatterplot with ozone concentrations as the response and temperature and wind speed as predictors. This will be a joint distribution. Try using *cloud()* from the *lattice* package. There are lots of slick options. What patterns can you make out? Now repeat the graphing but condition on month. What patterns do you see now? (For ease of readability, you can make the variable month a factor with each level named. For really fancy plotting, have a look at the library *ggplot2*.)

5. From the *graphics* library, construct a conditioning plot using *coplot()* with ozone concentrations as the response, temperature as a predictor, and wind speed as a conditioning variable. How does the conditioning plot attempt to hold wind speed constant?

   (a) Consider all the conditioning scatterplots. What common patterns do you see? What does this tell you about how ozone concentrations are related to temperature with wind speed held constant?
   (b) How do the patterns differ across the conditioning scatter plots? What does that tell you about interaction effects: how do the relationship between ozone concentrations and temperature differ for different wind speeds?

6. Construct an indicator variable for missing data for the variable Ozone. (Using *is.na()* is a good way.) Applying *table()*, cross-tabulate the indicator against month. What do you learn about the pattern of missing data? How might your earlier analyses using the conditioning plot be affected? (If you want to percentage the table, *prop.table()* is a good way.)

7. Write out the conventional parametric regression model that seems to be most consistent with what you have learned from the conditioning plot. Try to justify all of the assumptions you are imposing.

8. Implement your regression model in R using *lm()* and examine the results. Look at the regression diagnostics using *plot()*. What do the four plots tell you about your model? How do your conclusions about the correlates of ozone concentrations learned from the regression model compare to the conclusions about the correlates of ozone concentrations learned from the conditioning plot?

Set 2

The purpose of this exercise is to give you some understanding about how the complexity of a fitting function affects the results of a regression analysis and how test data can help.

1. Construct the training data as follows. For your predictor: $x = rep(1:30, times = 5)$. This will give you 150 observations with values 1 through 30. For your response: $y = rnorm(150)$. This will give you 150 random draws from the standard normal distribution. As such, they are on the average independent of x. This is the same as letting $y = 0 + 0x + \varepsilon$, which is nature's data generation process.

2. Plot the response against the predictor and describe what you see. Is what you see consistent with how the data were generated?

3. Apply a bivariate regression using *lm()* Describe what overall conclusions you draw from the output. The linear functional form is the "smoothest" possible relationship between a response and a predictor.

4. Repeat the linear regression with the predictor as a factor. Apply the same R code as before but use *as.factor(x)* instead of x. This is a linear basis expansion of x. The set of indicator variables for x (one for each value of x) when used as predictors, leads to the "roughest" possible relationship between a response and a predictor. (Technically, you are now doing a multiple regression.) Each value

Fig. 1.13 For predictors X and Z, and a binary response coded as *blue* or *red*, an overlaid decision boundary derived from a logistic regression (N = 100: 45 *reds* and 55 *blues*.)

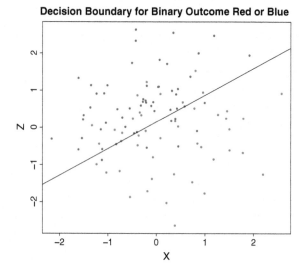

of the predictor can have its own estimate of the conditional mean. (In this case, you know that those conditional means are 0.0 in nature's "generative process.") Compare the R^2 and the adjusted R^2 from the *lm()* output and to the output from #3. What can you say about overfitting. Is there evidence of it here?

5. Construct 1/0 indicator variables for x-indicator variables whose t-values are greater than 1.64. (The *ifelse()* command is a good way to do this.) Apply *lm()* again including only these indicator variables as predictors. What do you find? (By chance, it is possible — but unlikely — that there is still nothing that is "statistically significant." If so, go back to step #1 and regenerate the data. Then pick up at step #3.)

6. Construct test data by repeating step #1. Because x is treated as fixed, you only need to regenerate y. Regress the new y on the subset of indicator variables you used in the previous step. What do you find? The results illustrate the important role of test data.

Set 3

The purpose of this exercise is to get you thinking about decision boundaries for classification problems. Figure 1.13 shows a decision boundary for a binary response coded as red or blue. The predictors are X and Z. The overlaid straight line is a decision boundary based on a logistic regression and values of X and Z for which response odds are $.5/(1 - .5) = 1.0$.

1. Should the observations above the decision be classified as blue or red? Why?
2. Should the observations below the decision be classified as blue or red? Why?
3. Suppose there were an observation with a z-value of 1 and an x-value of −1, but with an unknown response. What would be your best guess: red or blue? Why?

4. Suppose there were an observation with a z-value of -1.5 and an x-value of .5, but with an unknown response. What would be your best guess: red or blue? Why?

5. Why do you think the decision boundary was located at odds of 1.0?

6. How many red observations are misclassified? (For purposes of this exercise, points that seem to fall right on the decision boundary should not be considered classification errors. They are a little above or a little below, but you cannot really tell from the plot.)

7. How many blue observations are misclassified? (For purposes of this exercise, points that seem to fall right on the decision boundary should not be considered classification errors. They are a little above or a little below, but you cannot really tell from the plot.)

8. What fraction of the blue observations is classified correctly?

9. What fraction of the red observations is classified correctly?

10. Which outcome is classified more accurately?

11. What fraction of all of the observations is classified correctly?

$$f(x) = x^3 + 2x^2 + x + 1$$

$$f'(x) = 3x^2 + 4x + 1$$

$$f''(x) = \boxed{6x + 4}$$

$$\frac{f''(x) - 4}{6} = x$$

$$-\frac{4}{6} x \cdot 4 + \frac{1}{2}$$

Chapter 2
Splines, Smoothers, and Kernels

2.1 Introduction

This chapter launches a more detailed examination of statistical learning within a regression framework. Once again, the focus is on conditional distributions. But for now, the mean function for a response variable is central. How does the mean vary with different predictor values? The intent is to begin with procedures that have much the same look and feel as conventional linear regression and gradually move toward procedures that do not.

2.2 Regression Splines

A "spline" is a thin strip of wood that can be easily bent to follow a curved line (Green and Silverman 1994: 4). Historically, it was used in drafting for drawing smooth curves. Regression splines, a statistical translation of this idea, are a way to represent nonlinear, but unknown, mean functions.

Regression splines are not used a great deal in empirical work. As we show later, there are usually better ways to proceed. Nevertheless, it is important to consider them, at least briefly. They provide an instructive transition between conventional parametric regression and the kinds of smoothers commonly seen in statistical learning settings. They also introduce concepts and concerns that will be relevant throughout this chapter and in subsequent chapters.

Recall the general expression for function estimation with a quantitative response variable Y.

$$Y = f(\mathbf{X}) + \varepsilon, \tag{2.1}$$

The original version of this chapter was revised: See the "Chapter Note" section at the end of this chapter for details. The erratum to this chapter is available at https://doi.org/10.1007/978-3-319-44048-4_10.

© Springer International Publishing Switzerland 2016
R.A. Berk, *Statistical Learning from a Regression Perspective*,
Springer Texts in Statistics, DOI 10.1007/978-3-319-44048-4_2

where $\mathbf{X}$ is a set of predictors, $f(\mathbf{X})$ is not specified, and ε can be nothing more than a residual or nothing less than a traditional disturbance term depending, respectively, on whether a level I or level II regression is being undertaken.

Regression splines are an algorithmic way to empirically arrive at a $f(\mathbf{X})$. For a level I analysis, one tries to show how $\mathbf{X}$ is related to Y. For a conventional level II analysis, one tries to estimate nature's true response surface. For the kind of level II analysis we are using, one estimates an approximation of that true response surface. That is, the estimation target is acknowledged to be an approximation the $f(\mathbf{X})$, not the true $f(\mathbf{X})$, but one attempts to get close to the true response surface. The most common estimator is ordinary least squares. That estimator is linear, and the loss function is quadratic.

For a piecewise linear basis, the goal is to fit the data with a broken line (or hyperplane) such that at each break point the left-hand edge meets the right-hand edge. When there is a single predictor, for instance, the fit is a set of straight line segments, connected end to end, sometimes called "piecewise linear."

2.2.1 Applying a Piecewise Linear Basis

Consider as an example a wonderfully entertaining paper in which Zelterman (2014) documents associations by state in the U.S. between the number of internet references to zombies and census features for those states. The number of zombie references was determined through a "Google search" state by state. Like Zelterman, we let y be the number of zombie references by state per 100,000 people. We let x be the average in each state of minutes per day spent watching cable TV. The values used here for both variables are total fabrications constructed for didactic purposes.

Figure 2.1 shows an example of a piecewise linear function constructed in three steps.[1] The first step is to decide where the break points on x will be. Based on prior market research, suppose there are known tipping points at 90 and 180 min of TV watching a day. At 90 min a day, viewers often become fans of zombies on TV and shows with related content. At 180 min a day, zombie saturation is reached. Break points are defined at $x = a$ and $x = b$ (with $b > a$) so that in Fig. 2.1, $a = 90$ and $b = 180$. Such break points are often called "knots."

The next step is to define two indicator variables to represent the break points. The first, I_a, is equal to 1 if x is greater than 90 and equal to 0 otherwise. The second, I_b, is equal to 1 if x is greater than 180 and equal to 0 otherwise. Both are step functions. We let x_a be the value of x at the first break point, and x_b be the value of x at the second break point (i.e. 90 and 180 respectively).

The final step is to define the mean function that allows for changes in the slope and the intercept:

$$f(x_i) = \beta_0 + \beta_1 x_i + \beta_2 (x_i - x_a) I_a + \beta_3 (x_i - x_b) I_b. \qquad (2.2)$$

---

[1] Using conventional multiple regression, Zelterman (2014: 40–41) finds more internet references to zombies in states with fewer Miss America winners and fewer shopping centers per capita. Who knew?

Fig. 2.1 A piecewise linear
function with two knots for
the number of zombie
references on the internet as
a function of minutes per day
watching cable TV

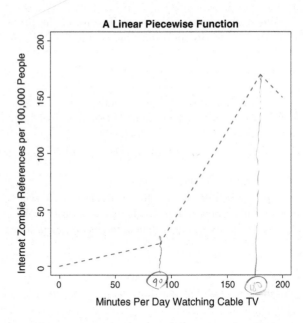

Looking back how linear basis expansions are defined in Eq. 1.17, it is apparent that
there are four transformations of X ($m = 1, 2, \ldots, 4$), each denoted by $h_m(X)$, in
which the first function of x is a constant. One has a set of predictors constructed
as a linear basis expansion of X. Equation 2.2 is, therefore, the mean function for a
conventional multiple regression with coefficient values that can be obtained from
ordinary least squares.

What exactly is the point of Eq. 2.2? Equation 2.2 is *not* a model representing how
the data were generated. But, it can be used as a mean function in a least squares
regression to help find fitted values that summarize associations in the data. Going
no farther, this can result in a level I analysis through which relationships in the data
are described.

For a level II analysis, Eq. 2.2 can play two related roles. First, it can represent
the mean function to be estimated. The approach taken here is that Eq. 2.2 is the
expression for the piecewise linear function that is a feature of a joint probability
distribution, but with no claims made about its correspondence to the truth. It is
the estimation target. When embedded in the population least squares framework
discussed in the last chapter, it can be viewed as the best (i.e., by least squares),
piecewise linear approximation of the true response surface and an appropriate estimation target. Second, used as the mean function in a least squares procedure applied
to training data, it is the mean function for the least squares estimator.

Whether for a level I or level II analysis, the piecewise linear function can be decomposed into its constituent line segments. The mean function for x less than a is

$$f(x_i) = \beta_0 + \beta_1 x_i. \tag{2.3}$$

In Fig. 2.1, β_0 is zero, and β_1 is positive.

For values of x greater than a but smaller than b, the mean function becomes

$$f(x_i) = (\beta_0 - \beta_2 x_a) + (\beta_1 + \beta_2)x_i. \tag{2.4}$$

For a positive β_1 and β_2, the line beyond $x = a$ is steeper because the slope is $(\beta_1 + \beta_2)$. The intercept is lower because of the second term in $(\beta_0 - \beta_2 x_a)$. This too is consistent with Fig. 2.1. If β_2 were negative, the reverse would apply.

For values of x greater than b, the mean function becomes,

$$f(x_i) = (\beta_0 - \beta_2 x_a - \beta_3 x_b) + (\beta_1 + \beta_2 + \beta_3)x_i. \tag{2.5}$$

For these values of x, the slope is altered by adding β_3 to the slope of the previous line segment. The intercept is altered by subtracting $\beta_3 x_b$. The sign and magnitude of β_3 determine by whether the slope of the new line segment is positive or negative and how steep it is. The intercept will shift accordingly. In Fig. 2.1, β_3 is negative and large enough to make the slope negative. The intercept is increased substantially.

Expressions like Eq. 2.2 are all one needs for a level I regression analysis. For a level II regression analysis, a credible data generating process also must be articulated. As before, we will generally employ a joint probability distribution as the "population" from which each observation is realized as a random, independent draw. Very often this approach is reasonable. But each level II regression analysis must be considered on a case by case basis. For example, if time is a predictor (e.g., month or year), there can be important conceptual complications as we will now see.

Figure 2.2 shows a three-piece linear regression spline applied to water use data from Tokyo over a period of 27 years.[2] The data were collected as part of a larger research project motivated by concerns about the provision of potable water to large metropolitan areas as human-induced climate change proceeds. Residential water use in 1000s of cubic feet is on the vertical axis. Year is on the horizontal axis. The locations of the break points were chosen using subject matter expertise about residential water use in Japan. The R code is shown in Fig. 2.3.

For a level I analysis, it is clear that water use was flat until about 1980, increased linearly until about 1996, and then flattened out again. The first break point may correspond to a transition toward much faster economic and population growth. The second break point may correspond to the introduction of more water-efficient technology. But why the transitions are so sharp is mysterious. One possibility is

---

[2]The data were provided by the Tokyo Municipal Water Works as part of a project funded by The Asian-Pacific Network for Global Change Research.

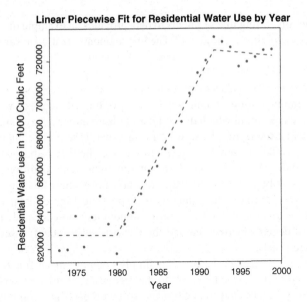

Fig. 2.2 A piecewise linear basis applied to water use in Tokyo by year

```
xa<-ifelse(year>1980,1,0)
xb<-ifelse(year>1992,1,0)
x1<-(year-1980)*xa
x2<-(year-1992)*xb
working<-data.frame(hhwater,year,xa,xb,x1,x2)
out1<-lm(hhwater~year+x1+x2,data=working)
plot(year,hhwater,xlab="Year",ylab="Residential
        Water use in 1000 Cubic Feet", main="Linear
        Piecewise Fit for Residential Water Use by Year",
        col="blue",pch=19)
lines(year,out1$fitted.values, lty="dashed",col="blue",lwd=3)
```

Fig. 2.3 R code for piecewise linear fit

that the break points correspond in part to changes in how the water use data were collected or reported.

In Fig. 2.2, the end-to-end connections between line segments work well with processes that unfold over time. But there is nothing about linear regression splines requiring that time be a predictor. For example, the response could be crop production per acre and the sole predictor could be the amount of phosphorus fertilizer applied to the soil. Crop production might increase in approximately a linear fashion until there is an excess of phosphorus causing of metabolic difficulties for the crops. At that point, crop yields might decline in roughly a linear manner.

More generally, fitting line segments to data provides an example of "smoothing" a scatterplot, or applying a "smoother." The line segments are used to summarize how x and y are related. The intent is to highlight key features of any association while removing unimportant details. This can often be accomplished by constructing fitted values in a manner that makes them more homogeneous than the set of conditional means of y computed for each unique value of x or binned values of x.[3]

Imagine a scatterplot in which the number of observations is large enough so that for each value of x there are at least several values of y. One could compute the mean of y for each x-value. If one then drew straight lines between adjacent conditional means, the resulting smoother would be an interpolation of the conditional means and as "rough" as possible. At the other extreme, imposing a single linear fit on all of the means at once would produce the "smoothest" fit possible. Figure 2.2 falls somewhere in between. How to think about the degree of smoothness more formally is addressed later. Effective degrees of freedom and the bias-variance tradeoff discussed in the last chapter are a start.

For a piecewise linear basis, one can simply compute mean functions such as Eq. 2.2 with ordinary least squares. With the regression coefficients in hand, fitted values are easily constructed. Indeed, many software packages compute and store fitted values on a routine basis. Also widely available are procedures to construct the matrix of regressors, although it is not hard to do so one term at a time using common transformation capabilities (See Fig. 2.3.). For example, the library *spline* has a procedure *bs()* that constructs a B-spline basis (discussed later) that can be easily used to represent the predictor matrix for piecewise linear regression.

In contrast to most applications of conventional linear regression, there would typically be little interest in the regression coefficients themselves; they are but a means to an end. The point of the exercise is to superimpose the fitted values on a scatterplot so that the relationship between y and x can be more effectively visualized. The story is in the visualization not the regression coefficients.

As already noted, for a level II analysis the estimation target is the same mean function in the population or joint probability distribution. But, with the longitudinal data, the inferential issues can be tricky. In particular, treating the data as independent, random realizations from a joint probability distribution does not work well. An obvious difficulty is that allowing year to be a random variable means that for any given dataset, some years might not be represented at all and some years might be represented more than once. In fact, the data were assembled with these particular years in mind; the data collection process took the specified years as given.

If in practice, year is treated as fixed, it probably makes sense to focus on a data generating process that also treats year as fixed. Then, one can imagine nature conditioning on year so that for each year, there is a probability distribution of water consumption values that in principle could be realized. The data on hand are realized from these conditional distributions. But after conditioning on year, are the water use observations realized independently? For example, if in one year average water

---

[3]For these data, there is only one value of y for each unique values of x. They may be treated as if they were means.

consumption increases, does that by itself have implications for the realized values of water consumption the next year? Without extensive subject-matter knowledge it is hard to know. Alternatively, it might be possible to specify a mean function that addressed possible dependence, but that would require a reconceptualization of how the data were realized.

There are significant complications if the break points were chosen through data snooping. For example, there is data snooping if the scatter plot for water consumption by year was examined to choose the best break point locations. Those locations become features of the regression specification itself so that the mean function specification could well be different with new realizations of the data (Leeb and Pötscher 2005, 2006, 2008). But, with the year treated as fixed, valid asymptotic inferences can be made to the same best, linear piecewise approximation, although conventional confidence intervals and tests are no longer valid, even asymptotically. If one assumes independence after conditioning on year, there can be valid asymptotic confidence intervals and tests using other procedures (Berk et al. 2010, 2014; Lockhart et al. 2014). However, the sample size here is very small. There are only 27 observations, and 4 degrees of freedom are used by the piecewise linear regression.[4]

The difficulties with a level II analysis may be even more fundamental. Nature's data generation process assumes, in effect, that history can repeat itself over and over, but we only get to see one random set of realized water consumption values from the joint probability distribution for the years in question. For Fig. 2.2, one must be comfortable assuming that Tokyo's water consumption values from 1970 to 1997 could have been different. Superficially, this may seem reasonable enough. But to be convincing, one would need to describe the ways in which nature makes this happen. In the absence of such an account, one has started down the slippery slope of assume-and-proceed statistics. It may be wise here to remain at level I.

2.2.2 Polynomial Regression Splines

Smoothing a scatterplot using a piecewise linear basis has the great advantage of simplicity in concept and execution. And by increasing the number of break points, very complicated relationships can be approximated. However, in most applications there are good reasons to believe that the underlying relationship is not well represented with a set of straight line segments. Another kind of approximation is needed.

Greater continuity between line segments can be achieved by using polynomials in x for each segment. Cubic functions of x are a popular choice because they strike a nice balance between flexibility and complexity. When used to construct regression splines, the fit is sometimes called "piecewise cubic." The cubic polynomial serves as a "truncated power series basis" in x.

---

[4]If there is dependence, one is in uncharted waters for post-model selection inference.

Unfortunately, simply joining polynomial segments end to end is unlikely to result in a visually appealing fit where the polynomial segments meet. The slopes of the two lines will often appear to change abruptly even when that is inconsistent with the data. Far better visual continuity usually can be achieved by constraining the first and second derivatives on either side of each break point to be the same.

One can generalize the piecewise linear approach and impose those continuity requirements. Suppose there are K interior break points, usually called "interior knots." These are located at $\xi_1 < \cdots < \xi_K$ with two boundary knots added at ξ_0 and ξ_{K+1}. Then, one can use piecewise cubic polynomials in the following mean function exploiting, as before, linear basis expansions of X:

$$f(x_i) = \beta_0 + \beta_1 x_i + \beta_2 x_i^2 + \beta_3 x_i^3 + \sum_{j=1}^{K} \theta_j (x_i - x_j)_+^3, \qquad (2.6)$$

where the "+" indicates the positive values from the expression inside the parentheses, and there are $K + 4$ parameters whose values need to be computed. This leads to a conventional regression formulation with a matrix of predictor terms having $K + 4$ columns and N rows. Each row would have the corresponding values of the piecewise cubic polynomial function evaluated at the single value of x for that case. There is still only a single predictor, but now there are $K + 4$ basis functions.

The output for the far-right term in Eq. 2.6 may not be apparent at first. Suppose the values of the predictor are arranged in order from low to high. For example, $x = [1, 2, 4, 5, 7, 8]$. Suppose also that x_j is located at an x-value of 4. Then, $(x - x_j)_+^3 = [0, 0, 0, 1, 27, 64]$. The knot-value of 4 is subtracted from each value of x, the negative numbers set to 0, and the others cubed. All that changes from knot to knot is the value of x_j that is subtracted. There are K such knots and K such terms in the regression model.

Figure 2.4 shows the water use data again, but with a piecewise cubic polynomial overlaid that imposes the two continuity constraints. The code is shown in Fig. 2.5. Figure 2.4 reveals a good eyeball fit, which captures about 95 % of the variance in water use. But, in all fairness, the scatterplot did not present a great challenge. The point is to compare Fig. 2.2 to Fig. 2.4 and note the visual difference. The linear piecewise fit also accounted for about 95 % of the variance. Which plot would be more instructive in practice would depend on the use to be made of the fitted values and on prior information about what a sensible $f(X)$ might be. This is a general point to which we will return many times. It can be very risky to rely on statistical summaries alone, such as fit statistics, to select the most instructive response surface approximation. Subject-matter knowledge, potential applications and good judgments need to play an important role.[5]

---

[5]This also is a good example of the problems one faces trying to adjust for the degrees of freedom used by the regression. There seems to be no way explicitly to introduce the constraints on the first and second derivatives, although they are built into fitting process. More is involved than the K estimates of θ_j.

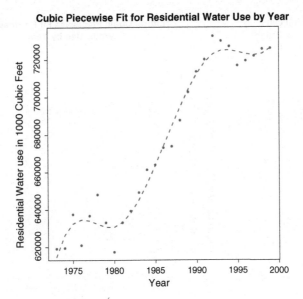

Fig. 2.4 A piecewise cubic basis applied to water use in Tokyo by year

```
library(splines)
cubic<-bs(year,knots=c(1980,1992))
out2<-lm(hhwater~cubic)
plot(year,hhwater,xlab="Year",ylab="Residential Water use
     in 1000 Cubic Feet", main="Cubic Piecewise Fit for
     Residential Water Use by Year",col="blue",pch=19)
lines(year,out2$fitted.values,lty="dashed",col="blue",lwd=3)
```

Fig. 2.5 R code for piecewise cubic fit

The regression coefficients ranged widely and, as to be expected, did not by themselves add any useful information. Any story was primarily in the fitted values. The issues for a level I and level II analysis are essentially the same as for a piecewise linear approach.

2.2.3 Natural Cubic Splines

Fitted values for piecewise cubic polynomials near the boundaries of x can be unstable because they fall at the ends of polynomial line segments where there are no continuity constraints, and where the data may be sparse. By "unstable" one means that a very few observations, which might vary substantially over random realizations of the

Fig. 2.6 A natural cubic
piecewise basis applied to
water use in Tokyo by year

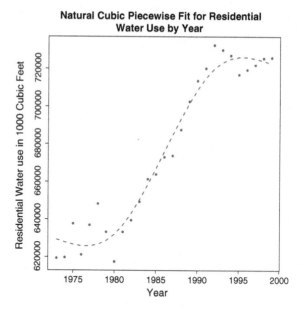

data, could produce rather different fitted values near the boundaries of x. As a result,
the plot of the fitted values near the boundaries might look somewhat different from
sample to sample.

Sometimes, constraints for behavior at the boundaries are added to increase stability. One common constraint imposes linearity on the fitted values beyond the
boundaries of x. This introduces a bit of bias because it is very unlikely that if data
beyond the current boundaries were available, the relationship would be linear. However, the added stability is often worth it. When these constraints are added, the result
is a "natural cubic spline."

Figure 2.6 shows again a plot of the water use data on year, but now with a smoother
constructed from natural cubic splines. The code can be found in Fig. 2.7. One can
see that the fitted values near the boundaries of x are somewhat different from the
fitted values near the boundaries of x in Fig. 2.4. The fitted values in Fig. 2.6 are
smoother, which is the desired result. There is one less bend near both boundaries,
but the issues for a level I or level II analysis have not changed.[6]

The option of including extra constraints to help stabilize the fit provides an
example of the bias–variance tradeoff discussed in the previous chapter, but for
piecewise cubic polynomials and natural cubic splines, the degree of smoothness
is primarily a function of the number of interior knots. In practice, the smaller the
number of knots, the smoother are the fitted values. A smaller number of knots
means that there are more constraints on the pattern of fitted values because there

---

[6]More generally, how one can formulate the boundary constraints is discussed in Hastie et al. (2009:
Sect. 5.2.1).

```
library(splines)
Ncubic<-ns(year,knots=c(1980,1992))
out3<-lm(hhwater~Ncubic)
plot(year,hhwater,xlab="Year",ylab="Residential Water use
        in 1000 Cubic Feet", main="Natural Cubic Piecewise
        Fit for Residential Water Use by Year",col="blue",pch=19)
lines(year,out3$fitted.values,lty="dashed",col="blue",lwd=3)
```

Fig. 2.7 R code for natural piecewise cubic fit

are fewer end-to-end, cubic line segments used in the fitting process. Consequently, less provision is made for a complex response surface.

Knot placement matters too. Ideally, knots should be placed where one believes, before looking at the data, the $f(X)$ is changing most rapidly. But it will often be very tempting to data snoop. In some cases, inspection of the data, coupled with subject matter knowledge, can be used to determine the number and placement of knots. Alternatively, the number and placement of knots can be approached as a conventional model selection problem. But that means determining a candidate set of models with different numbers of knots and different knot locations. That set could be very large. Absent subject matter information, knot placement has been long known to be a difficult technical problem, especially when there is more than one predictor (de Boors 2001). The fitted values are related to where the knots are placed in a very complicated manner. Fortunately, methods discussed later sidestep the knot number and location problem.

Even if a good case for a small number of candidate models can be made, one must be careful about taking any of their fit measures too literally. There will often be several models with rather similar values, whatever the kind of fit statistic used. Then, selecting a single model as "best" using the fit measure alone may amplify a small numerical superiority into a large difference in the results, especially if the goal is to interpret how the predictors are related to the response. Some call this "specious specificity." Also, one must be a very careful not to let small differences in the fit statistics automatically trump subject matter knowledge. The risk is arriving at a model that may be difficult to interpret, or effectively worthless. Finally, one has introduced the demanding complications that come with model selection. All is well for a level I analysis. But moving to a level II analysis can introduce difficult problems already mentioned. Toward the end of the chapter, we will consider an empirical example in which a split sample approach is very helpful for valid statistical inference.

In summary, for level II regression splines of the sort just discussed, there is no straightforward way to arrive at the best tradeoff between the bias and the variance because there is no straightforward way to determine knot location. A key implication is that it is very difficult to arrive at a model that is demonstrably the "best." Fortunately, there are other approaches to smoothing that are more promising. A broader point is that we have begun the transition from models to black box algorithms. As the substantive role for fitted values has become more prominent, the substantive role for regression coefficients has becomes less prominent.

2.2.4 B-Splines

In practice, data analyses using piecewise cubic polynomials and natural cubic splines are rarely constructed directly from polynomials of x. They are commonly constructed using a B-spline basis, largely because of computational convenience.[7] A serious discussion of B-splines would take us far afield and accessible summaries can be found in Gifi (1990: 366–370) and Hastie et al. (2009: 186–189). Nevertheless several observations are worth making even if they are a bit of a detour.

The goal is to construct a piecewise fit from linear basis expansions of x with nice numerical properties. B-splines meet this test. They are computed in a recursive manner from very simple functions to more complex ones.

For a set of knots, usually including some beyond the upper and lower boundaries of x, the recursion begins with indicator variables for each neighborhood defined by the knots. If a value of x falls within a given neighborhood, the indicator variable for that neighborhood is coded 1, and coded 0 otherwise. For example, if there is a knot at an x-value of 2 and the next knot is at an x-value of 3, the x-values between them constitute a neighborhood with its own indicator variable coded 1 if the value of x falls in that neighborhood (e.g., $x = 2.3$). Otherwise the coded value is 0. In the end, there is a set of indicator variables, with values of 1 or 0, depending on the neighborhood. These indicator variables define a set of degree zero B-splines.

Figure 2.8 is an illustration with interior knots at -2, -1, 0, 1, and 2. With five interior knots, there are four neighborhoods and four indicator variables. Using indicator variables as regressors will produce a step function when y is regressed on x; they are the linear basis expansion for a step function fit. The steps will be located at the knots and for this example, the mean function specification will allow for four levels, one for each indicator variable. With a different set of knots, the indicator variables will change.

As usual, one of the indicator variables is dropped from any regression analysis that includes an intercept. The deleted indicator becomes the baseline. In R, the procedure *lm()* automatically drops one of the indicator variables in a set if an intercept is included.

Next, a transformation can be applied to the degree zero B-splines (See Hastie et al. 2009: 186–189). The result is a set of degree one B-splines. Figure 2.9 shows the set of degree one B-splines derived from the indicator variables shown in Fig. 2.8.

---

[7]But there can be lots of options, depending on the application. For example, there are special issues when the intent is to smooth a 2-dimensional surface. An excellent discussion can be found in Wood (2006: Sect. 4.1).

Fig. 2.8 Degree zero
B-splines

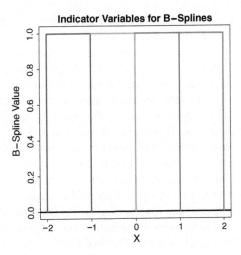

Fig. 2.9 Degree one
B-splines

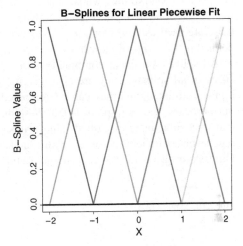

The triangular shape is characteristic of degree one *B*-splines, and indicates that the values for each spline are no longer just 0 or 1, but proportions in-between as well.

In Fig. 2.9, each new basis function is color coded. Starting from the left, the blue line maps x onto a set of *B*-spline values. From x-values of -2 to -1, the *B*-Spline values decline from 1 to 0 but are 0 for the rest of the x-values. These *B*-spline values would be the first column in a new predictor matrix. For x-values between -2 and 0, the green upside down V indicates that the *B*-spline values are between 0 and 1, but equal to 0 otherwise. These *B*-spline values would be the second column in a new predictor matrix. The same reasoning applies to the purple and red upside down Vs and to the yellow line. In the end, there would be six columns of *B*-spline values with the sixth column coded to have no impact because it is redundant, given other five columns. That column is not shown inasmuch as it has B-spline values that are 0 for all x-values.

Degree one B-splines are the basis for linear piecewise fits. In this example, regressing a response on the B-spline matrix would produce a linear piecewise fit with four slopes, one for each neighborhood defined by the indicator variables. For different numbers and locations of knots, the piecewise fit would vary as well.

A transformation of the same form can now be applied to the degree one B-splines. This leads to a set of degree two B-splines. A set of such B-splines is shown in Fig. 2.10. As before, each new basis function is color coded, and the shapes are characteristic. For this illustration, there is now a matrix having seven columns with one redundant column coded as all 0s. Should the B-spline matrix be used in a regression analysis, a piecewise quadratic fit would be produced. There would be one quadratic function for each neighborhood defined by the indicator variables.

The same kind of transformation can then be applied to the degree two B-splines. The result is a set of degree three B-splines. Figure 2.11 shows the set of degree three color-coded splines, whose shapes are, once again, characteristic. The regressor matrix now contains eight columns with one redundant column coded as all 0s. When these are used as regressors, there will one cubic function for each neighborhood defined by the original indicator variables.

All splines are linear combinations of B-splines; B-splines are a basis for the space of all splines. They are also a well-conditioned basis because they are not highly correlated, and they can be computed in a stable and efficient manner. For our purposes, the main point is that B-splines are a computational device used to construct cubic piecewise fitted values. No substantive use is made of the associated regression coefficients because they too are just part of the computational machinery. Our trek toward black box algorithms continues.

Fig. 2.10 Degree two
B-splines

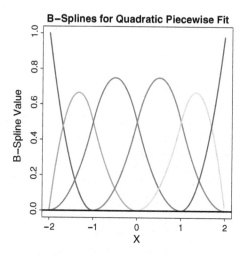

Fig. 2.11 Degree three
B-splines

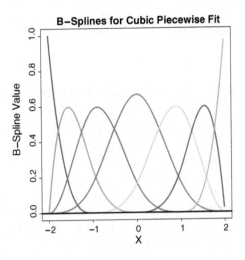

2.3 Penalized Smoothing

The placement of knots, the number of knots, and the degree of the polynomial are subject to manipulation by a data analyst. For a level I regression analysis, the goal is to arrive at an instructive fit of the data. Is one learning what one can about associations in the data? For a level II regression analysis, the goal is to estimate a useful approximation of the true response surface. Beyond documenting associations of various kinds, do the fitted values provide helpful information that might help guide future decisions?

Whether for a level I or level II analysis, the data analyst is engaged in "tuning." Therefore, the placement of knots, the number of knots, and the degree of the polynomial can seen as "tuning parameters." Unlike the usual parameters of a regression model, they typically are of little substantive interest. More like dials on a piece of machinery, they are set to promote good performance.

There are at least two problems with the tuning parameters for regression splines. First, there are at least three of them so that the tuning process can be quite complicated. For example, should one increase the number of knots or the degree of the polynomial? Usually, the only guidance is sketchy craft lore. Second, there is little or no formal theory to justify the tuning. To many, the tuning process feels like a "hack." The entire process is at least inelegant.

A useful alternative is to alter the fitting process itself so that the tuning is accomplished automatically, guided by clear statistical reasoning. One popular approach is to combine a mathematical penalty with the loss function to be optimized. The penalty imposes greater losses as a mean function becomes more complicated. For greater complexity to be accepted, the fit must be improved by an amount that is larger than the penalty. The greater complexity has to be "worth it." This leads to a very popular approach called "penalized regression."[8]

2.3.1 Shrinkage and Regularization

To get a feel for penalized regression, consider a conventional regression analysis with an indicator variable as the sole regressor. If its regression coefficient equals zero, the fitted values will be a straight line, parallel to the x-axis, located at the unconditional mean of the response. As the regression coefficient increases in absolute value, the resulting step function will have a step of increasing size. The difference between the conditional means of Y when the indicator is 0 compared to the conditional means of Y when the indicator is 1 is larger. In language we have begun to use, the fit becomes more rough. Or in still other language, the fit is more complex. In short, the larger the regression coefficient the rougher the fitted values.

For a level I regression analysis, less complexity can mean that important features of the fitted values are overlooked. More complexity can complicate unnecessarily interpretations of the fitted values. For a level II regression analysis, less complexity means that a smoother approximation of the true response surface is being estimated, which can increase bias with respect to nature's true response surface. More complexity can increase the variance of estimates of that response surface. We have the bias-variance tradeoff once again, and we are once again seeking a Goldilocks solution. The fitted values should not be too rough. The fitted values should not be too smooth. They should be just right.

Popular Goldilocks strategies are sometimes called "shrinkage" (Hastie et al. 2009: Sect. 3.4) and sometimes called "regularization" (Hastie et al. 2009: Chap. 5). In the context of statistical learning, both are tools for trying to address the bias-variance tradeoff. But it can be helpful to think of shrinkage as a special case of regularization in which the loss function for a conventional linear regression is altered to include a penalty for complexity. We will see in later chapters that regularization can apply to a much wider range of procedures and take many different forms. For now, we focus on shrinkage.

A number of proposals have been offered for how to control the complexity of the fitted values by constraining the magnitude of regression coefficients (See Ruppert et al. 2003: Sect. 3.5 for a very accessible discussion.). Two popular suggestions are:

1. constrain the sum of the absolute values of the regression coefficients to be less than some constant C (sometimes called an L_1-penalty); and

---

[8] Suppose the error sum of squares for a given amount of fitted value complexity is 1000. Ordinarily, an increase in the complexity of the fitted values that reduces the error sum of squares to less than 1000 would accepted. But suppose there is a penalty of 100. Now the penalized error sum of squares is 1100. Still, the error sum of squares threshold remains at 1000. Improvement in the fit has to overcome the penalty of 100.

2. constrain the sum of the squared regression coefficients to be less than some constant C (sometimes called an L_2-penalty).

The smaller the value of C is, the smaller the sum. The smaller the sum, the smaller is the typical magnitude of the regression coefficients. The smaller the typical magnitude of the regression coefficients, the smoother the fitted values. In part because the units in which the regressors are measured will affect how much each regression coefficient contributes to the sum, it can make sense to work with standardized regressors.[9] Often, very little interpretive weight is carried by the regression coefficients in any case if interest centers on the fitted values. The intercept does not figure in either constraint and is usually addressed separately.

For a level I analysis, both constraints can impose different amounts of smoothness in the fitted values. Description of the relationships between the response and the predictors can be affected. For a level II analysis, both constraints lead to shrinkage methods. The regression coefficients can be "shrunk" toward zero, making the fitted values more homogeneous. The population approximation is altered in the same fashion. When the intent is to represent the true response surface, one is prepared to introduce a small amount of bias into the estimated regression coefficients in trade for a substantial reduction in their variance so that the same is true of the fitted values.

One also can recast some measures of fit discussed in the last chapter within a shrinkage framework. The total number of regression coefficients to be estimated can serve as a constraint and is sometimes called an L_0-penalty. Maximizing the adjusted R^2, for example, can be seen as minimizing the usual error sum of squares subject to a penalty for the number of regression coefficients in the model (Fan and Li 2006).

Shrinkage methods can be applied with the usual regressor matrix or with smoother matrices of the sort we introduced earlier. For didactic purposes, we start within a conventional multiple regression framework and p predictors.

2.3.1.1 Ridge Regression

Suppose that for a conventional fixed X regression, one adopts the constraint that the sum of the p squared regression coefficients is less than C. This constraint leads directly to ridge regression. The task is to obtain values for the regression coefficients so that

$$\hat{\beta} = \min_{\beta} \left[\sum_{i=1}^{n} (y_i - \beta_0 - \sum_{j=1}^{p} x_{ij}\beta_j)^2 + \lambda \sum_{j=1}^{p} \beta_j^2 \right]. \tag{2.7}$$

In Eq. 2.7, the usual expression for the error sum of squares has a new component. That component is the sum of the squared regression coefficients multiplied by a

---

[9] For example, 3.2 additional years of age may count the same as smoking 11.4 additional cigarettes a day. They may both be equal to one standard deviation of their respective predictors.

constant λ. When Eq. 2.7 is minimized in order to obtain $\hat{\beta}$, the sizes of the squared regression coefficients are taken into account. This is an L_2 penalty.

For a given value of λ, the larger the $\sum_{j=1}^{p} \beta_j^2$ is, the larger the increment to the error sum of squares. The $\sum_{j=1}^{p} \beta_j^2$ can be thought of as the penalty function. For a given value of $\sum_{j=1}^{p} \beta_j^2$, the larger the value of λ is, the larger the increment to the error sum of squares; λ determines how much weight is given to the penalty. In short, $\sum_{j=1}^{p} \beta_j^2$ is what is being constrained, and λ imposes the constraint. C is inversely related to λ. The smaller the value of C, the larger is the value of λ.

It follows that the ridge regression estimator is

$$\hat{\beta} = (\mathbf{X}^T\mathbf{X} + \lambda\mathbf{I})^{-1}\mathbf{X}^T\mathbf{y}, \qquad (2.8)$$

where $\mathbf{I}$ is a $p \times p$ identity matrix. The column of 1s for the intercept is dropped from $\mathbf{X}$. β_0 is estimated separately.

In Eq. 2.8, λ plays same role as in Eq. 2.7, but can now be seen as a tuning parameter. It is not a feature of a population or a stochastic process. Its role is to help provide an appropriate fit to the data and can be altered directly by the data analyst. As such, it has a different status from the regression coefficients, whose values are determined through the minimization process itself, conditional upon the value of λ.

The value of λ is added to the main diagonal of the cross-product matrix $\mathbf{X}^T\mathbf{X}$, which determines how much the estimated regression coefficients are "shrunk" toward zero (and hence, each other). A λ of zero produces the usual least squares result. As λ increases in size, the regression coefficients approach zero, and the fitted values are smoother. In effect, the variances of the predictors are being increased with no change in the covariances between predictors and the response variable. This is easy to appreciate in the case of a single predictor. For a single predictor, the regression coefficient is the covariance of the predictor with the response divided by the variance of the predictor. So, if the covariance is unchanged and the variance is increased, the absolute value of the regression coefficient is smaller.

In ridge regression, the regression coefficients and fitted values obtained will differ in a complicated manner depending on the units in which the predictors are measured. It is common, therefore, to standardize the predictors before the estimation begins. However, standardization is just a convention and does not solve the problem of the scale dependent regression coefficients. There also can be some issues with exactly how the standardization is done (Bing 1994). In practice, the standardized regression coefficients are transformed back into their original units when time comes to interpret the results, but that obscures the impact of the standardization on Eq. 2.7. The penalty function has the standardized coefficients as its argument.

In whatever manner the value of λ is determined, a valid level I analysis may be undertaken. What varies is the smoothness of the fitted values from which descriptive summaries are constructed. For a level II analysis, if the value of λ is determined before the data analysis begins, one can resurrect a conventional "true model" approach. For reasons already addressed, that seems like a bad idea. Moreover, the shrinkage is a new source of bias. Using the "wrong model" perspective, one is estimating in an asymptotically unbiased manner an approximation of the true response surface determined by the value of λ.

If the value of λ is determined as part of the data analysis, there are significant complications for level II analysis. A key issue is how the value of λ is chosen. Ideally, there are training data, evaluation data, and test data as described in the last chapter. Using the training data and the evaluation data, one option is trial and error. Different values of λ are tried with the training data until there is a satisfactory fit in the evaluation data by some measure such as mean squared error. With modern computing power, a very large number of potential values can be searched very quickly. Once a value for λ is determined, a level II analysis properly can be undertaken with the test data, although if the degrees of freedom are used in the calculations, there are complications (Dijkstra 2011). If all one cares about is a level I analysis, one can simply search over all the data at once for a value of λ that leads to good results in statistical and subject-matter terms. However, it will be useful to keep in mind how much searching has been done. It is easy to get carried away by complex results that are essentially a byproduct of noisy data. After a lot of searching, complex results that come as a surprise need to be very cautiously interpreted.

If there are no evaluation and test data and the dataset is too small to partition, there are the fallback options noted in the last chapter such as cross-validation. The value of λ is chosen to maximize some cross-validation measure of fit. But no matter what the method, search for the best values of λ can lead to overfitting, especially if the searching is very extensive. In cross validation, for example, the training data are reused many times.[10]

One must also be careful with how ridge regression results are interpreted. Even within the wrong model perspective, the regression coefficient values are regularized to achieve a desirable set of fitted values. Features of the fitted values are driving the results, and regression coefficients are but a means to that end. For both level I and level II analyses, it is not entirely clear why a better fit of the data implies more instructive regression coefficients. For example, in a properly implemented randomized experiment, average treatment effect estimates are unbiased and have causal interpretations even though the overall fit may be poor. Also, there is nothing especially compelling about the L_2 ridge penalty. Other kinds of defensible penalties exist that can produce very different results.

---

[10]Suppose in training data with 100 observations there are 15 observations that are by chance anomalous and affect the regression results. About 15% of the observations in random splits of the data will be composed of these observations. So, in split after split, the regression results will be affected in a similar way. Yet, in real test data, that 15% might not be represented at all or at least no nearly so commonly. In other words, one is held captive to whatever features characterize the training data, even if those features are essentially noise. This is why cross-validation needs to be justified asymptotically. In all fairness, split samples can have less extreme versions of the same problems.

2.3.1.2 A Ridge Regression Illustration

Perhaps an example will help fix these ideas. The data come from a survey of 95 respondents in which a key question is how various kinds of social support may be related to depression.[11] There are 19 predictors and for this illustration, we will work with three: (1) "emotional" — a "summary of 5 questions on emotional support availability," (2) "affect" — a "summary of 3 questions on availability of affectionate support sources," and (3) "psi" — a "summary of 3 questions on availability of positive social interaction." The response "BDI," which stands for Beck depression inventory, is a 21-item inventory based on self-reports of attitudes and symptoms characteristic of depression (Beck et al. 1961). We are treating the data as random realizations so that the predictors and the response are random variables. No doubt the model is misspecified by conventional criteria. We adopt, therefore the best linear approximation approach, and the usual output from *lm()* takes the following form.

```
Call:
lm(formula = BDI ~ emotional + affect + psi, data =
socsupport)

Residuals:
    Min      1Q  Median      3Q     Max
-14.141  -5.518  -0.764   3.342  32.667

Coefficients:
             Estimate Std. Error t value Pr(>|t|)
(Intercept)  31.5209     5.0111   6.290 1.09e-08 ***
emotional     0.2445     0.3458   0.707  0.48133
affect       -0.4736     0.4151  -1.141  0.25693
psi          -1.6801     0.5137  -3.270  0.00152 **
---
Signif. codes:  0 *** 0.001 ** 0.01 * 0.05 . 0.1  1

Residual standard error: 8.6 on 91 degrees of freedom
Multiple R-squared:  0.216, Adjusted R-squared:  0.1901
F-statistic: 8.355 on 3 and 91 DF,  p-value: 5.761e-05
```

Consider first a level I analysis. The predictors "affect" and "psi" are negatively related to depression, and "emotional" is positively related to depression. As is often the case with constructed scales, it is difficult to know how substantively important the regression coefficients are. How big is big, and how small is small? For example, psi ranges from 5 to 15, and BDI ranges from 0 to 48. For each additional psi point, the average of the depression scale is about 1.7 points smaller. Even over the range of psi, the full range of BDI is not covered. Moreover, how does one translate variation

---

[11] The data, named *socsupport*, can be obtained as part of the *DAAG* library in R.

Fig. 2.12 Ridge regression results as a function of the log of the ridge penalty λ for each of the three predictors

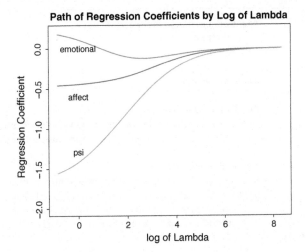

in any of the variables into *clinical* importance? How many points make a clinical difference?

For level II analysis, one has in principle an estimate of a best linear approximation of the true response surface as a property of the joint probability distribution responsible for the data. But, we know far too little about how the data were collected to make such a case one way or another. What joint probability distribution are we talking about? And were the data actually realized independently? If these problems could be resolved, proper estimation, confidence tests, and statistical tests can follow with sandwich estimates of the standard errors and an asymptotic justification. In this case, one would again reject the null hypothesis of 0.0 for the psi regression coefficient but not for the other regression coefficients. Still, with only 91 residual degrees of freedom it is not clear if one can count on the asymptotics.[12]

The conventional least squares estimates provide a benchmark for ridge regression results. Using the same mean function, Fig. 2.12 shows how the regression coefficients change as the ridge penalty is given more weight. When the ridge penalty is ignored, one has the ordinary least squares estimates. But as the ridge penalty gets larger, all three coefficients are shrunk toward zero in a proportional manner. The larger the coefficient, the greater the shrinkage. For λ values greater than about 1100 (i.e., approximately e^7), all three coefficients are effectively zero, and all three arrive at zero together. This is a characteristic of ridge regression. The code is provided in Fig. 2.13.

But what value of λ should be used? Figure 2.13 shows with the red dotted line how the average mean-squared error from a tenfold cross-validation changes with

---

[12]Several different forms of sandwich standard errors can be estimated with hccm() in the *car* library. There is little formal guidance on which to use. One might as well work with the default.

```
### Get Data and Ridge Software
library(DAAG)
library(glmnet)
data(socsupport)
attach(socsupport)

### Least Squares
X<-as.matrix(data.frame(emotional,affect,psi)) # Needs a matrix
out1<-lm(BDI~emotional+affect+psi,data=socsupport) # OLS results

### Ridge Regression
out2<-glmnet(X,BDI,family="gaussian",alpha=0) # Ridge results
plot(log(out2$lambda),out2$beta[2,],ylim=c(-2,.2),type="l",
     col="blue",lwd=3,xlab="log of Lambda", ylab="Regression
     Coefficient", main="Path of Regression Coefficients by
     Log of Lambda")
lines(log(out2$lambda),out2$beta[1,],type="l",col="red",lwd=3)
lines(log(out2$lambda),out2$beta[3,],type="l",col="green",lwd=3)
text(0,0,"emotional",cex=1.5)
text(0,-.6,"affect",cex=1.5)
text(0,-1.3,"psi",cex=1.5)
```

Fig. 2.13 R code for a least squares analysis and a ridge regression plot of coefficients as a function or λ

the log of λ.[13] The band around the average mean squared error is constructed as plus or minus two standard deviations computed from the 10 cross-validation folds. The blue vertical line shows the value of the log of λ for which the average mean squared error is the smallest. A logged value of λ equal to 1 does about as well as one can do. Looking back at Fig. 2.12, the regression coefficient for psi is shrunk from about -1.6 to about -1.0, affect is shrunk from about $-.5$ to about $-.4$, and the regression coefficient for emotional support is shrunk from about .25 to near 0.0. The regression coefficients and, consequently, the fitted values, have been regularized. But none of the regression coefficients are shrunk to exactly 0.0. The sequence of 3s across the top of the graph means that for each value of the log of λ, no predictors are dropped; all three predictors are retained in the regression.[14]

---

[13]The "canned" code from *glmnet* was used much as in the R documentation. Note that the regression coefficients are transformed back into their original units.

[14]In the output object from *glmnet()*, the 3 s are labeled "df", presumably for degrees of freedom. But the documentation makes clear that df is actually the number of predictors. In conventional linear regression, the degrees of freedom is usually taken to be the number of predictors plus 1 for the intercept. As noted in Chap. 1, when the value of λ is determined empirically, more degrees of freedom are used than the number of parameters to be estimated in the regression mean function. Moreover, one can get degrees of freedom that is not in integers (Dijkstra 2011). In short, the number of predictors should not be confused with the degrees of freedom used.

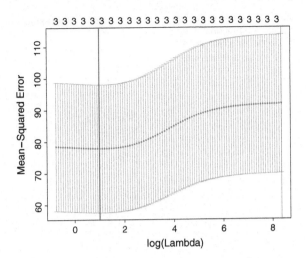

Fig. 2.14 Using cross-validation to choose the value of λ in ridge regression

Now what? Shrinkage is motivated by level II concerns, so the level I least squares analysis stands. For a level II analysis, the estimation target is the exact same ridge formulation with the selected value of λ as a feature of the joint probability distribution responsible for the data. It is not apparent why the ridge estimation target would be of interest. And even it it were, any level II interpretations must confront the model selection complications produced by the large number of cross-validation exercises undertaken (i.e., the default is 100). Estimates of the ridge regression approximation will be biased, even asymptotically. Confidence intervals and statistical tests will be invalid. It is with good reason that no statistical tests are provided by the software (Fig. 2.14).

In summary, the greatest substantive payoff from this mental health application probably comes from the level I analysis using ordinary least squares. The level II analysis from the least squares results would have been more persuasive had there been good reason to treat the data as random realizations from a substantively meaningful joint probability distribution or finite population. A larger sample would have helped too. Finally, there seems to be little that was gained applying the ridge regression formulation. One has to buy the focus on regression coefficients, the use of the L_2 penalty, and a lambda selected by cross-validation. And why was shrinkage a good idea to begin with in a very shaky level II setting? Perhaps the major take-home message is that ridge regression showcases some importance concepts and tools, but will not likely to be a useful data analysis procedure. We need to do better.

2.3.1.3 The Least Absolute Shrinkage and Selection Operator (LASSO)

Suppose that one proceeds as in ridge regression but now adopts the constraint that the sum of the absolute values of the regression coefficients is less than some constant. Just like for ridge regression, all of the predictors usually are standardized

Fig. 2.15 Lasso regression
results as a function of the
log of the ridge penalty λ for
each of the three predictors

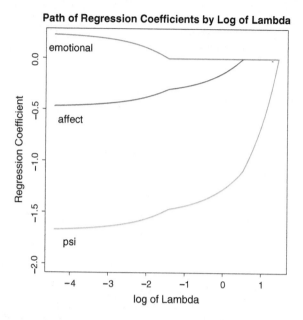

for the calculations, but the regression coefficients are transformed back into their
original units when time comes to interpret the results. The L_1 constraint leads
to a regression procedure known as the lasso[15] (Tibshirani 1996) whose estimated
regression coefficients are defined by

$$\hat{\beta} = \min_{\beta} \left[\sum_{i=1}^{n} (y_i - \beta_0 - \sum_{j=1}^{p} x_{ij}\beta_j)^2 + \lambda \sum_{j=1}^{p} |\beta_j| \right]. \qquad (2.9)$$

Unlike the ridge penalty, the lasso penalty leads to a nonlinear estimator, and
a quadratic programming solution is needed. As before, the value of λ is a tuning
parameter, typically determined empirically, usually through some measure of fit
or prediction error. Just as with ridge regression, a λ of zero yields the usual least
squares results. As the value of λ increases, the regression coefficients are shrunk
toward zero.

2.3.1.4 A Lasso Regression Illustration

Using the same data as for the ridge regression analysis, Fig. 2.15 shows that in
contrast to ridge regression, the regression coefficients are not shrunk proportionately.
(The code is provided in Fig. 2.16.) The regression coefficients are shrunk by a

---

[15]LASSO is sometimes written as "lasso," Lasso," or "LASSO."

```
### lasso Results
out3<-glmnet(X,BDI,family="gaussian",alpha=1)  # lasso
plot(log(out3$lambda),out3$beta[2,],ylim=c(-2,.2),type="l",
    col="blue",lwd=3,xlab="log of Lambda", ylab="Regression
    Coefficient", main="Path of Regression Coefficients by
    Log of Lambda")
lines(log(out3$lambda),out3$beta[1,],type="l",col="red",lwd=3)
lines(log(out3$lambda),out3$beta[3,],type="l",col="green",lwd=3)
text(-4,.1,"emotional",cex=1.5)
text(-4,-.6,"affect",cex=1.5)
text(-4,-1.8,"psi",cex=1.5)
```

Fig. 2.16 R code for lasso regression plot of coefficients as a function or λ

Fig. 2.17 Using cross-validation to choose the value of λ in lasso regression

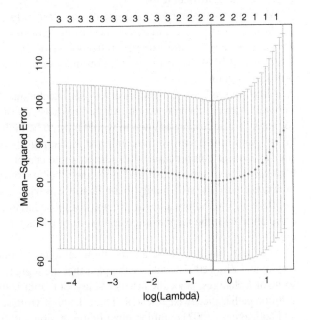

constant factor λ (Hastie it al. 2009: 69) so that some are shrunk relatively more than others as λ increases. But for a sufficiently large λ, all are shrunk to 0.0. This is a standard result that allows Hastie and his colleagues (2009: Sect. 3.4.5) to place ridge regression and the lasso in a larger model selection context. The lasso performs in a manner that has some important commonalities with model selection procedures used to choose a subset of regressors. When a coefficient value of 0.0 is reached, that predictor is no longer relevant and can be dropped.

Figure 2.17 shows how. We learn that a logged value for λ of about $-.4$ leads to the smallest average mean-squared error in the tenfold cross-validation. Looking back at Fig. 2.15, the predictor emotional has been shrunk to 0.0 and plays no role in the fitted values. On the top margin of the plot, one can see that the number of predictors has been reduced from three to two. A form of model selection has been implemented. The other two predictors remain active with psi still dominant. As the value of λ reaches about 2.5, the affect predictor is dropped as well. In practice, one would likely settle on the two predictors that are not shrunk to 0.0 and then use them in an ordinary least squares analysis. That is, the lasso chooses the predictors, but the analysis meant to inform subject-matter concerns is done with conventional least squares regression. Once a preferred set of regressors is chosen, the motivation for a fitting penalty is far less compelling.

Unfortunately, the lasso does not solve any of the level II difficulties that undermined the level II analysis with ridge regression. The main difference is in the use of an L_1 penalty rather than an L_2 that can make the lasso a useful, variable selection tool. But as before, this creates very difficult problems for estimation, confidence intervals, and statistical tests.

Were one just going to make use of the fitted values, logged $\lambda = -.4$ would produce the best performing results according to the cross-validation mean squared error and ideally, by the true generalization error that it is meant to approximate. There would be no need to revert to ordinary least squares. But all of the level II problems remain.

Although the lasso is certainly a very slick technique, it is unlikely in practice to find the "correct" mean function. At the very least, all of the regressors responsible for nature's true response function would have to be in the data set (how would you know?) and in the real world, combined as the regression mean function specifies (i.e., as a linear combination). In addition, there can be empirical obstacles such as high correlations among the predictors and whether some predictors that should be included contribute sufficiently to the fit after covariance adjustments to be retained. In effect, the predictors that survive are just those having a sufficiently large partial correlation with the response, given the set of predictors being empirically considered.

The lasso has generated an enormous amount of interest among statisticians. Rosset and Zhu (2007) consider the path that the regression coefficients take as the value of λ changes, place the lasso in a class of regularization processes in which the solution path is piecewise linear, and then develop a robust version of the lasso. Wang and colleagues (2007) combine quantile regression with the lasso to derive another robust model selection approach. Zou (2006) has proposed an adaptive version of the lasso when correlations between predictors are high so that unimportant coefficients are shrunk more aggressively. Zou and Hastie (2005) combine the ridge and lasso penalties and call the results "elastic net." Thus,

$$\hat{\beta} = \min_{\beta} \left[\sum_{i=1}^{n} (y_i - \beta_0 - \sum_{j=1}^{p} x_{ij}\beta_j)^2 + \lambda_1 \sum_{j=1}^{p} |\beta_j| + \lambda_2 \sum_{j=1}^{p} \beta_j^2 \right]. \qquad (2.10)$$

Elastic net can earn its keep in settings where the lasso stumbles: when the number of predictors is larger than the number of observations (which is common with microarray data) and when there are high correlations between predictors. Elastic net is a feature of *glmnet()* in R, and there are some promising extensions available in the R procedure *c060()* (Sill et al. 2014).

But, much of the work on the lasso has been directed toward model selection as an end in itself (Fan and Li 2006; Fan and Lv 2008; Meinshausen and Bühlmann 2006; Bühlmann and van de Geer 2011; Lockhart et al. 2014). There are a host of complications associated with model selection briefly noted in the last chapter. There are also many unsolved problems that can make real applications problematic. But perhaps most important here, a discussion model selection as a freestanding enterprise would take us far afield. Our emphasis will continue to be how to get good fitted values.[16]

In summary, ridge regression and lasso regression introduce the very important idea of penalized fitting and show some ways in which regularization can work. As the value of λ is increases, the regression coefficients are shrunk toward 0.0, and the fitted values become less rough. In the process, bias can be traded against variance with the hope of reducing generalization error in the fitted values. But with our focus on a set of inputs and their fitted values, the lasso is essentially a linear regression and is not even as flexible as regression splines; the linear mean function is very restrictive. We can do a lot better, and we will. The lasso can also be used as a model selection tool, but that is peripheral to our discussion.[17]

However, one point about model selection may be worth making. Before proceeding with model/variable selection, there needs to be ample justification. The dataset should have too many predictors for the number of observations available. Collinearity between predictors should be no worse than modest. And, the coefficients associated with the predictors should be sparse. In practice, whether these conditions are sufficiently met can be very difficult to ascertain. 9|6

2.4 Smoothing Splines

For the spline-based procedures considered earlier, the number and location of knots had to be determined a priori or by some measure of fit. We now consider an alternative that does not require a priori knots. A key feature of this approach is to effectively saturate the predictor space with knots and then protect against overfitting by constraining the impact the knots can have on the fitted values. The influence that knots

---

[16]Should one be interested in model selection per se, there are at least two other visible players within the penalized regression perspective: The Danzig Selector (Candes and Tao 2007; Gareth and Radchenko 2007; Liu et al. 2012) and the Regularization and Derivative Expectation Operator — RODEO — (Lafferty and Wasserman 2008). As mentioned earlier, model selection is sometimes called variable selection or feature selection.

[17]Lasso regularization is an example of "soft thresholding" because the regression coefficients gradually arrive at 0. Backward stepwise regression selects predictors by "hard thresholding" because regression coefficients, or functions of regression coefficients, smaller than some value are abruptly dropped from the analysis.

have can be diluted; the initial number of knots does not have to change but the impact of some can be shrunk to zero. We are proceeding in the same spirit as ridge regression and the lasso, but we are allowing for nonlinear associations between X and Y and introducing a different kind of penalty function.

We begin by returning to the wrong model perspective in which the predictors and the response are random variables. For a single predictor and a quantitative response variable, there is a function $f(X)$ with two derivatives over its entire surface. This is a common assumption in the statistical learning literature and in practice does not seem to be particularly restrictive. The goal is to minimize a penalized error sum of squares of the form

$$\text{RSS}(f, \lambda) = \sum_{i=1}^{N} [y_i - f(x_i)]^2 + \lambda \int [f''(t)]^2 dt, \qquad (2.11)$$

where λ is, as before, a tuning parameter. The first term on the right-hand side captures how close the fitted values are to the actual values of y. It is just the usual error sum of squares. The second imposes a cost for the complexity of the fit, much in the tradition of penalized regression, where t is a placeholder for the unknown function. The integral quantifies the roughness penalty, and λ once again determines the weight given to that penalty in the fitting process.[18] At one extreme, as λ increases without limit, the fitted values approach the least squares line. Because no second derivatives are allowed, the fitted values are as smooth as they can be. At the other extreme, as λ decreases toward zero, the fitted values approach an interpolation of the values of the response variable. For a level I analysis, the larger the value of λ, the smoother the representation of the association between X and Y. For a level II analysis, the estimation target is the smoothing splines function with the empirically determined values of λ as a feature of the joint probability distribution. When for a level II analysis one is trying to construct fitted values that usefully approximate the true response surface, if λ is larger, the smoother fitted values will likely lead to more bias and less variance. If λ is smaller, the rougher fitted values will likely lead to less bias and more variance. The value of λ can be used in place of the number of knots to tune the bias-variance tradeoff.

Equation 2.11 can be minimized with respect to the $f(x)$, given a value for λ. Hastie et al. (2009: Sect. 5.4) explain that a unique solution results, based on a set of natural cubic splines with N knots.[19] In particular,

$$f(x) = \sum_{j=1}^{N} N_j(x)\theta_j, \qquad (2.12)$$

---

[18]The second derivative at a given point will be larger the more rapidly the function is changing at that location. The integral is, in effect, the sum of such second derivatives. When the integral is larger, the function is rougher.

[19]There will be fewer knots if there are less than N distinct values of x.

where θ_j is a set of weights, $N_j(x)$ is an N-dimensional set of basis functions for the natural cubic splines being used, and j stands for the number of knots, of which there can be a maximum of N.

Consider the following toy example, in which x takes on values 0 to 1 in steps of .20. In this case, suppose $j = 6$, and Eq. 2.12, written as $f(x) = \mathbf{N}\theta$, then takes the form of

$$f(x) = \begin{pmatrix} -.267 & 0 & 0 & -.214 & .652 & -.429 \\ .591 & .167 & 0 & -.061 & .182 & -.121 \\ .158 & .667 & .167 & -.006 & .019 & -.012 \\ 0 & .167 & 0.667 & .155 & .036 & -.024 \\ 0 & 0 & .167 & .596 & .214 & .024 \\ 0 & 0 & 0 & -.143 & .429 & .714 \end{pmatrix} \begin{pmatrix} \theta_1 \\ \theta_2 \\ \theta_2 \\ \theta_4 \\ \theta_5 \\ \theta_6 \end{pmatrix}. \tag{2.13}$$

Equation 2.11 can be rewritten using a natural cubic spline basis and then the solution becomes

$$\hat{\theta} = (\mathbf{N}^T\mathbf{N} + \lambda\mathbf{\Omega}_N)^{-1}\mathbf{N}^T\mathbf{y}, \tag{2.14}$$

with $[\mathbf{\Omega}_N]_{ij} = \int N_j''(t)N_k''(t)dt$, where the second derivatives are for the function that transforms x into its natural cubic spline basis. $\mathbf{\Omega}_N$ has larger values where the predictor is rougher, and given the linear estimator, this is where the fitted values can be rougher as well. The penalty is the same as in Eq. 2.11.

To arrive at fitted values,

$$\hat{\mathbf{y}} = \mathbf{N}(\mathbf{N}^T\mathbf{N} + \lambda\mathbf{\Omega}_N)^{-1}\mathbf{N}^T\mathbf{y} = \mathbf{S}_\lambda\mathbf{y}, \tag{2.15}$$

where $\mathbf{S}_\lambda$ is a smoother matrix. For a given value of λ, we have a linear estimator of the fitted values.

Equation 2.14 can be seen as a generalized form of ridge regression. With ridge regression, for instance, $\mathbf{\Omega}_N$ is an identity matrix. In practice, N is replaced by a basis of B-splines that is used to compute the natural cubic splines.

The requirement of N knots may seem odd because it appears to imply that for a linear estimator all N degrees of freedom are used up. However, for values of λ greater than zero, the fitted values are shunk toward a linear fit, and the fitted values are made more smooth. Less than N degrees of freedom are being used.

As with the number of knots, the value of λ can be determined a priori or through model selection procedures. One common approach is based on N-fold (drop-one) cross-validation, briefly discussed in the last chapter. The value of λ is chosen so that

$$\text{CV}(\hat{f}_\lambda) = \sum_{i=1}^{N}[y_i - \hat{f}_i^{(-i)}(x_i)]^2 \tag{2.16}$$

is as small as possible. In standard notation, $\hat{f}_i^{(-i)}(x_i)$ is the fitted value with case i removed. Using CV to select λ can be automated to find a promising balance between the bias and the variance in the fitted values. The same reasoning can be used with an in-sample estimate of CV called the generalized cross-validation statistic (GCV), which is computed as,

$$\text{GCV} = \frac{1}{N} \sum_{i=1}^{N} \left[\frac{y_i - \hat{f}(x_i)}{1 - \text{trace}(\mathbf{S})/N} \right]^2, \quad (2.17)$$

where $\mathbf{S}$ is the smoother (or hat) matrix as before. Whether the CV or GCV is used, all of the earlier caveats apply. For a level II analysis, we are back in the model selection business with all of its complications. For example, the trace in Eq. 2.17 is not a proper expression for the degrees of freedom expended by the smoother.

2.4.1 A Smoothing Splines Illustration

To help fix all these ideas, we turn to an application of smoothing splines. Figure 2.18 shows four smoothed scatterplots based on Eqs. 2.11 and 2.12. The R code can be found in Fig. 2.19.

Each plot in Fig. 2.18 has the number of users of a particular server (centered) over time.[20] Time is measured in minutes. The penalty weight is *spar*, which can be thought of as a monotonic and standardized function of λ that is ordinarily set at a value from 0 to 1. The data, available in R — see Fig. 2.19 — constitute a time series of 100 observations. Because the documentation in R does not explain how the data were collected, we proceed with a level I regression analysis.[21]

The number of users connected to the server varies dramatically over time in a highly nonlinear manner. Because details of the nonlinearity probably would have been unanticipated, an inductive approach available with smoothing splines is appropriate. For Fig. 2.18, there are four different plots with four different values of *spar*. The quality of the fitted values changes dramatically. But there is no right answer. For a level I analysis, the goal is description. The value of *spar* depends heavily on subject-matter expertise and how the results might be used.

It could be very misleading to automatically choose the value of *spar* by some overall measure of in-sample fit. The fitted values are responding to both signal and noise. For example, is the dip around minute 40 to be taken seriously? It would seem to be "real" when *spar* is .4 or .6, but not when *spar* is .8 or 1. Someone very familiar with the setting in which the data were collected and more generally knowledgeable about patterns of server use would need to make that call.

For a level II analysis, one might want to consider the bias-variance tradeoff and in the absence of test data, set the value of *spar* using some approximation of out-of-sample performance. For these data, the default leave-one-out cross-validation

---

[20]The plotted fitted values vary around the mean of the response. More will be said about this later.
[21]The procedure *gam()* in the library *gam* was used.

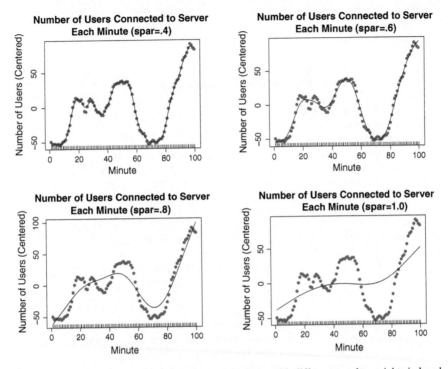

Fig. 2.18 Penalized smoothing splines for use by minute with different penalty weights indexed by the tuning parameter *spar*

selects a value of 8.5. But it is difficult to know what "out-of-sample" means. The data on hand are a sample of exactly what? To what does "out-of-sample" refer? Moreover, cross-validation is probably not a sensible procedure for time series data because cross-validation breaks up the temporal sequence of the data.[22]

More generally, the issues surrounding a level II analysis are largely the same as those addressed for ridge regression and the lasso. If the value of λ (or the equivalent) is chosen before before the data analysis begins, one can proceed as described in Chap. 1 with the response surface approximation perspective. If the value of λ is chosen as part of the data analysis, one is engaging in model selection. With true test data or split samples, there may be a framework in which to proceed, but the longitudinal nature of the data would have to be maintained.[23]

---

[22]When there is an empirical determination of spar, the *gam* procedure reports the degrees of freedom used, not spar. With a little trial and error, however, one can figure out what the value of spar is.

[23]For example, one might have another dataset for the same 100 min at the same time the next day. If day to day variation is essentially noise, one might well have valid test data.

```
# Data
data(WWWusage)
Minute<-1:100
NumUsers<-WWWusage
internet<-data.frame(NumUsers,Minute)

# Smoothing Splines
library(gam)
par(mfrow=c(2,2))
out<-gam(NumUsers~s(Minute, spar=.4),data=internet)
plot(out,xlab="Minute",ylab="Number of Users (Centered)",
    main="Number of Users Connected to Server
    Each Minute (spar=.4)", col="blue", pch=19,
    residuals=T)

out<-gam(NumUsers~s(Minute, spar=.6),data=internet)
plot(out,xlab="Minute",ylab="Number of Users (Centered)",
    main="Number of Users Connected to Server
    Each Minute (spar=.6)",col="blue",pch=19,
    residuals=T)

out<-gam(NumUsers~s(Minute, spar=.8),data=internet)
plot(out,xlab="Minute",ylab="Number of Users (Centered)",
    main="Number of Users Connected to Server
    Each Minute (spar=.8)",col="blue",pch=19,
    residuals=T)

out<-gam(NumUsers~s(Minute, spar=1.0),data=internet)
plot(out,xlab="Minute",ylab="Number of Users (Centered)",
    main="Number of Users Connected to Server
    Each Minute (spar=1.0)",col="blue",pch=19,
    residuals=T)
```

Fig. 2.19 R code for penalized smoothing splines

2.5 Locally Weighted Regression as a Smoother

Thus far, the discussion of smoothing has been built upon a foundation of conventional linear regression. Another approach to smoothing also capitalizes on conventional regression, but through nearest neighbor methods. We start with those.

2.5.1 Nearest Neighbor Methods

Consider Fig. 2.20 in which the ellipse represents a scatter plot of points for values for X and Y. There is a target value of X, labeled x_0, for which a conditional mean $\bar{y}_0$ is to be computed. There may be only one such value of X or a relatively small number of such values. As a result, a conditional mean computed from those values alone risks being very unstable. One possible solution is to compute $\bar{y}_0$ from observations with values of X close to x_0. The rectangle overlaid on the scatterplot illustrates a region of "nearest neighbors" that might be used. Insofar as the conditional means for Y are not changing systematically within that region, a useful value for $\bar{y}_0$ can be obtained. For a level I description, the conditional mean is a good summary for Y derived from the x-values in that neighborhood. If that conditional mean is to be used as an estimate in a level II analysis of the true response surface, it will be unbiased and likely be more stable than the conditional mean estimated only for the observations with $X = x_0$. In practice, however, some bias is often introduced because Y actually does vary systematically in the neighborhood. As before, one hopes that the increase in the bias is small compared to the decrease in the variance.

A key issue is how the nearest neighbors are defined. One option is to take the k closest observations using the metric of X. For example, if X is age, x_0 is 24 years old, and k is 10, the ten closest x-values might range from 23 to 27 years of age. Another option is take some fixed fraction f of the observations that are closest to x_0. For example, if the closest 25 % of the observations were taken, k might turn out to be 30, and the age-values might range between 21 and 29. Yet another option is to vary either k or f depending on the variability in Y within a neighborhood. For example, if there is more heterogeneity that is likely to be noise, larger values of k or f can be desirable to improve stability. For any of these approaches, the neighborhoods will likely overlap for different target values for X. For another target value near x_0, some near neighbors will likely be in both neighborhoods. There also is no requirement that the neighborhood be symmetric around x_0.

Fig. 2.20 A conditional mean $\bar{Y}_0$ for X_0, a target value of X

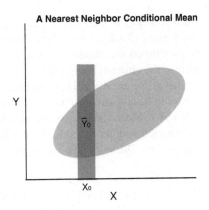

Fig. 2.21 Interpolated
conditional means

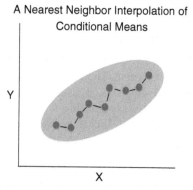

A Nearest Neighbor Interpolation of
Conditional Means

Suppose now that for each unique value of x, a nearest neighbor conditional mean for y is computed using one of the approaches just summarized. Figure 2.21 shows a set of such means connected by straight lines. The pattern provides a visualization of how the means of y vary with x. As such, the nearest neighbor methods can been seen as a smoother.

The values k or f are often referred to as the "bandwidth," "window," or "span" of a neighborhood. The larger the values of k or f, the larger the size of the neighborhood, and Fig. 2.21 will change in response. Larger neighborhoods will tend to make the smoothed values less variable. If the smoothed values are to be treated as level II estimates of the true response surface, they will likely be more biased and more stable. Smaller neighborhoods will tend to make the smoothed values more variable. If the smoothed values are to be treated as level II estimates of the true response surface, they will likely be less biased and less stable.

2.5.2 Locally Weighted Regression

Nearest neighbor methods can be effective in practice and have been elaborated in many ways (Ripley 1996; Shakhnarovich 2006). In particular, what if within each neighborhood the conditional means of Y vary systematically? At the very least, there is information being ignored that could improve the estimate of $\bar{y}_0$.

Just as in conventional linear regression, if Y is related to X in a systematic fashion, there can be less variation in the regression residuals than around the neighborhood mean of Y. More stable estimates can follow. The idea of applying linear regression within each neighborhood leads to a form of smoothing based on locally weighted regressions. The smoother commonly is known as "lowess".[24]

---

[24]Lowess is sometimes said to stand for locally weighted scatter plot smoothing. But Cleveland, who invented the procedure (Cleveland 1979), seems to prefer the term "local regression" known as "loess" (Cleveland 1993: 94).

We stick with the one predictor case a bit longer. For any given value of the predictor x_0, a polynomial regression is constructed only from observations with x-values that are nearest neighbors of x_0. Among these, observations with x-values closer to x_0 are weighted more heavily. Then, $\hat{y}_0$ is computed from the fitted regression and used as the smoothed value of the response y at x_0. The process is repeated for all other values of x.

Although the lowess polynomial is often of degree one (linear), quadratic and cubic polynomials are also used. It is not clear that much is gained in practice using the quadratic or cubic form. In some implementations, one can also employ a degree zero polynomial, in which case no regression is computed, and the conditional mean of y in the neighborhood is used as $\hat{y}_0$. This is just the nearest neighbor approach except for the use of distance weighting. Perhaps surprisingly, the lowess estimator is linear for a given value of k or f (Hastie et al. 2009; Sect. 6.1.1).

The precise weight given to each observation depends on the weighting function employed. The normal distribution is one option. That is, the weights form a bell-shaped curve centered on x_0 that declines with distance from x_0. The tricube is another option. Differences between x_0 and each value of x in the window are divided by the length of the window along x. This standardizes the differences. Then the differences are transformed as $(1 - |z|^3)^3$, where z is the standardized difference. Values of x outside the window are given weights of 0.0. As an empirical matter, most of the common weighting functions give about the same results, and there seems to be no formal justification for any particular weighting function.

As discussed for nearest neighbor methods, the amount of smoothing depends on the value of k or f. For f, proportions between .25 and .75 are common. The larger the proportion of observations included, the smoother are the fitted values. The span plays the same role as the number of knots in regression splines or λ in smoothing splines. Some software also permits the span to be chosen in the units of the regressor. For example, if the predictor is population size, the span might be defined as 10,000 people wide.

More formally, each local regression at each x_0 is constructed by minimizing the weighted sum of squares with respect to the intercept and slope for the $M \leq N$ observations included in the window. Thus,

$$\text{RSS}^*(\beta) = (\mathbf{y}^* - \mathbf{X}^*\beta)^T \mathbf{W}^* (\mathbf{y}^* - \mathbf{X}^*\beta). \qquad (2.18)$$

The asterisk indicates that only the observations in the window are included. The regressor matrix $\mathbf{X}^*$ can contain polynomial terms for the predictor, should that be desired. $\mathbf{W}^*$ is a diagonal matrix conforming to $\mathbf{X}^*$, with diagonal elements w_i^*, which are a function of distance from x_0. This is where the weighting-by-distance gets done.

The overall algorithm then operates as follows.

1. Choose the smoothing parameter such as bandwidth, f, which is a proportion between 0 and 1.
2. Choose a point x_0 and from that the ($f \times N = M$) nearest points on x.

3. For these *M* nearest neighbor points, compute a weighted least squares regression line for *y* on *x*.
4. Construct the fitted value $\hat{y}_0$ for that single x_0.
5. Repeat Steps 2 through 4 for each value of *x*. Near the boundary values of *x*, constraints are sometimes imposed much like those imposed on cubic splines and for the same reasons.
6. To enhance visualization, connect adjacent $\hat{y}$s with straight lines.

There is also a robust version of lowess. After the entire fitting process is completed, residuals are computed in the usual way. Weights are constructed from these residuals. Larger residuals are given smaller weights and smaller residuals larger weights. Using these weights, the fitting process is repeated. This, in turn, can be iterated until the fitted values do not change much (Cleveland 1979) or until some predetermined number of iterations is reached (e.g., three). The basic idea is to make observations with very large residuals less important in the fitting.

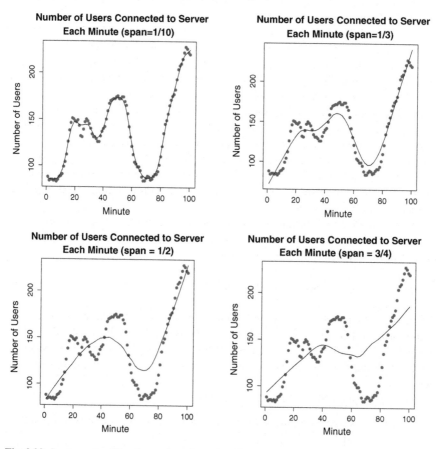

Fig. 2.22 Lowess smoothing for use by minute for different spans

Whether the "robustification" of lowess is useful will be application-specific and depend heavily on the window size chosen. Larger windows will tend to smooth the impact of outlier residuals. But because the scatterplot being smoothed is easily plotted and examined, it is usually easy to spot the possible impact of outlier residuals and, if necessary, remove them or take them into account when the results are reported. In short, there is no automatic need for the robust version of lowess when there seem to be a few values of the response that perhaps distort the fit.

Just as with penalized smoothing splines, a level I analysis is descriptive. A level II analysis can entail estimation of a response surface approximation of the same form and with the same values of the tuning parameters as used for the training data. That approximation can also be used to provide estimates of the true response surface that are subject to the same sort of bias-variance tradeoffs discussed earlier.

2.5.2.1 A Lowess Illustration

Figure 2.22 repeats the earlier analysis of server use, but applies lowess rather than smoothing splines. The results are much the same over a set of different spans. The fraction for each reported span is the proportion of observations that define a given neighborhood. (See Fig. 2.23 for the R code.)

```
# Data
data(WWWusage)
Minute<-1:100
NumUsers<-WWWusage

# Lowess
par(mfrow=c(2,2))
scatter.smooth(Minute,NumUsers,xlab="Minute",ylab="Number of
     Users", main="Number of Users Connected to Server
     Each Minute (span=1/10)", span=1/10,pch=19,col="blue")
scatter.smooth(Minute,NumUsers,xlab="Minute",ylab="Number of
     Users", main="Number of Users Connected to Server
     Each Minute (span=1/3)", span=1/3, pch=19, col="blue")
scatter.smooth(Minute,NumUsers,xlab="Minute",ylab="Number of
     Users", main="Number of Users Connected to Server
     Each Minute (span = 1/2)", span=1/2, pch=19, col="blue")
scatter.smooth(Minute,NumUsers,xlab="Minute",ylab="Number of
     Users", main="Number of Users Connected to Server
     Each Minute (span = 3/4)", span=3/4, pch=19,col="blue")
```

Fig. 2.23 R code lowess smooth

Figure 2.22 was produced in R by *scatter.smooth().*[25] One can also proceed with *loess()*, which has more options and separates the plotting from the fitting. Both procedures require that the span (or an equivalent turning parameter) be hard coded although there have been proposals to automate the tuning, much as done for smoothing splines (Loader 2004: Sect. 4).

In summary, lowess provides a good, practical alternative to smoothing splines except that the span is not determined automatically (at least in R). Otherwise, it has pretty much the same strengths and weaknesses, and performance will be similar. For example, the same issues arise about whether the dip in use at about minute 40 is "real." Or even if it is, whether the dip is substantively or practically important. The lower lefthand plot in Fig. 2.22 may be the most instructive rendering for these data.

2.6 Smoothers for Multiple Predictors

The last set of figures is only the most recent example in which the limitations of a single predictor are apparent. Many more things could be related to server use than time alone. We need to consider smoothers when there is more than one predictor.

In principle, it is a simple matter to include many predictors and then smooth a multidimensional space. However, there are three significant complications in practice. The first problem is the curse of dimensionality addressed in the last chapter. As the number of predictors increases, the space the data need to populate increases as a power function. Consequently, the demand for data increases very rapidly, and one risks data that are far too sparse to produce a meaningful fit. There are too few observations, or those observations are not spread around sufficiently to provide the support needed. One must, in effect, extrapolate into regions where there is little or no information. To be sensible, such extrapolations would depend on knowing the $f(X)$ quite well. But it is precisely because the $f(X)$ is unknown that smoothing is undertaken to begin with.

The second problem is that there are often conceptual complications associated with multiple predictors. In the case of lowess, for example, how is the neighborhood near x_0 to be defined (Fan and Gijbels 1996: 299–300)? One option is to use Euclidian distance. But then the neighborhood will depend on the units in which predictors happen to be measured. The common practice of transforming the variables into standard deviation units solves the units problem, but introduces new problems. When does it make substantive sense to claim that two observations that are close in standard deviations are close in subject-matter units?

---

[25]The plots produced by *scatter.smooth()* are not centered around the mean of the response, but whether the plot is centered or not should have no effect on an interpretation of the relationship between Y and X unless variation relative to the mean of Y matters. It also might if the actual values of the approximate response surface were important (e.g., in forecasting).

Consider a simple case of two predictors. Suppose the standard deviation for one predictor is five years of age, and the standard deviation for the other predictor is two years of education. Now suppose one observation falls at x_0's value of education, but is five years of age higher than x_0. Suppose another observation falls at x_0's value for age, but is two years higher in eduction than x_0. Both are one standard deviation unit away from x_0 in Euclidian distance. But do we really want to say they are equally close to x_0?

Another approach to neighborhood definition is to use the same span (e.g., .20) for both predictors, but apply it separately in each direction. Why this is a better definition of a neighborhood is not clear. And one must still define a distance metric by which the observation in the neighborhood will be weighted.

The third problem is that gaining meaningful access to the results is no longer straightforward. When there are more than two predictors, one can no longer graph the fitted surface in the usual way. How does one make sense of a surface in more than three dimensions?

2.6.1 Smoothing in Two Dimensions

Given the problems just summarized, the step from a single predictor to two predictors can be challenging. But there are extensions of the single-predictor setting that can work well and that introduce some tools that will be important as we move to applications with more than two predictors. We will proceed drawing heavily on an empirical example.

A key issue in the study of climate is cyclical variation in rainfall for areas on the Pacific rim. An important driver is measured by the Southern Oscillation Index (SOI), which is the difference in sea level barometric pressure between Tahiti and Darwin, Australia. Negative values are associated with a phenomenon called "El Niño." Positive values are associated with a phenomenon called "La Niña." Both are connected to patterns of rainfall in ways that are not well understood.

The illustrative data we will use has 101 observations. Predictors are year from 1900 to 2001 and the average yearly SOI. Average yearly rainfall in Australia is the response. The data are shown in Fig. 2.24, and the code is shown in Fig. 2.25.[26]

Much as in the case of conventional multiple linear regression, the goal is to fit a surface to the data. Rainfall is the response. Year and SOI are the predictors. Unlike conventional linear regression, no model is imposed. In particular, the correct fit is not assumed to be a plane produced by a linear combination of year and SOI. A smoothing splines formulation for a single predictor is applied, but the single predictor is the product of year and SOI, just as one might represent an interaction effect between the two. The product variable is smoothed and then plotted in the 2-dimensional predictor space.

---

[26]The data can be obtained from the *DAAG* library under the name *bomsoi*.

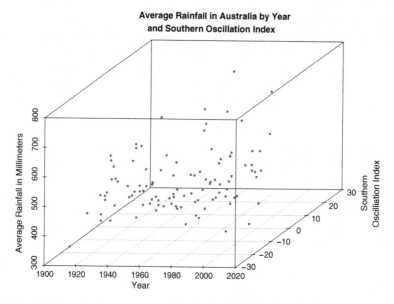

Fig. 2.24 A 3-dimensional scatter plot of rainfall in Australia as a function year and the southern oscillation index

```
library(DAAG)
data(bomsoi)
attach(bomsoi)
library(scatterplot3d)
scatterplot3d(Year,SOI,avrain,xlab="Year", ylab="Southern
              Oscilliation Index",zlab="Average Rainfall in
              Millimeters", main="Average Rainfall in Australia
              by Year and Southern Oscillation Index",pch=19,
              color="blue")
```

Fig. 2.25 R code for the 3-D scatter plot

Figure 2.26 shows the result for the Australian rainfall data from 1900 to 2001.[27] Values of the tuning parameter range from .2 to 1.0. As before, larger values of spar produce smoother surfaces. Any one of the values (or some other) could be preferred,

[27]The procedure used was *gam* in the *gam* library. There is an alternative implementation of *gam* in the *mgcv* library, written by Simon Wood, that has a very large number of somewhat daunting options. For example, there are several rather different ways to smooth a nonadditive function of two predictors. Documentation is extensive, but challenging in spots. Fortunately, the defaults seem to work well and yielded much the same results as shown in Fig. 2.26.

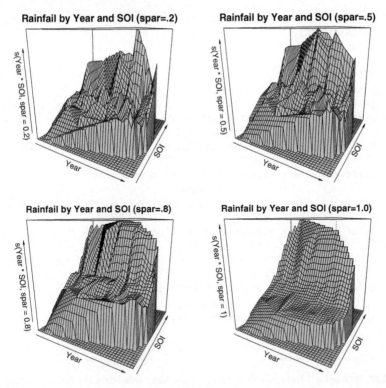

Fig. 2.26 3-Dimensional scatter plot of rainfall in Australia as a function of year and the southern oscillation index

but a spar-value of 1.0 was chosen using leave-one-out cross-validation. The label on the vertical axis shows the expression by which the fitted values were computed.[28]

Within a level I analysis, there is a modest increase in rainfall over the time period with most of that increase occurring early. Rainfall increases when the SOI is larger, but the relationship is highly nonlinear. The association is especially pronounced for larger values of the SOI. For some smaller values of spar, the surface is "torqued." The relationship between SOI and rainfall is substantially stronger in some years than others. For example, with spar = .2, the strongest association is in the 1980s. However, with only 101 observations spread across the 2-dimensional predictor space, there are relatively few observations behind such results. That may be reason enough to

---

[28]The use of the * operator means multiplication. (See Fig. 2.27.) Year is multiplied by SOI. Currently, the plotting procedure "knows" when it sees * that the plotting surface should be in 2-D predictor space. If one does the multiplication in advance and uses the product as a predictor, *gam* produces the same fit and summary statistics. But the plot treats the product as the vector it is. The procedure does not "know" that the vector is the product of two predictors. Figure 2.26 shows the results as perspective plots. Contour plots would convey much the same information with more numerical detail but in a less easily understood visual format. Computations in *gam* are undertaken using cubic smoothing splines with B-splines the behind-the-scenes workhorse as usual.

```
library(DAAG)
data(bomsoi)
attach(bomsoi)
llbrary(gam)
library(akima)
par(mfrow=c(2,2))
out1<-gam(avrain~s(Year*SOI,spar=.2),data=bomsoi,
                    family=gaussian)
plot(out1,theta=30, main="Rainfail by Year and SOI (spar=.2)",
        col="light blue")
out2<-gam(avrain~s(Year*SOI,spar=.5),data=bomsoi,
                    family=gaussian)
plot(out2, theta=30, main="Rainfail by Year and SOI (spar=.5)",
        col="light blue")
out3<-gam(avrain~s(Year*SOI,spar=.8),data=bomsoi,
                    family=gaussian)
plot(out3, theta=30, main="Rainfail by Year and SOI (spar=.8)",
        col="light blue")
out4<-gam(avrain~s(Year*SOI,spar=1),data=bomsoi,
                    family=gaussian)
plot(out4, theta=30, main="Rainfall by Year and SOI (spar=1.0)",
        col="light blue")
```

Fig. 2.27 R code for 3-Dimensional smooth of Australian rainfall data as a function of year and the southern oscillation index

prefer the fitted values with spar $= 1.0$ and provides a small-scale object lesson about the curse of dimensionality.

Much as in several earlier analyses, a level II analysis would be very challenging. The data are longitudinal with year as one of the predictors. In the same fashion as the Tokyo water use data, the data collection conditions on year. As a result, the data may be best considered as random realizations from a set of conditional distributions. But then, we still have to rely on a theory of how nature is able to repeat the rainfall patterns for a given set of years. Perhaps this could be worked out by researchers steeped in climate science, but for now at least, no level II analysis will be attempted.

2.6.2 The Generalized Additive Model

Moving beyond two predictors usually requires a different strategy. A more practical and accessible means needs to be found to approximate a response surface when the predictor space is greater than two. One approach is to resurrect an additive formulation that in practice can perform well.

The Generalized Additive Model (GAM) is superficially an easy extension of the Generalized Linear Model (GLM). GAM tries to circumvent the curse of dimensionality by assuming that the conditional mean of the response is a linear combination of functions of the predictors. Thus, the generalized additive model with p predictors can be written as

$$Y = \alpha + \sum_{j=1}^{p} f_j(\mathbf{X}_j) + \varepsilon, \tag{2.19}$$

where α is fixed at the mean of Y. We once again minimize the penalized regression sum of squares (PRSS) but with respect to all the p f_j's (Hastie et al. 2009: 297):

$$\text{PRSS}(\alpha, f_1, f_2, \ldots, f_p) = \sum_{i=2}^{N} \left(y_i - \alpha - \sum_{j=1}^{p} f_j(x_{ij}) \right)^2 + \sum_{j=1}^{p} \lambda_j \int f_j''(t_j)^2 dt_j. \tag{2.20}$$

Equation 2.20 is a generalization of single-predictor smoothing splines that allows for a different value of λ_j for each function in the linear combination of functions; there are p values for λ that need to be specified in advance or more typically, determined as part of the data analysis. The pth second derivatives correspond to the pth function only.[29]

In the same manner as the generalized linear model, the generalized additive model permits several different link functions and disturbance distributions. For example, with a binary response, the link function can be the log of the odds (the "logit") of the response, and the disturbance distribution can be logistic. This is analogous to logistic regression within the generalized linear model. But, there are no regression coefficients associated with the predictors. Regression coefficients would just scale up or scale down the functions of predictors. Whatever impact they would have is absorbed in the function itself. In other words, the role of the regression coefficients cannot be distinguished from the role of the transformation and therefore, the regression coefficients are not identified.

Each predictor can have its own functional relationship to the response. Because these functions are usually estimated using single-predictor smoothers of the sort addressed earlier, the term nonparametric is commonly applied despite the a priori commitment to an additive formulation. Alternatively, all of the functions may be specified in advance with the usual linear model as a special case.

All of the common regression options are available, including the wide range of transformations one sees in practice: logs, polynomials, roots, product variables (for interaction effects), and indicator variables. As a result, GAM can be parametric as well and in this form, is really no different from the generalized linear model. The parametric and nonparametric specifications can be mixed so that some of the

---

[29]The notation t_j is a placeholder for the unknown jth function.

functions are derived empirically from the data, and some are specified in advance.
Then the model is often called semiparametric.

One can use for GAM the same conception of "holding constant" that applies to
conventional linear regression. Suppose that for a conventional regression analysis
each of the predictors is transformed in a known manner. With least squares, each
transformed predictor is covariance adjusted; the relationship between a given transformed predictor and the response is determined with the linear dependence between
that transformed predictor and all other transformed predictors removed. One would
like to do the same thing when each transformation is not known. But there can be
no covariance adjustments until the transformations are determined, and there can
be no transformations until each predictor is covariance adjusted. The backfitting
algorithm provides a solution.

2.6.2.1 A GAM Fitting Algorithm

The backfitting algorithm is a common way to estimate the functions and coefficient
α in Eq. 2.20 (Hastie et al. 2009: Sect. 9.1.1) using the following steps.

1. Initialize with $\hat{\alpha} = \frac{1}{N} \sum_1^N y_i$, $\hat{f}_j \equiv 0$, $\forall i, j$. Each function is given initial values
   of 0.0, with α fixed at the mean of y.
2. Cycle: $j = 1, \ldots, p, 1, \ldots, p, \ldots$,

$$\hat{f}_j \leftarrow S_j \left[\{y - \hat{\alpha} - \sum_{k \neq j} \hat{f}_k(x_{ik})\}_1^N \right].$$

$$\hat{f}_j \leftarrow \hat{f}_j - \frac{1}{N} \sum_{i=1}^N \hat{f}_{ij}$$

   Fitted values from all predictors but predictor j are linearly combined and subtracted from the response. A smoother S_j is applied to the resulting "residuals."
   The result is a new set of fitted values for predictor j. These fitted values are then
   centered. All of the other predictors are cycled through one at a time in the same
   manner until each of the p predictors has a revised set of fitted values.
3. Repeat Step 2 until $\hat{f}_j$ changes less than some small, pre-determined amount. In
   the process, adjustments are made for nonlinear dependence between predictors.

The backfitting algorithm is quite general and quite fast. A wide variety of
smoothers can be applied and in the past have been. For example, both lowess and
penalized smoother splines are available in R. A range of smoothing basis functions
can be employed as well (Wood 2006: Sect. 4.1). Some procedures also permit the
use of functions of two predictors at a time, so that the smoothed values represent a
surface rather than a line, just as in Fig. 2.26; one can work with a linear combination

of bivariate smoothed values. Excellent implementations in R include the procedure *gam( )* in the *gam* library and the procedure *gam( )* in the *mgcv* library.[30]

So what's not to like? The linear combination of smooths is not as general as a smooth of an entire surface, and sometimes that matters. Looking back at the El Niño example, the response surface was "torqued." The nonlinear function along one predictor dimension varied by the values of the other predictor dimension. This is a generalization of conventional interaction effects for linear regression in which the slope for one predictor varies over values of another predictor. The generalized additive model does not allow for interaction effects unless they are built into the mean function as product variables; interaction effects are not arrived at inductively. This is no different from conventional linear regression.

2.6.2.2 An Illustration Using the Generalized Additive Model

Although population counts from the U.S. census are highly accurate, they are certainly not perfect. In the absence of perfection, small differences between the actual number of residents in an area and the counted number of residents in that area can have very important consequences for definitions of voting districts, the number of elected representatives a county or state can have, and the allocations of federal funds. Beginning with the 1980 U.S. census, there were particular concerns about population undercounts in less affluent, minority-dominated voting districts.

The data we will now use come for a study by Ericksen, Kadane and Tukey (1989) that sought correlates of census undercounts. Sixty-six geographical areas were included, 16 being large cities. The other geographical units were either the remainder of the state in which the city was located or other states entirely. Sampling was purposive.

We use the following variables:

1. Undercount — the undercount as a percentage of the total count;
2. Minority — the percentage of residents who are Black or Hispanic;
3. Language — the percentage of residents who have difficulty with English;
4. Housing — the percentage of residential buildings that is small and multi-unit; and
5. Crime — reported crimes per 1000 residents.

The first variable is the response. The others are predictors thought to be related to census undercounts. No doubt there are any number of other predictors that subject-matter experts would claim should have been included. For example, we know nothing about the census enumeration procedures or the race and gender of enumerators.

---

[30]There are some important differences in the computational details, output, plotting facility, and ease of use, many of which boil down to personal taste. From Hastie et al. (2009), it is natural to work with the *gam* library. From Wood (2006), it is natural work with the *mgcv* library. Both references provide important background because the documentation in R is not meant to teach the material and makes reference to terms and concepts that may be unfamiliar.

We also know nothing about any efforts by local authorities to encourage residents to cooperate. By conventional criteria, the mean function is misspecified.

Using the procedure *gam( )* in the library *mgcv*, we applied the generalized additive model to the data. An examination of the tabular output indicated that nearly 80 % of the deviance was accounted for. There was also lots of other information, much like that provided for conventional linear regression, and if there had been predictors that were not smoothed (e.g., factors), their regression coefficients would have been displayed. For each smoothed predictor, the effective degrees of freedom was reported, although as noted earlier, an inductively determined value of λ makes those values suspect. Still, large values for the effective degrees of freedom indicate that a function is more complex.

Figure 2.28 shows how the predictors are related to the response. (See Fig. 2.29 for the R code.) For each graph, the response is centered around $\hat{\alpha}$, and there are rug plots just above the horizontal axes. Also shown are the response values after

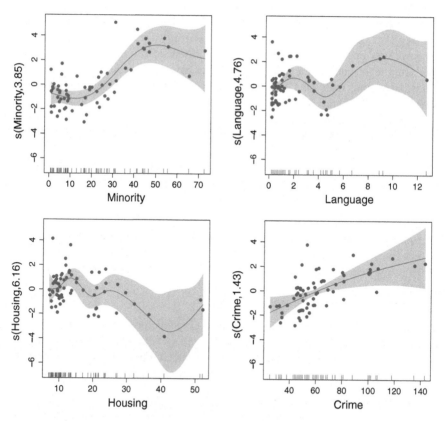

Fig. 2.28 Correlates of the estimated undercount percentage for the U.S. 1980 census (The predictor is on each *horizontal* axis, the centered fitted values are on each *vertical* axis, the *shaded* areas are error bands, rug plots are shown, and $N = 66$.)

```
library(car)
data(Ericksen)
library(mgcv)

# make better variable names plotting
attach(Ericksen)
City<-as.numeric(ifelse(city=="city",1,0))
Minority<-minority
Language<-language
Housing<-housing
Crime<-crime
Undercount<-undercount
temp<-data.frame(Undercount,Crime,Housing,Language,Minority,City)

# GAM from mgcv
out<-gam(Undercount~s(Minority)+s(Language)+s(Housing)+
         s(Crime)+City,data=temp,family=gaussian)
par(mfrow=c(2,2))
plot(out,residual=T,cex=1,pch=19,shade=T,
     shade.col="light blue",col="blue")
```

Fig. 2.29 R code for undercount analysis

adjustments consistent with the earlier discussion of holding constant. The vertical axis label includes the effective number of degrees of freedom used by the particular smoothed function, determined by tuning the equivalent of λ_j with the GCV statistic. For example, there are a little more than six degrees of freedom used by the housing variable and a little more than one degree of freedom used by the crime variable. The former is highly nonlinear. The latter is very nearly linear. The four values for effective degrees of freedom (or alternatively, spar) were determined by an automated search over values of the generalized cross-validation statistic.

There are also shaded areas representing plus and minus two standard errors for the fitted values. Were one doing a level II analysis, they are supposed to convey uncertainty in the estimates. But it is difficult to know what to make of this rendering of uncertainty. Constant disturbance variance is assumed, there is almost certainly bias in the estimated fitted values (Wood 2006, Sect. 4.4.1), and model selection by the GCV statistic makes any conventional level II analysis problematic. As discussed in the first chapter, the consequences of model selection are far more weighty than just some additional uncertainty to contend with. Perhaps the major take-away is that the "error bands" widen dramatically where the data are most sparse. Fitted values in those regions need very careful scrutiny and perhaps have no interpretive value.

In general, all four predictors show positive relationships with the size of the undercount in regions where the data are not sparse. For example, the relationship with the percentage of residents having problems with English is positive until the value exceeds about 2%. The relationship then becomes negative until a value of about 5% when the relationship turns positive again. But there is no apparent substantive explanation for the changes in the slope, which are based on very few observations. The twists and turns could be the result of noise or neglected predictors, but with so little data, very little can be concluded. The changing width of the shaded area makes the same point.

Do any of the estimated relationships matter much? The observed values for the undercount can serve as an effective benchmark. They range from a low of −2.3% to a high of 8.2%. Their mean is 1.9%, and their standard deviation is 2.5%. Where the data are not sparse, each predictor has fitted values that vary by at least 1 percentage point. Whether changes variable by variable of a percentage point or two matter would need to be determined by individuals with subject-matter expertise. But perhaps more telling is what happens when the four fitted relationships are combined in a linear fashion to arrive at fitted values. Fitted values range from little below −1% to about 7.5%, and as Fig. 2.30 shows, there is a substantial number of areas with fitted undercounts greater than 4%. Moreover, the distribution tends to decline over positive values up to about 4%, after which there is an uncharacteristic increase. One might have expected continuing declines in the right tail. At least from a policy point of view, it might be instructive to know which geographical areas fall on the far right of the histogram. In short, insofar as the observed variability in the undercount matters, so does the variability in the fitted values.

Ignoring the data snooping for a moment, does one have the makings of a level II analysis? One would need clarification on what the estimation target is. In addition,

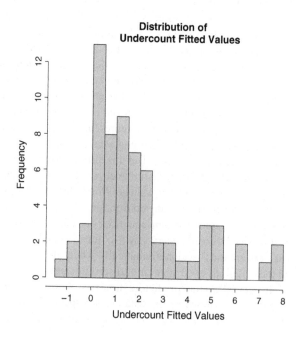

Fig. 2.30 Histogram of the undercount percentage fitted values from the GAM procedure (N = 66)

the data are not a probability sample of anything, and one would be hard pressed to provide some reasonable joint probability distribution responsible for the data. These present significant challenges before one gets to the data analysis.

2.7 Smoothers with Categorical Variables

Smoothers can be used with categorical variables. When a predictor is categorical, however, there is really nothing to smooth. A binary predictor can have only two values. The "smoother" is then just a straight line connecting the two conditional means of the response. For a predictor with more than two categories, there is no way to order the categories along the predictor axis. Any imposed order would imply assigning numbers to the categories. How the numbers were assigned could make an enormous difference in the resulting fitting values, and the assigned numbers necessarily would be arbitrary. Consequently, the categories are reconfigured as indicator variables.

When the response is categorical and binary, smoothing can be a very useful procedure. All of the earlier benefits apply. In addition, because it is very difficult to see much in a scatterplot with a categorical response, a smoother may be the only way to gain some visual leverage on what may be going on. However, the earlier caveats apply too.

Within the generalized additive model (GAM), the analysis of binary response variables can be seen as an extension of binomial regression from the generalized linear model (GLM). The right hand side is a linear combination of predictor functions. The left hand side is the response transformed by a link function to logit units (i.e., the log of the odds). What is different is that the functions of each predictor are unknown.

2.7.1 An Illustration Using the Generalized Additive Model with a Binary Outcome

We consider again the low birthweight data, but now the response is binary: low birthweight or not. A birthweight is low when it is less than 2.5 kg. The following predictors are used:

1. Age — in years;
2. Mother's weight — in pounds;
3. Uterine — presence of uterine irritability; and
4. Smoke — whether the mother smokes.

Using the defaults in *gam* (in the library *mgcv*), about 9 % of the deviance can be attributed to the four predictors. Consider first the role of the two binary predictors. When the mother smokes, the odds of a low birthweight baby are multiplied by

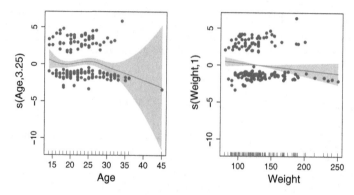

Fig. 2.31 A GAM analysis of a new born low birthweight as a function of background character-
istics of mothers (The mother's age and weight are on the *horizontal* axes, the centered fitted logits
are on the *vertical* axes, and the *shaded* area represents error bars. $N = 189$)

```
library(mgcv)
library(MASS)
data(birthwt)
attach(birthwt)

# Rename and Clean up variables
Low<-as.factor(low)
Age<-age
Weight<-(lwt)
Uterine<-as.factor(ifelse(ui==1,"Yes","No"))
Smokes<-as.factor(ifelse(smoke==1,"Yes","No"))
temp<-data.frame(Low,Age,Weight,Uterine,Smokes)

# Apply GAM
out<-gam(Low~s(Age)+s(Weight)+Uterine+Smokes,family=binomial,
                data=birthwt)
par(mfrow=c(1,2))
plot(out,se=T,residuals=T,pch=19,col="blue",shade=T,
     shade.col="light blue")
```

Fig. 2.32 R code for low birthweight analysis

2.32. When the mother has uterine irritability, the odds of a low birthweight baby are
multipled by 2.05. Both are exponentiated regression coefficients like those that can
be obtained from a logistic multiple regression.[31] In practical terms, both associations
are likely to be seen as substantial.

---

[31] The regression coefficients are usually reported with the response in logit units. They are part of
the routine tabular output from *gam()*.

Fig. 2.33 Histogram of the fitted values in proportion units for low birthweight GAM analysis ($N = 189$)

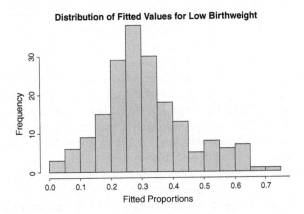

Distribution of Fitted Values for Low Birthweight

Figure 2.31 (code in Fig. 2.32) shows the smoothed plots for the mother's age and weight. The units on the vertical axis are logits centered on the mean of the response in logit units. Weight has a linear relationship with the logit of low birth weight. The relationship between age and the logit of birth weight is roughly negative overall, but positive between about the age of 20 and 25. Yet, to the eye, both relationships do not appear to be strong, and the impression of a negative relationship with age is driven in part by one observation for a woman who is 45 years old. However, looks can be deceiving. When the logit units are transformed into probability units,[32] the difference in the proportion of low birthweight babies can be about .30 greater when a mother of 35 is compared to a mother of 25. A similar difference in the proportion of low birthweight babies is found when women weighing around 100 pounds are compared to women weighing around 200 pounds.[33]

GAM output can include two kinds of fitted values for binary response variables: the linear combination of predictors in logit units and fitted proportions. The former can be useful for diagnostic purposes because many of the conventional regression diagnostics apply. One has an additive model in logit units. The latter are useful for interpretation as approximate values of the response surface.

Figure 2.33 is a histogram of the fitted values in proportion units. One can see that substantial variation is found between different cases. Fitted proportion ranges from a little above 0.0 to nearly .80. Some prefer to see the proportions as probabilities, but such interpretations require a clear and credible explanation of the stochastic process by which the fitted values are produced. In effect, one is moving from a level I to a level II analysis.

The formulation we have favored that depends on a joint probability distribution may work as a start, but we know so little about how the data were collected that

---

[32]How to transform logits into probabilities and interpret them properly will be discussed in later chapters. There can be subtle issues.

[33]The relationship reported in Chap. 1 was rather different. In Fig. 1.2, the relationship between birthweights and mothers' weights was generally positive. But for that analysis, the mother's weight was the only predictor. Conditioning on other predictors makes a difference.

making a credible case would be very difficult. For example, perhaps these births occurred in a medical facility for women with difficult pregnancies. If women there are all served by the same medical staff, birthweights may not be independently realized. How a given pregnancy proceeds may affect how subsequent pregnancies are handled. The estimation process introduces further problems. Empirical determination of λ means that model selection is in play. There might be work-arounds were there real test data or if the dataset is large enough to be split into three subsets.

The default output included the usual information in the standard format about the statistical tests undertaken. The plots came with error bands. The issues raised are the same as just addressed. If the value of λ (or its equivalent) were determined before the GAM analysis began, one could at least in principle proceed with the formulation derived for response surface approximations, although a lot of hard thinking would be required to pin down the reality to which the generating joint probability distribution applies. However, the value of λ was determined empirically as part of the fitting process. We are again put in harm's way by model selection. It is difficult to know what properties the regression coefficients and fitted values have as estimates. One is probably best off sticking with a level I analysis unless there are real test data or the dataset is large enough to subdivide.

2.8 An Illustration of Statistical Inference After Model Selection

Significant parts of the discussion in this chapter have emphasized the risks in a level II analysis when penalty weights are determined empirically as part of the data analysis. For readers who rely on "statistical significance" to extract subject-matter conclusions, the tone may be disappointing and even annoying. As a possible corrective, consider now a level II analysis that perhaps can be properly be defended.

Figure 2.34 in a rendering of the overall inferential strategy introduced in Chap. 1. Tuning is done working back and forth between training data and evaluation data. Once the procedure is tuned, test data are used to get an honest performance assessment. It can then be possible in an additional step to get a sense of the uncertainty in any honest performance assessment. That process is based on bootstrap resampling and is discussed in a bit more detail below, with more to follow in later chapters.

There are two kinds of honest assessments. If the goal is to estimate *generalization error*, results determined with the help of evaluation data are fixed. Using GAM as an example, the values of λ and the associated functions of the predictors are set. Fitted values determined from the x-values for all cases in the test data are then compared to the actual values of Y in the test data using a statistic such as MSE. If the goal is to estimate *expected prediction error*, matters are more complicated because tuning implies model selection. Perhaps the safest approach is to treat the values of any tuning parameters as fixed once they are determined with the help of evaluation data. Then the procedure is applied to the test data. Again using GAM as

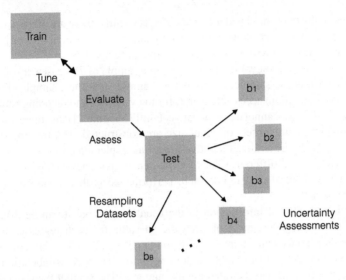

Fig. 2.34 A split sample approach for a level II analysis that includes tuning with an evaluation sample, assessment with a test sample, and uncertainty addressed with bootstrap resampling

an illustration, with the values of λ fixed, the response function for each predictor is estimated again, and one or more measures of fit are computed. All results are then honest with respect to data snooping for the given set tuning parameter values.

Uncertainty in test data performance assessment can be addressed with a nonparametric bootstrap. A total of B samples with replacement are drawn from the test data. Whether for generalization error or expected prediction error, a performance assessment is undertaken in each bootstrap sample. The distribution of performance assessments over samples from the test data can be used to characterize some forms of uncertainty — details to follow.

Let's see how this can play out. The data, available in R, are taken from the U.S. Panel Study of Income Dynamics (PSID). Funded by the National Science Foundation, the study began in 1968 and has been going for nearly 45 years. Households are followed over time and as the children of those households leave and form their own households, they are followed as well. New households are added when needed and feasible. Topics addressed in the survey have expanded over the years to include more than economic well-being: health, child development, time use and others (McGonagle et al. 2012). The data available in R are on married women in 1975. (See the code in Fig. 2.35.)

Given the sampling design, it may be reasonable to treat each observation in the dataset as a random realization from a joint probability distribution. In this case, the population is real and finite, but very large. The response is whether a married woman is in the labor force (even if unemployed). Predictors include (1) the wife's age, (2) family income excluding the wife's income in thousands of dollars, (3) whether the wife attended college, (4) whether the husband attended college, and (5) the number of children in the household under 6 years of age. Clearly, there are other potentially important predictors such as the wife's health and the local availability of jobs. We are working within the wrong model perspective once again.

The R code used is shown in Fig. 2.35. With a sample of 753 cases, it is practical to construct a training sample, an evaluation sample, and a test sample. The code starts by providing more accessible names for the variables and recoding some stray observations — one cannot have negative family income. Then, three randomly chosen, disjoint, data subsets of equal size are constructed. The training data are analyzed using the generalized additive model as implemented in *gam()* from the *mgcv* library. Several different values for the penalty parameters (i.e., *sp*) are tried beginning the smallest at .01. For each, performance is then assessed using the evaluation data.[34]

There is a wealth of information in the usual output, but it can be difficult to arrive at an overall assessment of what the *sp* value for each regressor function should be. For binary outcomes, a "confusion table" can be a very effective overall assessment tool. A confusion table is nothing more than a cross-tabulation of the actual binary outcome and the fitted binary outcome. The smaller the proportion of cases misclassified, the better the fitted values perform.

Confusion tables will play a key role in later chapters, and there are a number of complications and subtleties. For now, we simply will classify a case as in the labor force if the fitted value in the response metric is greater than .50 and not in the labor force if the fitted value in the response metric is equal to or smaller than .50. The marginal distribution of labor force participation provides a baseline for the GAM fitted values. Nearly 57 % of the sample are in the labor force. Applying the Bayes classifier to the marginal distribution, classification error is minimized if all cases are classified as in the labor force. The proportion misclassified is then .43. How much better can be done using the predictors and good values for *sp*?

Regardless of the *sp* values tried, performance was modest. In the training data, about 10 % of the deviance could be attributed to the five predictors with the mis-classification proportion a little less than .33. Improvement over the baseline was noticeable, but not dramatic.

For the *sp* values tried, out-of-sample performance did not vary much. Confusion tables from the evaluation data were all rather similar. For each, the misclassification proportion was about .36. Because the functions for both smoothed predictors were essentially straight lines, smaller *sp* values did not improve the fit enough to overcome the loss of degrees of freedom. Therefore, the values of *sp* for both quantitative predictors were set to the relatively large value 1.0.[35]

---

[34]The evaluation data provide out-of-sample performance measures, but with each new *sp* value, the out-of-sample benefits decline a bit. The model is being tuned to the evaluation data so that the fitting responds to both its random and systematic variation. Nevertheless, the evaluation data are very instructive. It was easy to see that with small values of *sp*, the overfitting in the training is substantial.

[35]Effectively the same results were obtained when the default of fitting by the GCV statistic was used.

```
## Set Up Data
library(car)
data(Mroz)
# Clean up labels and stray observations
Participates<-Mroz$lfp # in labor force
Age<-Mroz$age # age
FamIncome<-ifelse(Mroz$inc < 0,0,Mroz$inc) # family income
WifeColl<-Mroz$wc # Wife college degree
HusColl<-Mroz$hc # husband colleage degree
Kids5<-Mroz$k5 # Number of kinds under 6
temp1<-data.frame(Participates,Age,FamIncome,
                  WifeColl,HusColl,Kids5)

# Construct 3 random disjoint splits
index<-sample(1:753,753,replace=F) # shuffle row numbers
temp2<-temp1[index,] # put in random order
Train<-temp2[1:251,] # training data
Eval<-temp2[252:502,] # evaluation data
Test<-temp2[503:753,] # test data

## Determine Value of spar
library(mgcv)
# Applications to Training Data
out1<-gam(Participates~s(Age,sp=.01)+s(FamIncome,sp=.01)+
          WifeColl+HusColl+Kids5,data=Train,family=binomial)
Tab<-table(out1$fitted.values>.5,
           Train$Participates) # Confusion table
Tab
(Tab[1,2]+Tab[2,1])/sum(Tab) # Proportion Misclassified

# Apply to Evaluation Data
out2<-predict(out1,newdata=Eval,type="response") # Fitted values
Tab<-table(out2>.5,Eval$Participates) # Confusion table
Tab
(Tab[1,2]+Tab[2,1])/sum(Tab) # Proportion Misclassified

## Get Honest Performance Estimate
# With best values for sp, apply to test data
out3<-gam(Participates~s(Age,sp=1)+s(FamIncome,sp=1)+
          WifeColl+HusColl+Kids5,data=Test,family=binomial)
Tab<-table(out3$fitted.values>.5,
           Test$Participates) # Confusion table
Tab
(Tab[1,2]+Tab[2,1])/sum(Tab) # Proportion Misclassified
```

Fig. 2.35 R code for a level II analysis of the PSID data

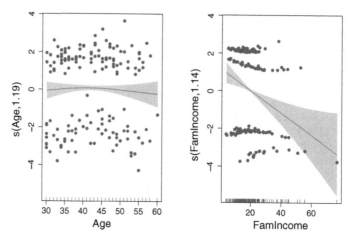

Fig. 2.36 Smoother estimates for age and family income in the test data (Fitted values in the units of centered log odds are on the *vertical* axes, predictors age and family income are on the *horizontal* axes, the *shaded* areas show error bands, and $N = 251$.)

The test data provide an antidote to model selection. Because the goal was to represent how the predictors were related to labor force participation, and no forecasting was anticipated, an estimate of expected prediction error was used as the performance yardstick. With the value of *sp* fixed at the "best" value, the generalized additive model was applied using the test data. Again, about 33 % of the cases were misclassified, and a little more than 10 % of the deviance could be attributed to the predictors. There was no evidence of meaningful overfitting. Among the three linear predictors, if a wife had attended college, the odds of labor force participation are multiplied by a factor of 3.3. A husband's college attendance hardly matter. For each additional child under six, the odds of labor force participation are multiplied by a factor of .20.[36]

Figure 2.36 shows in the test data the relationships between labor force participation and the two smoothed predictors. The near-linearity is apparent. Age has virtually no relationship with labor force participation, although there is a hint of decline for wives over 50. Family income (excluding the wife's income) has a very strong effect. The odds increase by a factor of about 3.9 when the lowest income households are compared to the highest. Lower income can dramatically increase a wife's labor force participation. So much for the level I analysis.

Thanks to the test data, it is relatively easy to move to level II. All of the results just reported from the test data can be used as asymptotically unbiased estimates for the population's same generalized additive model with the same sp values. But, there is considerable uncertainty to address. Although original sample had 753 observations,

---

[36]The number of children under 6 ranged from 0 to 2. With only 3 predictor values, smoothing was not an option.

Fig. 2.37 Average bootstrap
fitted values and
Point-By-Point Error bands
for the labor force analysis
using 200 nonparametric
bootstrap samples
($N = 251$)

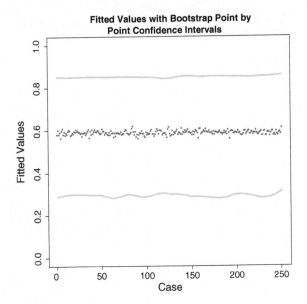

the test sample had only 251, and that is the relevant sample size. Still, some use can be made of the nonparametric bootstrap with the test sample.

The bootstrap will be addressed in some depth in later chapters. For now, take on faith that Fig. 2.37 shows the bootstrapped point-by-point error bands around the average of the fitted values over 200 bootstrap samples. As such, they can be viewed as legitimate asymptotic estimates of point-by-point 95 % confidence intervals.

But confidence intervals around what? If the estimation target is the true response surface, the error bands are not confidence intervals. Because the estimates include bias, the error bands only capture the variance around the biased estimates. If the estimation target is an approximation of the true response surface, one has asymptotically valid confidence intervals around estimates of that approximation surface.

The major message from Fig. 2.37 that the wiggle around the fitted values is very large: approximately plus or minus .25. This is consistent with the small improvement in fit compared to the marginal Bayes classifier. It is also consistent with the small fraction of the deviance that could be attributed to the predictors and with the modest sample size.

A key implication is that the estimates of classification error can vary widely as well. Figure 2.38 shows a histogram of the proportion of cases misclassified over the 200 bootstrap samples. Although of the estimates cluster between .35 and .40, estimates range from about .28 to .45. Yet, the estimated probability of a misclassification proportion of less than the marginal Bayes classifier of .43 is about .98. Even the very weak model is likely to be an improvement. And there is more good news. The stronger relationships reported — for the wife attending college, the number of

Fig. 2.38 Bootstrap
distribution of proportion
misclassified over 200
bootstrap samples
($N = 251$)

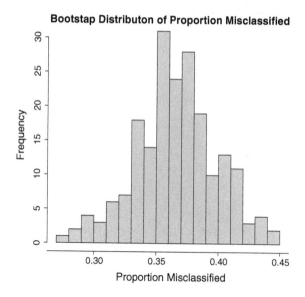

children under 6 and family income — all have reported p-values far smaller than
.05 for a proper two-tailed test and a null hypothesis of no relationship.[37]

Still, there are at least three important caveats. First, the split sample approach
comes at a price. Working with fewer observations split by split means that all level II
results are less precise than had a full sample procedure been used (Faraway 2014). A
more subtle point is that for smoothers and statistical learning more generally, more
complex associations can be found with larger samples. In the case of smoothing
splines, a smaller value for λ may be justified in a substantially larger sample. For
a level I regression analysis, richer descriptions can follow. For a level II analysis,
there can be a reduction in bias if there is focus on the true response surface and true
conditional relationships.

Second, all of the statistical inference is asymptotic. A sample of 251 is probably
large enough so that the inference is not misleading, but there is no way to know
for sure. It is at least encouraging that the bootstrap distribution of the estimated
misclassification error when examined with normal QQ plot (*qqnorm()*), showed no
troubling departures from normality. The same can be said about the distributions of
fitted values from which each of the error bands were constructed.[38] The sample of
251 may well be large enough for our purposes.

---

[37]These come from the standard *gam()* output. This is playing somewhat fast and loose. Ideally,
the test should use a standard error estimate taking into account that the predictors are random
variables. In principle, some version of the sandwich should apply. Alternatively, a nonparametric
bootstrap could be used. One would resample the test data and obtain empirical distributions for
each regression coefficient. Statistical tests or confidence intervals could follow. But with p-values
so small, it is very likely that the test results would be confirmed.

[38]A random subset of 25 were examined.

Third and more fundamentally, the thought experiment behind the nonparametric bootstrap envisions random samples from a population, or realizations from a joint probability distribution, with the model and value of sp already known. This is consistent with conventional statistical inference. But, one might also wonder about uncertainty caused by the random data splitting. A very different thought experiment is implied, and its relevance can be argued. In principle, one could address that uncertainty by wrapping the entire analysis, including the sample splitting, in a nonparametric bootstrap.

There is also a need to briefly address again the role of all level II analyses. This example works because the way the data were assembled comports well with the joint probability distribution formulation. Other examples can work without real random sampling when a credible case can be made from subject matter knowledge, past research and an examination of the data on hand. For example, suppose as a criminal justice researcher, one wanted to study probation failures, and suppose one had access to data over several years on all individuals released on probation in a large city. Such data could have well over 100,000 observations. One can certainly imagine a joint probability distribution for the outcomes and predictors of interest as a product of the social processes determining how individuals do on probation. But, over time that joint probability distribution could well change as new laws are passed, new administrative regulations are promulgated, and the mix of convicted offenders varies. To what time interval does the data on hand apply?

There is no definitive way to address this question, but knowledge of the setting and surrounding circumstances can be very helpful. For example, have there been any important changes in the governing statutes? One can also make some headway using the data. It would be a simple matter to look at subsets of the data for several months at a time. Is there evidence that the joint probability distribution responsible for the data is changing in ways that matter? For example, is the fraction of the offenders being convicted for drug crimes increasing substantially? If key features of the data appear to be stable over the period the data were collected, the data may be seen as realized from a single joint probability distribution. One might also infer that the joint probability distribution changes slowly so that forecasts made for new cases in the not-too-distant future may be valid. As with all real data analyses, it is difficult to know for sure, but one properly can capitalize on the balance of evidence.

More difficult would be making the case that the observations were realized independently. Sometimes there are co-offenders for a given crime, and some crimes can be serial in nature. One might want to use the data to see how common both were for different kinds of crimes. For many crimes, both may be relatively rare. In addition, it may be possible to condition on certain predictors so that most dependence is removed, although that may lead to a revision of the plain vanilla, joint probability distribution approach. We will have a lot more to say about these issues in later chapters. Level II analyses with statistical learning can be a challenge.

Fig. 2.39 2-Dimensional vector spaces that change the roles of variables and observations (The *left* figure has observations in variable space, and the *right* figure has variables in observation space.)

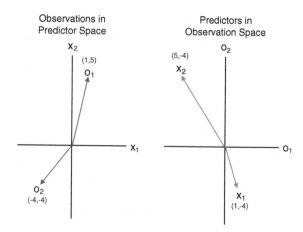

2.9 Kernelized Regression

In this chapter, much has been made of linear basis expansions as a way to make better use of the information a set of predictors contains. But each kind of expansion retained a matrix structure in which rows were observations and columns were variables. There is a very different and powerful way to transform the data from observations located in variable space to variables located in observation space. The result can be a kernel matrix that with some regularization can form a new kind of predictor matrix for a wide range of regression applications.[39]

Figure 2.39 illustrates how one can represent observations in variable space or variables in observation space. O_1 and O_2 are observations, and X_1 and X_2 are variables. The arrows represent vectors. Recall that vectors are lines with direction and length. We use them here primarily as a visualization tool.

The left plot shows observations in variable space and is the way one normally thinks about a scatter plot. There are two observations in a space defined by two predictors. The right plot shows variables in observation space, and is one way to think about kernels. There are two predictors in a space defined by two observations. For example, in the plot on the left, O_1 has a value of 1 for X_1 and a value 5 for X_2. In the plot on the right, X_1 has a value of 1 for O_1 and a value of -4 for O_2. In practice, there would be many more predictors and many more observations.

But why bother with predictors in observation space? Thinking back to the discussion of linear basis expansions in Chap. 1, kernels can alter the number of dimensions in which the values of a response variable are located. By increasing the number of dimensions, one may find good separation more easily. This is an important rationale for working with kernels. Kernels also have other desirable properties that can

---

[39]In statistics, there are other meanings of "kernel" such as when the term is used for localized estimators (Hastie et al. 2009: Sect. 6.6.1). In computer science, "variables" are sometimes called "feature vectors" that are located in "input space."

Fig. 2.40 R code inner products of **X**

```
              X # The predictor matrix

                  V1 V2 V3
          Ilene   1  2  3
          Jim     4  2  0
          Ken     1  0  0
          Linda   5  3  5
          Mary    3  2  4


          # Cross Product Matrix t(X)%*%X

                  V1 V2 V3
              V1  52 31 40
              V2  31 21 29
              V3  40 29 50


          # Kernal Matrix X%*%t(X)

          Ilene Jim Ken Linda Mary
  Ilene     14   8   1    26   19
  Jim        8  20   4    26   16
  Ken        1   4   1     5    3
  Linda     26  26   5    59   41
  Mary      19  16   3    41   29
```

make them a very handy tool. These will be considered as the discussion of kernels proceeds.[40]

Consider Eq. 2.21, a very simple predictor matrix **X** with five rows and three columns. Rows and columns are labeled. The rows are people and the columns are variables that are features of those people. Linear basis expansions of the sort we have considered so far could be applied to all three predictors or a subset.

$$
\mathbf{X} = \begin{pmatrix}
 & V1 & V2 & V3 \\
Ilene & 1 & 2 & 3 \\
Jim & 4 & 2 & 0 \\
Ken & 1 & 0 & 0 \\
Linda & 5 & 3 & 5 \\
Mary & 3 & 2 & 4
\end{pmatrix}. \tag{2.21}
$$

Figure 2.40 shows the **X** matrix, and the results from two different forms of matrix multiplication. The first is $\mathbf{X}^T\mathbf{X}$, which produces the usual sum of cross products, a symmetric matrix that plays such an important role in the ordinary least squares

---

[40] Adam Kapelner and Justin Bleich helped extensively with the exposition of kernels. They deserve much of the credit for what clarity there is. Lack of clarity is my doing.

estimator. Its main diagonal contains for each variable the sum of its squared values. For example, value of 21 in the second row and second column is the sum of the squared values of V2. The off-diagonal elements contain for each pair of variables their sum of element by element products, called inner products. The result is a scalar. For example, the value of 40 in the first row and third column and also in the third row and the first column results from $(1 \times 3) + (4 \times 0) + \cdots + (3 \times 4)$.

The second matrix is derived from $\mathbf{X}$ by computing $\mathbf{XX}^T$. It too is symmetric. There are again sums of squared values or sums of cross-products, but the roles of variables and observations are switched. The main diagonal now contains for each *person* the sum of that person's squared values over the three variables. For example, Linda's diagonal value is 59: $5^2 + 3^2 + 5^2$. The off-diagonal elements are the sums of cross products for *person* pairs over the three variables. For example, the sum of cross products for Jim and Ilene is $(4 \times 1) + (2 \times 2) + (3 \times 0) = 8$. As before, these are sums of cross-products that result in a scalar.

Notice that this matrix has 5 columns rather than 3. Were one to use the matrix columns as a set of predictors, there would be 5 regressors. The response variable values would now reside in a 5-D predictor space, not a 3-D predictor space. The number of dimensions has been increased by 2.

$\mathbf{XX}^T$ is often called a "linear kernel" and can be viewed as a similarity matrix (Murphy 2012: 479). The off-diagonal elements can be measures of the association between the different rows of $\mathbf{X}$. One can learn which observations are more alike over the full set of variables. In this example, a close look at $\mathbf{X}$ indicates that Mary and Linda have the most similar values for V1, V2, and V3, and from the kernel matrix, the value of 41 is the largest off-diagonal element. A kernel matrix is conventionally denoted by $\mathbf{K}$.

There are many kinds of kernels constructed with different kernel functions denoted in general by $\kappa(x, x')$. The notation x and x' means one row and another row, although it can also mean a row with itself in which case, each sum of cross products is non-negative (i.e., $\kappa(x, x') \geq 0$). Any kernel matrix, $\mathbf{K}$, is symmetric (i.e., $\kappa(x, x') = \kappa(x', x)$). For regression applications, it is common to work with Mercer kernels for which $\mathbf{K}$ is positive semi-definite.

The preference for Mercer kernel begins with $\mathbf{X}$. Imagine linear basis expansions for the full set of predictors each represented by $h(x)$. For Mercer kernels, $\kappa(x, x') = \langle h(x), h(x') \rangle$, which means the inner products of the expansions are contained in Mercer kernels (Hastie et al. 2009: Sect. 12.3.1).[41] There is no need the know the actual expansions because for regression applications one can proceed directly with the kernel. This is a very convenient computational shortcut, which means that in practice, model specification is usually a choice between different kinds of kernels

---

[41] Imagine a predictor $\mathbf{X}$ expanded so that each original column can now be many columns defined by some linear basis expansion (e.g., polynomials or indicator variables). In this context, the inner product means multiplying two rows (i.e. vectors) of the expanded predictor so that a scalar is produced. As before, it is just the sum of cross products. More generally, if there are two (column) vectors v_1 and v_2, the inner product is $v_1^T v_2$. The outer product is $v_1 v_2^T$, which results in a matrix. The same reasoning applies when a vector is multiplied by itself.

without much regard for the implied basis expansions. More will be said about kernels in the chapter on support vector machines.[42]

However, there are several complications. Because the kernel function requires that all elements in $\mathbf{X}$ be numeric, categorical predictors are a problem. At best, they can be transformed into 1/0 indicator variables, but the gap between a 1 and a 0 is arbitrary. And actually, the problem is more general. $\mathbf{K}$ depends on the units in which each column of $\mathbf{X}$ is measured. With different units, there are different kernels even when the kernel function is the same. Standardization of each column of $\mathbf{X}$ is, therefore, a common practice. But the common units chosen are effectively arbitrary and make it difficult to understand what the similarities mean. Two rows that are the much alike in standard deviation units, may be very different in their original units, which is how one normally thinks about those rows. One should always ask, therefore, "similar with respect to what?"

A second complication is that a kernel matrix is necessarily $N \times N$. Therefore, some form of dimension reduction is required in a regression setting. Regularization is required. Options include using a subset of $\mathbf{K}$'s principal components as regressors or a form penalized regression. For example, the latter can lead to a ridge regression approach. In the notation of Hastie et al. (2009: Sect. 12.3.7),

$$\hat{f}(x) = h(x)^T \hat{\beta} = \sum_{i=1}^{N} \hat{\alpha}_i K(x, x_i), \tag{2.22}$$

and

$$\hat{\alpha} = (K(x, x_i) + \lambda \mathbf{I})^{-1} \mathbf{y}. \tag{2.23}$$

Equation 2.22 shows the fundamental equivalence between regressors as basis functions and regressors as columns of $\mathbf{K}$. Equation 2.23 shows how the new regression coefficients $\hat{\alpha}$ for $\mathbf{K}$ are computed. Equation 2.23 is a close cousin of conventional ridge regression.

With $\hat{\alpha}$ in hand, the fitted values can follow as usual as long as one remembers to use $\mathbf{K}$ not $\mathbf{X}$. For fitted values from *new* observations, the same reasoning carries over, but the new observations $\mathbf{Z}$ need to be "kernelized" (Exterkate et al. 2011: Sect. 2.2). A prediction kernel is constructed as $\kappa(x, z') = \langle h(x), h(z') \rangle$ not as $\kappa(x, x') = \langle h(x), h(x') \rangle$. That is, the inner products are undertaken with respect to $\mathbf{X}$ and $\mathbf{Z}$, not with respect to $\mathbf{X}$ itself. For the linear kernel one computes $\mathbf{X}\mathbf{Z}^T$ rather than $\mathbf{X}\mathbf{X}^T$. That is,

$$\hat{f}(x, z) = \sum_{i=1}^{N} \hat{\alpha}_i K(x, z_i). \tag{2.24}$$

---

[42]There is a lot of very nice math involved that is actually quite accessible if it is approached step by step. For readers who want to pursue this, there are many lectures taught by excellent instructors that can be viewed for free on the web. These are generally more helpful than formal textbook treatments because the intuitions behind the math are often well explained. A good example is the lecture by MIT professor Patrick Winston "Lecture 16 – Learning: Support Vector Machines."

Also as before, λ in Eq. 2.23 is a tuning parameter whose value needs to be specified in advance or determined empirically. This leads to a third complication. Often it is desirable for λ to be large because, in effect, one starts with N predictors (much like for smoothing splines). But, empirically determining a sensible value for λ can be challenging, as we will soon see. There are usually additional tuning parameters.

A fourth complication is that kernel matrices produce a new kind of black box. In Eq. 2.22, for example, the regressors are columns of $\mathbf{K}$ not columns of $\mathbf{X}$, and the estimated regression coefficients in Eq. 2.23 are $\hat{\alpha}$ not $\hat{\beta}$. It is a bit like trying to make sense of the regression coefficients associated with B-splines. Moreover, only in very special cases is it practical to work backwards from $\mathbf{K}$ to $h(x)$. The linear expansions of $\mathbf{X}$ typically are not accessible. As before, therefore, the story will be in the fitted values.

Finally, there many different kinds of kernels, and several different kinds of Mercer kernels that can be used in practice (Murphy 2012: Sect. 14.2; Duvenaud et al. 2013). Because of the black box, it is very difficult to know which kernel to use. The decision is usually based on experience with particular subject-matter applications and craft lore. We turn to two kernels that are popular for regression analysis.

2.9.1 Radial Basis Kernel

The bottom matrix in Fig. 2.40 is an example of a linear basis kernel. Formally, it is relatively easy to work with, but is not used much because there are other kernels that usually perform better. A good example is the radial basis kernel that is sometimes characterized as an "all purpose" kernel. Perhaps its most important departure from the linear kernel is that row comparisons are made initially by subtraction not multiplication. With each variable standardized and $\|.\|$ denoting the Euclidian distance (i.e. the "norm"), the radial basis kernel is defined by the function

$$k(x, x^{'}) = exp(-\sigma \|x - x'\|^2), \tag{2.25}$$

where $\|x - x'\|^2$ is the squared Euclidian distance between two rows.

The first step is to compute the sum of squared *differences*. For the second and third row of our toy $\mathbf{X}$, one has for the sum of squared differences: $(4 - 1)^2 + (2 - 0)^2 + (0 - 0)^2 = 13$. The sum of squared differences is multiplied by $-\sigma$ and then exponentiated. For the radial basis kernel, otherwise known as the Gaussian radial basis kernel (Murphy 2012: Sect. 14.2.1), σ is a scale parameter specifying the spread in the kernel values. The kernel matrix $\mathbf{K}$ is always symmetric and $N \times N$. If the scale parameter σ happens to be 0.5, the value in $\mathbf{K}$ for the second and third row of

```
library(kernlab)

# Radial Basis Kernel

tune<-rbfdot(sigma=.5)
kernelMatrix(tune,X)
An object of class "kernelMatrix"
          Ilene       Jim         Ken        Linda        Mary
Ilene 1.0000e+00 1.2341e-04 1.5034e-03 2.7536e-05 8.2085e-02
Jim   1.2341e-04 1.0000e+00 1.5034e-03 1.3710e-06 2.0347e-04
Ken   1.5034e-03 1.5034e-03 1.0000e+00 1.3888e-11 6.1442e-06
Linda 2.7536e-05 1.3710e-06 1.3888e-11 1.0000e+00 4.9787e-02
Mary  8.2085e-02 2.0347e-04 6.1442e-06 4.9787e-02 1.0000e+00

# ANOVA Basis Kernel

tune<-anovadot(sigma=2.0,degree=2)
kernelMatrix(tune,X)
An object of class "kernelMatrix"
          Ilene       Jim         Ken        Linda        Mary
Ilene 9.000000 1.000000 1.0007e+00 1.8407e-02 1.2898e+00
Jim   1.000000 9.000000 1.0007e+00 7.3263e-02 1.2810e+00
Ken   1.000671 1.000671 9.0000e+00 2.3195e-16 4.5014e-07
Linda 0.018407 0.073263 2.3195e-16 9.0000e+00 7.3444e-02
Mary  1.289748 1.288986 4.5014e-07 7.3444e-02 9.0000e+00
```

Fig. 2.41 R code for radial basis and ANOVA basis kernels

X is $e^{(13 \times -.5)} = .0015034$. The top matrix in Fig. 2.41 follows in the same manner.[43]

The diagonal entries of the radial basis kernel are always 1 ($e^0 = 1$), and the off-diagonal entries are between 0 and 1. Because radial kernels build on Euclidian distances, they can be viewed as similarity matrices. With a smaller distance between a pair observations, there is greater similarity. Thanks to the negative sign the associated with σ, a larger kernel value then conveys greater similarity.

When the value of σ is larger, the off-diagonal kernel values become smaller, so their measured similarities are reduced. The rows become more heterogeneous, which is consistent with the idea a larger scale value. In language we used earlier, the bandwidth, span, or window has gotten smaller. A more complex set of fitted values can be accommodated. Consequently, σ typically is treated as a tuning parameter.

[43]For consistency, the kernel expressions and notation are the same as in the documentation for *kernlab* (Karatzoglou et al. 2004), the excellent library containing the kernel procedures used. In some expositions, λ is used instead of σ and then $\lambda = \frac{1}{2\sigma^2}$, where σ is another constant. In that form, the radial basis kernel commonly is called the Gaussian radial basis kernel. Note that this λ is not the same λ as in Eq. 2.23.

Radial basis kernels have proved to be useful in a wide variety of applications but for regression, there can be a better choice (Karazolou et al. 2004: Sect. 2.4).

2.9.2 ANOVA Radial Basis Kernel

The ANOVA radial basis kernel builds on the radial basis kernel. Using common notation for the ANOVA kernel,

$$k(x, x') = \left(\sum_{k=1}^{p} exp(-\sigma(x^k - x'^k)^2) \right)^d, \qquad (2.26)$$

where x^k and x'^k are the two values for predictor k, p is the number of predictors in X, and σ is again a scale parameter typically used for tuning. As before, larger values of σ allow for a more complex fit.[44] The values for d are usually 1, 2, or 3. Because the computations begin with differences that after being transformed are added together, the calculations are linear when $d = 1$, and one has a linear, additive effects expression. When $d = 2$, one has an expression with products that can be seen as two-way interaction variables. By the same reasoning, when $d = 3$, one has three-way interaction variables. In practice, d is treated as a tuning parameter along with σ.[45] Larger values for d allow for a more complex set of fitted values.

The lower matrix in Fig. 2.41 shows the results for the same predictor matrix X when σ is set to 2.0 and d is set to 2. Because there are 3 predictors in X, the main diagonal elements are all equal to 9 (i.e., $(1 + 1 + 1)^2$). Off-diagonal elements no longer have an upper bound of 1.0.

2.9.3 A Kernel Regression Application

In a regression context, the radial kernel and the anova kernel can be used as predictor matrices that replace X in a regression analysis. Both kernels provide a very rich

---

[44]The computational translation is a little tricky. These are the steps for any given entry i, j in K. (1) As before, one does an element by element subtraction of observations i and j over each of the predictors. These are rows in X. (2) Square each of the differences. (3) Multiply each of these squared differences by minus σ. (4) Exponentiate each of these products. (5) Sum the exponentiated products. (6) Raise the sum to the power of d.

[45]To illustrate, consider X with three predictors. For the pair of observations from, say, the first and second row of X and $d = 1$, the sum of differences is $(x_{11} - x_{21})^2 + (x_{12} - x_{22})^2 + (x_{13} - x_{23})^2$. This is linear and additive in the squared differences. For $d = 2$, the result is $[(x_{11} - x_{21})^2 + (x_{12} - x_{22})^2 + (x_{13} - x_{23})^2]^2$. All of the terms are now products of two squared differences, which are two-way interaction effects. For $d = 3$, the result is $[(x_{11} - x_{21})^2 + (x_{12} - x_{22})^2 + (x_{13} - x_{23})^2]^3$. All of the terms are now products of three squared differences, which are three-way interaction effects. Hence the name ANOVA kernel.

menu of complicated transformations that are directly given to the fitting machinery. One hopes that $\mathbf{K}$ can find relationships with the response that $\mathbf{X}$ cannot. Complicated nonlinear relationships are in play through what is effectively a nonparametric formulation.

As usual, "nonparametric" can be used in different ways. What one means for kernelized regression is that the regression structure is not meant to be a model of anything. The regression structure is just part of an algorithm linking input to outputs. There are regression coefficients for the columns in $\mathbf{K}$, but they have no subject-matter interpretation. Just as for smoothing splines, the goal is to interpret and use the relationship between inputs and outputs.

The heavy emphasis on fitted values has meant that for kernel regression, ways to visualize how inputs are related to outputs are not as well developed. Some of the visualization procedures discussed in later chapters could be applied, but at least in R, they have not been applied yet. Where kernel regression method can shine is in forecasting.

A natural question, therefore, is what kernel methods estimate. Kernel regression methods can be used to estimate an approximation of the true response surface as a feature of nature's joint probability distribution. That approximation has the same structure, and same values for the tuning parameters used with the training data. The fitted values from the data can be taken as biased (even asymptotically) estimates of the true response surface. In short, a level II analysis has the same features as a level II analysis for smoothing splines. And as before, one has to make a credible case that a level II analysis is justified.

Even if the choice of kernel is made before looking at the data, in practice the kernel's parameters will be tuned, and the regularization parameter will be tuned as well. So, here too the data snooping issues have been addressed. One is usually in the model selection business once again.

Consider Eqs. 2.22 and 2.23. What may look to be a simple application of ridge regression is not so simple. There are three tuning parameters, two for the ANOVA kernel and one for the regularization, that typically need to be determined empirically. A first impulse might be to use some in-sample fit measure such as the GCV statistic. A search is undertaken over values of the tuning parameters. Their values are determined by the best fit value. However, any credible in-sample fit statistics should take the effective degrees of freedom (EDF) into account because the effective degrees of freedom is changing as the values of the tuning parameters are varied. If the effective degrees of freedom is ignored, a better fit may result simply from more degrees of freedom being used in the fitting process. This matters even for a level I analysis because the data analyst could be faced with unnecessarily complicated fitted values that will be challenging to interpret.

Yet, as discussed in Chap. 1, even the idea of an effective degrees of freedom (or effective number of parameters) in such a setting is being questioned. What does the effective degrees of freedom mean when there is tuning? In practice, therefore, a sensible level I analysis requires a careful examination of the fitted values and plots of the actual response values against the fitted values. Subject-matter knowledge can be critical for determining which sets of fitted values are most instructive. In short, the level I concerns for conventional ridge regression carry over but now with more tuning parameters to specify.

For a level II analysis, we are again faced with model section implications that can introduce challenging problems for statistical inference. Rather than using some in-sample fit statistics, why not employ cross-validation? The issues are tricky. A kernel matrix is $N \times N$, and the tuning is done with respect to the full kernel matrix. Yet, cross-validation necessarily fits subsets of the data, each with fewer than N observations. Tuning could be quite different, and with respect to the full kernel matrix, misleading. Probably the best cross-validation approach is N-fold because for each pass through the data only one observation is lost.

Alternatively, one might employ a split sample strategy. As before, the training and evaluation samples are exploited to determine the values for the tuning parameters. The kernel regression coefficients $\hat{\alpha}$ from the training sample are used to obtain fitted values in the evaluation data, from which one or more performance measures are computed. With the values of the tuning parameters determined, the test data can be employed to obtain honest performance assessments. But one is still faced with a smaller N than had the data not be split. If one is prepared to settle for working with and tuning for a kernel fit based on a substantially smaller sample, a split sample approach can work well. The new estimation target is test sample version.

There are apparently no fully satisfactory procedures currently in R that implement the kind of penalized kernel regression shown Eqs. 2.22 and 2.23.[46] But with split samples and the *kernelMatrix()* procedure from the library *kernlab* to construct the requisite kernels, it is relatively easy to write a "one-off" R-script that implements a version of Eqs. 2.23 and 2.24 cycling through the training data many times using different sets of values for σ, d, and λ.[47] Each set of $\hat{\alpha}$ is then used to produce fitted values in the evaluation data. Once acceptable tuning parameter values are determined, they are used to compute a penalized kernel ridge regression in the test data.

To see how this plays out, suppose one wanted to analyze variation in the gross domestic earnings for movies made in the United States immediately after the movie opens. There are data on 471 movies for which one has the following regressors: (1) the budget for making each movie, (2) the number of theaters in which it opened, and (3) opening day's earnings. The response is gross domestic earnings over the next 24 months. These data were randomly split into a training sample, an evaluation sample, and a test sample of equal sizes. The performance criterion was mean squared error.

From the search over the movie training data and evaluation data, σ was a chosen to be 10, d was chosen to be 2.0, and λ was chosen to be 3. There were several sets

---

[46]There is in the *CVST* library a procedure with which to do penalized kernel ridge regression. However, the documentation is very spare, and the references cited often do not seem germane. It is, therefore, very difficult to know what the underlying code is really doing, and some of the output is problematic.

[47]The library *kernlab()* was written by Alexandros Karatzoglou, Alex Smola, and Kurt Hornik. It is has an excellent collection of functions for working with kernels in a wide variety of ways.

Fig. 2.42 Domestic gross sales in million of dollars by the fitted values from a penalized kernel regression using the test data (N = 157)

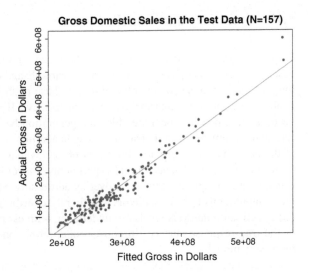

of tuning parameters that performed approximately as well, and the among those, the set with the smallest tuning parameter values for the kernel and the largest value for penalty parameter was selected. There seemed to be no reason to unnecessarily use up degrees of freedom.

A kernel regression with the same number of observations and tuning parameters values was used with the test data. In the same spirit as expected prediction error, a plot of the observed response values against the fitted response values for the test data is shown in Fig. 2.42. Overlaid is the least squares line from which the R^2 of .92 was computed. Overall, the scatterplot has a sensible pattern although the fitted values do not track some of the highest or lowest gross sales as well. This means that if the goal is to represent very soon after a movie is released its gross domestic sales over the next two years, the results look promising except for the few "flops" and "blockbusters." It is easy to capture those response values too with a more complex set of fitted values (e.g. with a σ of 20, a d of 3, and a λ of 1), but that leads to unrealistic measures of fit (e.g., an R^2 of .99).

For a level II analysis, the estimation target is the kernel regression approximation of the true response surface with the same values for the tuning parameters. If one can define a substantively relevant joint probability distribution or finite population from which each observation was independently realized, the test data results can provide an asymptotically unbiased estimates. And much as in the previous example, one can then apply a nonparametric bootstrap to the test data and obtain information on the uncertainty built into the R^2 of .92.

2.10 Summary and Conclusions

Regression splines and regression smoothers can be very useful level I tools for describing relationships between a response variable and one or more predictors. As long as one is content to "merely" describe, these methods are consistent with the goals of an exploratory data analysis. Moving to a level II analysis can be challenging because there needs to be a credible data generation backstory consistent with the formal requirements of statistical inference. In addition, when model selection is part of the data analysis, there are significant obstacles that in practice can be difficult to overcome. In the absence of real experiments, a level III analysis will depend, as usual, on a compelling interpretive overlay addressing why one should believe that the manipulation of given predictors will alter the distribution of the response. And all three regression analysis levels are undertaken with estimates of an approximation of the true response surface. In conventional terms, one is working misspecified regression models.

Experience suggests that for most datasets, it does not make a great difference which brand of smoother one uses. The dominant factor is usually the values of λ or other tuning parameters that determine smoothness and the bias-variance tradeoff. Less clear is how their values are best determined. Most methods emphasize some measure of generalization error. This is certainly sensible given the empirical focus on fitted values. But fitted values with low generalization error do not necessarily make scientific or policy sense. Moreover, any overall measure of out-of-sample performance can neglect that performance will usually be better for some predictors than others. Often a subset of predictors are of special interest, and it is on their performance that a useful evaluation should rest. These complications and others suggest that it can be a mistake to automatically defer to default tuning values or default tuning procedures. There is no substitute for subject-matter expertise and a careful examination of a wide range of data analysis output. Judgment matters. It is very important to avoid what a number of philosophers and social scientists call "statisticism" (Finch 1976; Lamiell 2013).

Finally, there are other smoothers that have not been discussed either because they perform best in a relatively narrow set of applications or because they are not yet ready for widespread use. An example of the former is wavelet smoothing (Hastie et al. 2009: Sect. 5.9). "Wavelet bases are very popular in signal processing and compression, since they are able to represent both smooth and/or locally bumpy functions in an efficient way — a phenomenon dubbed time and frequency localization" (Hasite et al. 2009: 175). An example of the latter is very recent work that applies trend filtering to nonparametric regression (Tibshirani 2015). The key idea is to define the fitting penalty a novel way, not using second derivatives, by a discrete differencing operator on the regression coefficients. The result is a smoother that adapts locally. It will fit a rougher function where the data are more rough and a smoother function where the data are more smooth.[48] In short, the book is not closed on smoothers, and readers interested in such procedure should at least skim the relevant journals from time to time.

For a wide range of problems, there are statistical learning techniques that arguably perform better than the procedures discussed in this chapter. They can fit the data better, are less subject to overfitting, and permit a wider range of information to be brought to bear. One price, however, is that the links to conventional regression analysis become even more tenuous. In the next chapter, we continue down this path.

Demonstrations and Exercises

Just as for the first chapter, these demonstrations and exercises emphasize the analysis of data. What substantive insights can be properly extracted? You may need to install some packages depending on what you have already installed. (Have you updated R and the procedures you will be using lately?)

Set 1: Smoothers with a Single Predictor

1. Load the dataset called airquality using the command *data(airquality)*. Attach the data with the command *attach(airquality)*. Use *gam()* from the *gam* library with Ozone as the response and Temp as the sole predictor. Estimate the following three specifications assigning the output of each to its own name (e.g., output1 for the first model).

```
gam(Ozone ~ Temp)
gam(Ozone ~ as.factor(Temp))
gam(Ozone ~ s(Temp))
```

The first model is the smoothest model possible. Why is that? The second model is the roughest model possible. Why is that? The third model is a compromise between the two in which the degree of smoothing is determined by the GCV statistic. (See the *gam()* documentation followed by the smoothing spline documentation.)

For each model, examine the numerical output and plot the fitted values against the predictor. For example, if the results of the first model are assigned to the name "output1," use *plot.gam (output1, residuals=TRUE)*. Also, take a look at the output object for the variety of gam features and output that can be accessed. Extractor functions are available.

Which model has the best fit judging by the residual deviance? Which model has the best fit judging by the AIC? Why might the choice of the best model differ depending on which measure of fit is used? Which model seems to be most useful

---

[48] The idea of allowing for locally varying complexity in fitted values is an old one. Fan and Gijbels (1992, 1996), who have made important contributions to the topic, attribute the idea to Breiman, Meisel and Purcell (1977).

judging by the plots? Why is that?

2. Using *scatter.smooth()*, overlay a lowess smooth on a scatterplot with the variable Ozone on the vertical axis and the variable Temp on the horizontal axis. Vary three tuning parameters: span: .25, .50, .75; degree: 0, 1, 2; family as Gaussian or symmetric. How do the fitted values change as each tuning parameter is varied? Which tuning parameter seems to matter most? (You can get the same job done with *loess()*, but a few more steps are involved.)

3. The relationship between temperature and ozone concentrations should be positive and monotonic. From the question above, select a single set of tuning parameter values that produces a fit you like best. Why do you like that fit best? If there are several sets of fitted values you like about equally, what it is about these fitted values that you like also?

4. For the overlay of the fitted values you like best (or select a set from among those you like best) describe how temperature is related to ozone concentrations.

Set 2: Smoothers with Two Predictors

1. From the library *assist* load the dataset TXtemp. Load the library *gam*. With mmtemp as the response and longitude and latitude as the predictors, apply *gam()*. Construct the fitted values using the sum of a 1-D smoothing spline of longitude and a 1-D smoothing spline of latitude. Try several different values for the degrees of freedom of each. You can learn how to vary these tuning parameters with *help(gam)* and *help(s)*. Use the *summary()* command to examine the output, and *plot.gam()* to plot the two partial response functions. To get both plots on the same page use *par(mfrow=c(2,1))*. How are longitude and latitude related to temperature? (If you want to do this in *gam()* in the *mgcv* library, that works too. But the tuning parameters are a little different.)

2. Repeat the analysis in 1, but now construct the fitted values using a single 2-D smoother of longitude and latitude together. Again, try several different values for the degrees of freedom. Examine the tabular output with *summary()* and the plot using *plot.gam()*. You will need to load the library *akima* for the plotting. How do these results compare to those using two 1-D predictor smooths? (For 2-D smoothing, the plotting at the moment is a little better using *gam* in the *mgcv* library.)

Set 3: Smoothers with More Than Two Predictors

1. Still working in *gam()*, build an additive model for mmtemp with the predictors longitude, latitude, year, and month. Use a lowess smooth for each. Try different spans and polynomial degrees. Again use the *summary()* and *plot.gam()* command. To get all four graphs on the same page use *par(mfrow=c(2,2))*. How is

temperature related to each of the four predictors?

2. Repeat the analysis just done using smoothing splines in *gam()*. See if you can tune the model so that you get very close to same graphs. Does it matter which kind of smoother you use? Why or why not? (Keep in mind that you tune *s()* differently from *lo()*.)

Set 4: Smoothers with a Binary Response Variable

1. From the *car* library, load the dataset *Mroz*. Using *glm()*, regress labor force participation on age, income, and the log of wages. From the library *gam*, use *gam()* to repeat the analysis, smoothing each of the predictors with the smoother of your choice. Note that labor force participation is a binary variable. Compare and contrast your conclusions from the two sets of results. Which procedure seems more appropriate here? Why?

Chapter 3
Classification and Regression Trees (CART)

3.1 Introduction

Recall that in stagewise regression, the results of a stage are fixed no matter what happens in subsequent stages. Earlier stages are not re-visited. Forward stepwise regression is not a stagewise procedure because all of the included regression coefficients are re-estimated as each new regressor is added to the model. In a similar fashion for backwards stepwise regression, all of the remaining regression coefficients are re-estimated as each additional regressor is dropped from the model.

If you look under the hood, conventional classification and regression trees (CART), also called decision trees in computer science, essentially a form of stagewise regression with predictors that are indicator variables. CART output is typically displayed in a tree-like structure, which accounts for how the technique is named. A defining feature of CART is the way in which predictors are transformed and selected.

Suppose one has a single quantitative response variable and several predictors. There is interest in $\hat{Y}|X$. The immediate task is to find the single best binary predictor from among a set of predictors, all of which may be numerical. To do this, two kinds of searches are undertaken. First, for each predictor, all possible binary splits of the predictor values are considered. For example, if the predictor is age in years, and there are age-values of 21 through 24, all possible splits maintaining order would be 21 versus 22–24, 21–22 versus 23–24, and 21–23 versus 24.

Ordinal predictors can be handled in the same fashion. For example, the possible answers to a questionnaire item might be "strongly agree," "agree," "can't say," "disagree," and "strongly disagree." Then, all possible binary splits of the data are considered with the order maintained i.e. in strength of agreement. Unlike conventional regression, ordinal predictors pose no special problems.

The original version of this chapter was revised: See the "Chapter Note" section at the end of this chapter for details. The erratum to this chapter is available at https://doi.org/10.1007/978-3-319-44048-4_10.

© Springer International Publishing Switzerland 2016
R.A. Berk, *Statistical Learning from a Regression Perspective*,
Springer Texts in Statistics, DOI 10.1007/978-3-319-44048-4_3

Closely related reasoning can be applied when a predictor is categorical. For instance, if the predictor is marital status with categories never married, married, and divorced, all possible splits would be never married versus married and divorced, married versus never married and divorced, and divorced versus never married and married. For categorical variables, there is no order to maintain.

How is the "best split" for each predictor defined? For quantitative response variables, the baseline is the response variable sum of squares. Each possible binary split of each predictor implies a different two-way partitioning of the data. For example, one partition might include all individuals under 25 years of age, and the other partition would then include all individuals 25 years of age or older. The response variable sum of squares is computed separately within each partition and added together. That sum will be equal to or less than the sum of squares for the response variable before the partitioning. The "best" split for each predictor is defined as the split that reduces the sum of squares the most.

With the best split of each predictor determined, the best split *overall* is determined as the second step. That is, the best split for each predictor is compared by the reduction in the sum of squares. The predictor with the largest reduction wins the competition. It is the predictor that when optimally split, leads to the greatest reduction in the sum of squares.

With the two-step search completed, the winning split is used to subset the data. In other words, the best split for the best predictor defines two subsets. For example, if the best split were to be 21–22 versus 23–24 years of age, all individuals 21–22 would form one subset, and all individuals 23–24 would form the other subset.

There are now two partitions of the original data, defined by best split within and between the predictors. Next, the same two-step procedure is applied to each partition separately; the best split within and between predictors for each subset is found. This leads to four partitions of the data, and once again, the two-step search procedure is undertaken separately for each. The recursive process can continue until there is no meaningful reduction in the sum of squares of the response variable. Then, the results are conventionally displayed as an inverted tree: roots at the top and canopy at the bottom.

As addressed shortly, the recursive partitioning results can be represented within a linear basis expansion framework. The basis functions are indicator variables defined by the best splits. With these determined, a regression of the response on the basis functions yields regression coefficients and fit statistics as usual. In practice, there is no need to translate the partitioning into a regression model; the partitioning results stand on their own as a regression analysis. Because the partitions are determined empirically from the data, the partitioning process introduces a form of model selection. This creates complications for any level II analysis.

The two-step search procedure is easily generalized to categorical response variables, but other performance measures are used rather than the sum of squares. Among the options to be discussed later is the deviance. The upside down tree display of key output remains.

There is a remarkably large number of tree-based statistical methods (Loh 2014). In this chapter, we consider Classification and Regression Trees (CART) introduced by Breiman, Friedman, Olshen, and Stone in 1984. CART has been in use for about 30 years (Breiman et al. 1984) and remains a popular data analysis tool. We will focus on CART as it has traditionally been implemented. There are some interesting refinements and extensions (Chaudhuri et al. 1995; Lee 2005; Chipman et al. 1998; Loh 2014; Su et al. 2004; Choi et al. 2005; Hothorn et al. 2006; Zeileis et al. 2008), and even some major reformulations (Grubinger et al. 2014). There are also CART-like procedures such as CHAID (Kass 1980) and C5.0 (Quinlan 1993), which has a computer science lineage. A discussion of these variants would take us some distance from the approach emphasized in here in part because they treat CART primarily as a stand-alone data analysis tool. CART sometimes can be an effective stand-alone procedure as well, but more important for our purposes, it has become an integral component of statistical learning algorithms discussed in subsequent chapters. A discussion of CART provides an essential foundation for understanding those algorithms.

Chapter 2 was devoted almost entirely to quantitative response variables. Equal time and more is now given to categorical, and especially binary, response variables. As noted earlier, procedures that assign observations to classes are sometimes called "classifiers." When CART is used with categorical response variables, it is an example of a classifier. One grows a classification tree.

Categorical response variables introduce a number of issues that either do not apply to quantitative response variables, or apply only at a high level of abstraction. We now need to get this material on the table in part because it applies to classifiers in addition to CART. We also emphasize again the differences between level I, level II and level III regression analyses and remind readers of the critical difference between explanation and forecasting.

This is a somewhat plodding, tedious chapter. An effort has been made to include only the material that is really needed. But that's a lot, and it is probably necessary to slog through it all.

3.2 The Basic Ideas

We begin with conceptual overview of the CART computational machinery. Mathematical details are provided later. For a binary response variable coded "A" or "B," and predictors X and Z, Fig. 3.1 is the three-dimensional scatterplot illustrating a simple classification problem as it might be attacked by CART. CART's algorithm is called "greedy" because it searches for the best outcome without looking back to past splits or forward to future splits. The algorithm lives only in the present.

The vertical red line at, say, $Z = 3$ produces the first partition. It represents the best split in a competition between all possible splits of X or Z. The A values tend to be concentrated to the left, and the B values tend to be concentrated to the right. The green horizontal line at $X = 5$ produces the subsequent partition of the left subset. It represents the best split of the left partition. The upper left corner is now homogeneous in A. This is an ideal outcome. The yellow horizontal line at $X = -2$

Fig. 3.1 A recursive
partitioning for a binary
response variable and
predictors X and Z (The
response is coded A or B.
The *red line* shows the first
partition. The *green* and
yellow lines show the next
two partitions.)

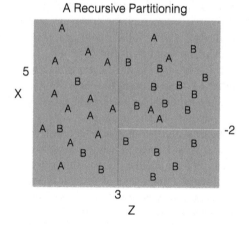

produces the best subsequent split of the right partition. The lower right corner is now homogeneous in B. This too is an ideal outcome. In principle, the lower left partition and the upper right partition would be further subdivided.

Figure 3.1 makes clear that CART constructs partitions with a series of straight-line boundaries perpendicular to the axis of the predictor being used. These may seem like serious constraints on performance. Why linear? Why perpendicular? They are simple to work with and can perform very well in practice.

The values at which the partitioning is done matter. For example, Fig. 3.1 reveals that cases with $Z \leq 3$ and $X > 5$ are always A. Likewise, cases with $Z > 3$ and $X \leq -2$ are always B. We are able describe all four conditional distributions of the binary response variable conditioning on the four partitions of X and Z. Within each partition, the proportion of A-values (or B-values) might be a useful summary statistic for the binary outcome. How do these proportions vary over the different partitions? We are still doing a regression analysis.

3.2.1 Tree Diagrams for Understanding Conditional Relationships

CART partitioning is often shown as an inverted tree. A tree visualization allows the data analyst to see how the data partitions were constructed and consider the conditional relationships implied. Explanation can be in play within a level I regression analysis.

Figure 3.2 is a simple, schematic illustration of an inverted tree. The full dataset is contained in the root node. The data are then broken into two mutually exclusive pieces. Cases with $X > C_1$ go to the right, and cases with $X \leq C_1$ go to the left. The latter are then in terminal node 1, which is not subject to any more subsetting; no meaningful improvements in fit can be made. The former are in an internal node that can be usefully subdivided further, and the internal node is partitioned again. Observations with $Z > C_2$ go to the right and into terminal node 3. Observations with $Z \leq C_2$ go to the left and into terminal node 2. Further subsetting is not productive.

Fig. 3.2 A simple CART
tree structure

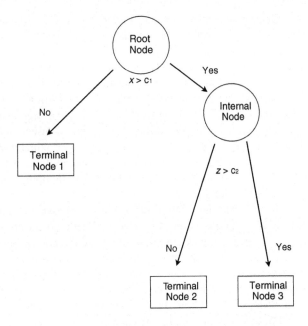

In this case, all splits beyond the initial split of the root node imply, in regression language, interaction effects. The right partition imposed at the internal node only includes observations with X-values that are greater than C_1. Consequently, the impact of Z depends on observations with $X > C_1$, which is an interaction effect.

When there is no natural order to a predictor's values, the partitioning criterion selected is usually represented by the name of the variable along with the values that go to the right (or left, depending on the software) side. For example, if ethnicity is a predictor and there are five ethnicities represented by the letters a though e, the software might represent the partitioning criterion for a given split as *ethnicity = ade*. All cases belonging to ethnic groups a, d, and e are being placed in the right-hand partition.

Splits after the initial split do not have to represent interaction effects. If an immediately subsequent partitioning of the data uses the same predictor (with a different breakpoint), the result is an additional step in the step function for that predictor. A more complicated nonlinear function results, but not an interaction effect. In practice, however, most partitions of the data represent interaction effects.

It is easy to translate Fig. 3.2 into linear basis expansions. One just defines all of the terminal nodes with indicator variables, each of which is a function of one or more predictors (including the constant term). Thus,

$$f(X, Z) = \beta_0 + \beta_1[(I(x \leq c_1)] \\ + \beta_2[I(x > c_1 \ \& \ z \leq c_2)] + \beta_3[I(x > c_1 \ \& \ z > c_2)]. \qquad (3.1)$$

One can see the importance of interaction effects whenever two or more predictors are needed to construct the indicator variable. Interaction effects need to be kept in mind when CART tree diagrams are interpreted.

The application of CART is always an opportunity for a level I analysis. For a level II analysis, we once again must treat the data as random realizations from a nature's joint probability distribution. The estimation target is a classification or regression tree, having the same structure as the tree derived from the data, but as a feature of the joint probability distribution. Consequently, CART fitted values can be used as estimates of the corresponding, approximate response surface. The same level II reasoning can be applied to regression equations for the terminal nodes, such Eq. 3.1. But because CART has built in data snooping, the level II opportunities are somewhat limited.

To illustrate these initial ideas, consider passenger data from the sinking of the Titanic.[1] What predictors are associated with those who perished compared to those who survived? Figure 3.3 shows the CART results as an inverted tree. Survived is coded as a 1, and perished is coded as a 0. In each terminal node, the left number is the count of those who perished, and the right number is the count of those who survived. If the majority perished, the node is colored red. If the majority survived, the node is colored blue. Figure 3.4 contains the code.[2]

For this analysis, predictors used include:

1. sex — the gender of the passenger;
2. age — age of the passenger in years;
3. pclass — the passenger's class of passage;
4. sibsp — the number of siblings/spouses aboard; and
5. parch — the number of parents/children aboard.

The first split on sex. Males are sent down the left branch. Females are sent down the right branch. The two subsequent splits for males are at ages of 9.5 years and 2.5 years. For males, there are three terminal nodes. For the older males, 136 survived and 600 did not. Because the majority did not survive, the node is labeled with a 0 for not surviving. For males, only those 2.5 years old or younger were likely to survive (i.e., 24 to 3). For females, the splits are much more complicated but can be considered with the same sort of reasoning. For example, most of the females traveling in first or second class survived, and the terminal node is given a label of 1 accordingly (i.e., 233 to 17). If one takes the cinematic account seriously, the results broadly make sense, and a level I analysis of the data has been undertaken.

It is challenging to make a credible case for a level II analysis. What is the joint probability distribution responsible for the data? It could perhaps be the joint probability distribution for passengers on ocean liners using as a response of whether or not each survived the passage. But much more specificity would be needed. For

---

[1] Thanks go to Thomas Cason who updated and improved the existing Titanic data frame using the Encyclopedia Titanica.

[2] The procedure *rpart()* is authored by Terry Therneau and Beth Atkinson. The procedure *rpart.plot()* is authored by Stephen Milborrow. Both procedures are superb.

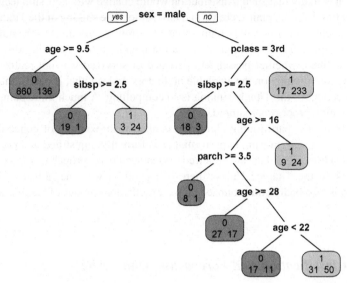

Fig. 3.3 A classification tree for the Titanic data: 1 = Survived, 0 = Perished (In each terminal node, the number who perished and the number who survived are shown, to the *left* and *right* respectively. In *red nodes*, the majority perished. In *blue nodes*, the majority survived. N = 1309)

```
### CART Code
library(PASWR) # To get the data
data(titanic3) # Load the data

library(rpart) # Load the CART library
library(rpart.plot) # Load the fancy plotting library

# Partition the data
out<-rpart(survived~sex+age+pclass+sibsp+parch, data=titanic3,
method="class")
#Plot the tree
prp(out,extra=1,faclen=10,varlen=15,cex=1.2,
    main="Classification Tree for Titanic Survivors",
    box.col=c("red","lightblue")[out$frame$yval])
```

Fig. 3.4 R code for the CART analysis of the Titanic data

example, it is likely that such a distribution would change with new ship technology and better training of captains, crews, and navigators. The sinking of the Titanic itself led to revisions of marine safety regulations governing such things as the number of lifeboats required on board. And even if a reasonable joint probability distribution could be defined, whether passengers perished or survived was not realized independently, conditioning on the available predictors. Indeed, that is part of the reason why the account of the Titanic sinking is so compelling. A much more complicated data realization process is required.

In addition, the partitioning algorithm is clearly an example of concerted data snooping. Therefore, in-sample performance is formally unjustified and potentially very misleading. Test data are required. What would be proper test data for the passengers on the Titanic? Unless there is a good answer, the fallback of cross-validation is also badly compromised. What exactly does an out-of-sample estimate mean?

3.2.2 Classification and Forecasting with CART

There is far more to the output from CART than a tree diagram. Indeed, perhaps the most important output is found in the terminal nodes. Suppose the response variable is binary, and the task is classification. Within each of the terminal nodes, the proportion of "successes" and proportion of "failures" can be calculated. These conditional proportions are often of significant descriptive interest as one kind of fitted values. For example, in Fig. 3.2 if the proportion of successes in terminal node 3 is .70, one can say for cases with $x > c_1$ and $z > c_2$ that the proportion of successes is .70. Analogous statements can be made about the other terminal nodes. For example, the proportion of success for cases with $x \leq c$ (terminal node 1) might be .25. Ideally, terminal node proportions will vary substantially, implying that the partitioning is making important distinctions between different kinds of cases. If one knows for any given case the value of x and the value of z, it really matters for the proportion of successes.

In addition, the conditional proportions can be used to attach class labels to terminal nodes that, in turn, can be assigned to observations. The class labels are a second kind of fitted value. If the majority of observations in a terminal node are As, all of the observations in that partition may be assigned to class A. If the majority of observations in a terminal node are Bs, all of the observations in that partition may be assigned to class B. These labels convey what is most typical in a terminal node and, therefore, is most typical for cases with a particular configuration of indicator variables. If all of the observations in a terminal node need to be placed into a single category, the terminal node class label provides the means. When CART is used in this manner, it is Bayes classifier, applied individually to each terminal node.

Think back to the discussion of logistic regression in Chap. 1. Recall that there were fitted proportions and fitted classes. Cases with fitted proportions that exceeded some threshold were assigned to one of the two classes. Cases with fitted proportions that did not exceed that threshold, or were equal to it, were assigned to the other class. Much the same is going on within each of the terminal nodes of classification trees, where by the Bayes classifier, the threshold is .50.

But why would anyone care about the class labels? The class labels can be critical if new data are provided that contain the same predictors but with the binary outcome unknown. The labels are a good guess for the unknown binary outcome for each case. Often, this plays out as forecasting. Suppose one knows that observations with certain values for predictors fall in a particular terminal node, and that the majority of observations in that partition have, say, the outcome category A. Then, new observations that fall in that terminal node, but for which the response is unknown, sensibly might be predicted to be A as well. If a level II analysis is credible, the class label can be thought of as a fitted value to be used for forecasting.

3.2.3 Confusion Tables

If CART assigns classes to observations, it is certainly fair to ask how good those assigned classes actually are. Instructive assessments can be obtained from "confusion tables," briefly introduced earlier, which cross-tabulate the observed classes against the classes that CART assigns. Ideally, the two will correspond much of the time. But that will be a matter of degree, and confusion tables can provide useful measures of fit. We will consider confusion tables many times in the pages ahead, but a few details are important to introduce now. For ease of exposition at this point, the categorical outcome variable is binary.

Table 3.1 shows an idealized confusion table. There are two classes for the response variable: success and failure. The letters in the cells of the table are cell counts. For example, the letter "a" is the number of observations falling in the upper-left cell. All of the observations in that cell are characterized by an observed class of failure and a predicted class of failure. When the observations are from training data used to build the tree, "predicted" means "assigned." They are a product of the CART fitting process. If the observations are from test data not used to build the tree, "predicted" means "forecasted." The difference between fitting and forecasting is critical in the next several chapters.

In many situations, a split-sample strategy can be employed so that the values of tuning parameters are determined by fitting performance in the evaluation data.

Table 3.1 A confusion table

	Failure predicted	Success predicted	Model error
Failure	a	b	$b/(a+b)$
Success	c	d	$c/(c+d)$
Use error	$c/(a+c)$	$b/(b+d)$	Overall error $= \frac{(b+c)}{(a+b+c+d)}$

Once a satisfactory tree has been grown and honestly assessed with the test data, it is ready for use when the outcome class is not known, but the predictor values are.

There are generally four kinds of performance assessments that are made from confusion tables.

1. The overall proportion of cases incorrectly classified is an initial way to assess performance quality. It is simply the number of observations in the off-diagonal cells divided by the total number of observations. If all of the observations fall on the main diagonal, CART has, by this measure, performed perfectly. None of the observations have an actual class that does not correspond to the fitted class. When no cases fall in the main diagonal, CART is a total failure. All of the observations have an actual class that does not correspond to the fitted class. Clearly, a low proportion for this "overall error" is desirable, but how good is good depends on the baseline for fitting skill when no predictors are used. The real issue is how much better one does once the information in the predictors is exploited. A lot more is said about this shortly.

2. The overall error neglects that it will often be more important to be accurate for one of the response variable classes than for another. For example, it may be more important to correctly diagnose a fatal illness than to correctly diagnose excellent perfect health. This is where the row proportions shown in the far right-hand column become critical. One conditions on the actual class outcome. For each actual class, the row proportion is the number of observations incorrectly fitted divided by the total of observations of that class. Each row proportion characterizes errors made by the statistical procedure. When the true outcome class is known, how common is it for the procedure to fail to identify it?

   The two kinds of model failures are often called "false positives" and "false negatives." Successes incorrectly called failures are false negatives. Failures incorrectly called successes are false positives.[3] The row proportions representing the relative frequency of procedure-generated false negatives and false positives should, ideally, be small. Just as for overall error, the goal is to do better using the information contained in the predictors than could be done ignoring that information. But, the exercise now is done for each row separately. It is common for the procedure to perform better for one outcome than the other.

3. The column proportions address a somewhat different question. One conditions on the fitted class and computes the proportion of times a fitted class is wrong. Whereas the row proportions help evaluate how well the CART algorithm has performed, the column proportions help evaluate how useful the CART results are likely to be if put to work. They convey what would happen if a practitioner

---

[3]Here, the use of the class labels "success" and "failure" is arbitrary, so which off-diagonal cells contain "false positives" or "false negatives" is arbitrary as well. What is called a "success" in one study may be called a "failure" in another study.

used the CART results to impute or forecast. One conditions on either predicted success or on predicted failure from which two different estimates of errors in use can be obtained. Just as for model errors, it is common for the errors in use to differ depending on the outcome. The goal is much the same as for model error: for each column, to be wrong a smaller fraction of the time than if the predictors are ignored.

4. The ratio of the number of false negatives to the number of false positives shows how the results are trading one kind of error for the other. For example, if b is 5 times larger than c, there are five false positives for every false negative. This means that the CART procedure produces results in which false negatives are five times more important than false positives; one false negative is "worth" five false positives. Ratios such as this play a key role in our discussion later about how to place relative costs on false negatives and false positives.

In summary, confusion tables are an essential diagnostic tool. We rely on them in this chapter and all subsequent ones. They also raise some important issues that are very salient in the pages ahead.

3.2.4 CART as an Adaptive Nearest Neighbor Method

Not only is CART an essential component of many statistical learning procedures, it has direct links to other methods that on the surface might seem to be totally unrelated. In particular, it can be instructive to think about CART within an adaptive nearest neighbor framework. The partitions shown in Fig. 3.1 can be viewed as neighborhoods defined by nearest neighbors. But unlike conventional nearest neighbor methods, CART arrives at those neighborhoods adaptively. Like all stagewise (and stepwise) procedures, CART data snoops.

Consider, for example, terminal node 3 in Fig. 3.2. Within that node, are all observations whose values of x are greater than c_1, and whose values of z are greater than c_2. For these observations, a conditional mean or proportion can be computed. In other words, the nearest neighbors for either of these summary statistics are defined as all cases for which $x > c_1$ and $z > c_2$. All of the observations for which this condition holds can be used to arrive at a single numerical summary for the response variable.

The neighborhood represented by the terminal nodes is adaptive in three senses. First, information from the response variable is used to determine the neighborhood. A measure of fit is exploited to arrive recursively at the terminal node neighborhood. Second, because a large number of predictors and break points are examined, a large number of potential neighborhoods are evaluated before an actual neighborhood is formed. Third, the terminal node neighborhoods that result can be defined by different sets of predictors and different sets of break points. Both are arrived at inductively by the CART algorithm. For example, a given predictor can help define one terminal node, but not another. Even when a given predictor is used to define more than one terminal node, it may enter at different stages of the partitioning and use different break points.

The terminal node neighborhoods can be constructed sequentially by where in the predictor space some step function for the response leads to the greatest difference in level. This follows from the desire to make the two resulting subsets as homogeneous as possible. Then, because for each split the single best predictor is chosen, each terminal node, and its implied neighborhood, can be defined using a subset of predictors. That is, one need not define nearest neighbors using the entire predictor space. This is in contrast to the multivariate lowess smoother discussed in the last chapter and is a way to fight back against the curse of dimensionality.

Within a level II analysis, there are also implications for the bias-variance tradeoff it fitted values are used to estimate the true response surface.[4] Suppose for a given terminal node a goal is to estimate the proportion of 1s for all observations in the terminal node neighborhood defined by a particular set of x-values. For example, suppose the binary response is whether a high school student graduates; graduation is coded as 1 and drop out is coded as 0. The terminal node neighborhood in question contains high school students, self-identified as Asian, who have family incomes in excess of $75,000. But suppose there is an omitted predictor variable. Even if it happened to be in the dataset, it would not be selected (e.g., the labor market for blue collar jobs). A more subtle error occurs when the correct predictor is chosen, but at the wrong breakpoint. (e.g., a grade point average < 2.0 rather than < 1.5). Because the neighborhood is not defined correctly, and there is a good chance that the estimated proportion will be biased with respect to the true response surface. A potential remedy is to further refine the terminal nodes by growing a larger tree. There is an opportunity for more predictors to determine the terminal node neighborhoods leading to a more homogeneous mixes of cases. But for a given sample size, a larger tree implies that on the average, there will be fewer cases in each terminal node. Although bias may be reduced, variance may be increased.

In summary, although smoothers, adaptive nearest neighbor methods, and CART come from very different traditions, they have important similarities. Additional and helpful connections between other statistical learning procedures will be addressed in subsequent chapters. We turn now to the CART details.

3.3 Splitting a Node

The first problem that the CART algorithm needs to solve is how to split each node using information contained in the set of predictors. For a quantitative predictor with m distinct values, there are $m - 1$ splits that maintain the existing ordering of values. So, $m - 1$ splits on that variable need to be evaluated. For example, if there are 50

---

[4]Recall that the response surface approximation itself can often be estimated in an asymptotically unbiased fashion.

distinct high school GPA scores possible, there are 49 possible splits that maintain the existing order. However, there are often algorithmic shortcuts that can capitalize, for instance, on ordering the splits by the size of the conditional mean or proportion. The same logic holds for ordinal predictors.

Order does not matter for categorical predictors. Consequently, a categorical variable with k categories has $(2^{k-1} - 1)$ possible splits. For example, if there are five ethnic group categories, there are 15 possible splits. Hence, although there are sometimes shortcuts here too, the computational burdens are generally much heavier for categorical variables. There are no order restrictions on how a categorical predictor is split.

Recall that starting at the root node, CART algorithm evaluates all possible splits of all predictor variables and picks the "best" single split overall. The best split of the variable selected is better than the best split of any other predictor. The data are then partitioned according to that best split. The same process is applied to all subsequent nodes until, at the extreme, all cases have been placed in a terminal node all their own. Because the final partitions do not overlap, each case can only be in one terminal node.

How is "best" to be formally defined? It is common to focus on the "impurity" of a node. Impurity is essentially heterogeneity. The goal is to have as little impurity (heterogeneity) overall as possible. Consequently, the best split is the one that reduces impurity the most. To help simplify the exposition that follows, assume a binary response variable coded 1 or 0. The term "success" is used to refer to outcomes coded 1 and the term "failure" to refer to outcomes coded 0.

A discussion of impurity can work using the proportions of successes and failures in a node or using the probabilities of a success or a failure for cases in that node. Most expositions favor probabilities and assume that they are known. There is really no didactic cost to this assumption.

Suppose that a dataset is realized from a joint probability distribution, so the concept of a probability can apply. Consider a given node, designated as node A. The impurity of node A is taken to be a nonnegative function of the probability that $y = 1$, written as $p(y = 1|A)$.

If A is a terminal node, ideally it should be composed of cases that are all equal to 1 or all equal to 0. Then $p(y = 1|A)$ would be 1.0 or 0.0. Intuitively, impurity is the smallest it can be. If half the cases are equal to 1 and half the cases are equal to 0, the probability is equal to .50. A is the most impure it can be because a given case is as likely to be a 1 as it is a 0.

One can more formally build on these intuitions. Let the impurity of node A be:

$$I(A) = \phi[p(y = 1|A)], \tag{3.2}$$

with $\phi \geq 0$, $\phi(p) = \phi(1 - p)$, and $\phi(0) = \phi(1) < \phi(p)$. In other words, impurity is nonnegative, and symmetrical with a minimum when A contains all 0s or all 1s, and a maximum when A contains half of each.[5]

There remains a need to define the function ϕ. For classification, three definitions have been used in the past: Bayes error, the cross-entropy function, and the Gini index. In order they are:

$$\phi(p) = \min(p, 1 - p); \tag{3.3}$$

$$\phi(p) = -p \, \log(p) - (1 - p) \, \log(1 - p); \tag{3.4}$$

and

$$\phi(p) = p \, (1 - p). \tag{3.5}$$

All three functions for impurity are concave, having minimums at $p = 0$ and $p = 1$ and a maximum at $p = .5$. Entropy and the Gini index are the most commonly used, and in CART generally give very similar results except when there are more than two response categories. Then, there is some reason to favor the Gini index (Breiman et al. 1984: 111). The Gini index is more likely to partition the data so that there is one relatively homogeneous node having relatively few cases. The other nodes are then relatively heterogeneous and have relatively more cases. For most data analyses, this is a desirable result. Entropy tends to partition the data so that all of the nodes for a given split are about equal in size and homogeneity. This is generally less desirable. But the choice between the two impurity functions can depend on the costs associated with classification errors, which is a topic addressed shortly.

One might legitimately wonder why CART does not directly minimize classification error. Direct minimization of overall classification error is discussed in some detail by Breiman and his colleagues (1984: Sect. 4.1). In part because classification error is not continuous, there can be several splits for a given stage minimizing classification error. In addition, minimizing classification error at each stage has a tendency, like entropy, to produce a tree structure that is often more difficult to interpret. For now, we focus on node impurity as just defined. However, direct minimization of classification error resurfaces as a useful consideration when boosting is considered in Chap. 6.

For real applications, the probabilities are not likely to be known. Suppose one uses data to estimate the requisite probabilities. It should be apparent by now that obtaining good estimates involves conceptual and technical complications, but for didactic purposes, assume that the complications have been effectually addressed.

Building on Zhang and Singer (1999; Chaps. 2 and 4), for any internal node, we focus on a potential left "daughter" node A_L, and a right "daughter" node A_R. We wish to evaluate the usefulness of a potential partitioning of the data. Table 3.2

---

[5]The use of I in Eq. 3.2 for impurity should not be confused with the use of I to represent an indicator variable. The different meanings should be clear in context.

Table 3.2 Counts used to determine the usefulness of a potential split (The cell entries are counts, with the first subscript for rows and the second subscript for columns)

	Failure	Success	Total
Left Node: $x \leq c$	n_{11}	n_{12}	$n_{1.}$
Right Node: $x > c$	n_{21}	n_{22}	$n_{2.}$
	$n_{.1}$	$n_{.2}$	$n_{..}$

provides the information needed. The entries in each cell are counts, with rows as the first subscript and columns as the second subscript.

As before, we let $y = 1$ if there is a success and 0 otherwise. The estimate of $p(y = 1|A_L)$ is given by $n_{12}/n_{1.}$. Similarly, the estimate $p(y = 1|A_R)$ is given by $n_{22}/n_{2.}$.

Consider calculations for entropy as an example. Entropy impurity for the left daughter is

$$I(A_L) = -\frac{n_{11}}{n_{1.}}\log(\frac{n_{11}}{n_{1.}}) - \frac{n_{12}}{n_{1.}}\log(\frac{n_{12}}{n_{1.}}). \tag{3.6}$$

Entropy impurity for the right daughter is

$$I(A_R) = -\frac{n_{21}}{n_{2.}}\log(\frac{n_{21}}{n_{2.}}) - \frac{n_{22}}{n_{2.}}\log(\frac{n_{22}}{n_{2.}}). \tag{3.7}$$

Imagine that for the left daughter there are 300 observations with 100 successes and 200 failures. It follows that the impurity is $-.67(-.40) - .33(-1.11) = .27 + .37 = .64$. Imagine now that for the right daughter there are 100 observations with 45 successes and 55 failures. The impurity is $-.55(-.60) - .45(-.80) = .33 + .36 = .69$.

To put these numbers in context, it helps to consider the smallest and largest possible values for the impurity. The greatest impurity one could obtain would be for 50 % successes and 50 % for failures. The computed value for that level of impurity would be .693. For proportions of 1.0 or 0.0, the value of entropy impurity is necessarily 0. In short, the minimum value is 0, and the maximum is a little more than .69. The closer one gets to 50–50, where the impurity is the greatest, the closer one gets to .693. The impurity numbers computed are rather close to this upper bound and reflect, therefore, substantial heterogeneity found in both daughter nodes. It is likely that this split would not be considered to be a very good one.

Once all possible splits across all possible variables are evaluated in this manner, a decision is made about which split to use. But the impact of a split is not just a function of the impurity of a node. The importance of each node must also be taken into account. A node in which few cases are likely to fall should be less important than a node in which many cases are likely to fall. The former probably will not matter much, but the latter probably will.

We define the improvement resulting from a split as the impurity of the parent node minus the weighted left and right daughter impurities. If this is a large number, entropy impurity is reduced substantially. More formally, the benefits of the split s for node A,

$$\Delta I(s, A) = I(A) - p(A_L)I(A_L) - p(A_R)I(A_R), \tag{3.8}$$

where $I(A)$ is the value of the parent impurity, $p(A_R)$ is the probability of a case falling in the right daughter node, $p(A_L)$ is the probability of a case falling in the left daughter node, and the rest is defined as before. The two probabilities can be estimated from information such as provided in Table 3.2; they are just the marginal proportions $n_1./n_{..}$ and $n_2./n_{..}$. They serve as weights.

$\Delta I(s, A)$ can be essentially the reduction in the deviance and thus, there is a clear link to the generalized linear model that can prove useful when different fitting procedures are compared. CART finds the best $\Delta I(s, A)$ for each variable. The variable and split with the largest value are then chosen to define the new partition. The same approach is applied to all subsequent nodes.

The CART algorithm can keep partitioning until there is one case in each node. There is then no impurity whatsoever. Such a tree is called "saturated." However, well before a tree is saturated, there will usually be far too many terminal nodes to interpret, and the number of cases in each will be quite small. The very small node sizes lead to very unstable results. Small changes in the data can produce trees with rather different structures and interpretations. One option is to prohibit the CART algorithm from constructing any terminal nodes with sample sizes smaller than some specified value. A second option is considered shortly. And we show in later chapters that there can be ways to work usefully with saturated trees, as long as there is a very large number of them.

3.4 Fitted Values

CART is a method to construct, using a predictors, a conditional distribution. Interest commonly centers on some measure of location. For classification problems, the conditional proportion is usually the measure. For regression problems, the measure is usually the conditional mean. Using linear basis expansions, explicit links to parametric regression can be made. It follows that most of the issues raised by parametric regression, and most of the concepts associated with parametric regression, carry over.

3.4.1 Fitted Values in Classification

As noted earlier, there are two kinds of classification fitted values for CART. First, within each terminal node, the proportion of observations for each of the classes are fitted values. They are conditional proportions that characterize the terminal node. For example, if the response variable is binary and the proportion of successes is .55, the fitted value for that terminal node is .55 (or .45 if one wants to focus on failures).

It can be useful to compare such fitted values across terminal nodes as part of a level I analysis.

If a level II analysis can be justified, the reasoning becomes more elaborate. One envisions the same neighborhoods in the joint probability distribution as found with the data. In each of those population neighborhoods, there are expectations for the proportion of successes. Those expectations are the estimation targets, and the in-sample proportions can be used as estimates. However, because the neighborhoods are a product of extensive data snooping, the quality of those estimates is unknown and possibly misleading. Having test data can really help. One "drops" the test data down the tree, and the fitted proportions will be asymptotically unbiased estimates of the tree-derived approximate response surface. Moreover, with the nonparametric bootstrap applied to the test data, asymptotically valid confidence intervals can be constructed around the estimates. An example using the bootstrap with CART is provided as part of the last exercise in this chapter.

The second kind of fitted values require an additional step: a class is assigned to each terminal node. As described above, the assigned class is determined by a majority vote (or a plurality if there are more than two response categories). Then within each terminal node, winning class is attached to each observation. The voting threshold (e.g., .50) has some of the features of a decision boundary, but only for one node at a time.

In-sample performance measures can follow directly. For any given terminal node, what proportion of the time is the assigned class the correct class? For example, if the proportion of successes in a terminal node is .90, the assigned class is "success," and that assigned class will be incorrect for 10 % of the observations in that node. The ideal real result would 0.0 %, which would follow if the terminal node were perfectly homogeneous. The issues are much the same as for the column calculations in confusion tables. How often is the assigned class wrong? One difference for terminal nodes is that the error rate for a terminal node is only for a subset of observations defined by a predictor neighborhood. Another difference is that a full confusion table cannot be constructed because for a given terminal node, only one class is assigned. The table would have one column and two rows.

But just as before, in-sample results can be misleading. It is better to work with test data with which the accuracy of assigned classes can be more honestly addressed. Better estimates of generalization error may be obtained, and once again, a non-parametric bootstrap can be applied to the test data to construct confidence intervals around the estimates of generalization error.

3.4.2 An Illustrative Prison Inmate Risk Assessment Using CART

A key issue for prison administrators is understanding which inmates are likely to place themselves and others in harm's way. Use of narcotics, assaults on prison

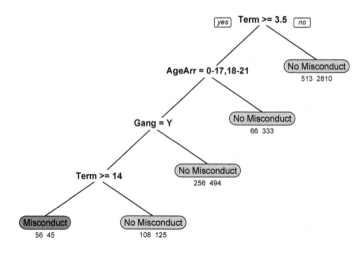

Fig. 3.5 CART recursive partitioning of the prison data (N = 4806)

guards, and homicides are examples. Although such events are relatively rare, they have very serious consequences. It follows that it would be very useful if such conduct could be anticipated. Then, for the high-risk inmates, preventive measures might be taken. For example, inmates from rival street gangs might be housed in different prisons. Low-risk inmates might be given far greater freedom to participate in job training and educational programs. A prerequisite, however, is a way to find effective predictors of misconduct in prison.

Using data from the administrative records of a large state prison system, Fig. 3.5 shows a classification tree suggesting which kinds of inmates are reported for some form of misconduct within 18 months of intake.[6] From Fig. 3.6, one can see that there are two tuning parameters. A relatively large minimum node sample size of 100 was imposed to stabilize the results and to keep the diagram very simple. More will be said soon about the complexity parameter *cp*, but a small value allows splits that do not reduce node impurity very much. According to the documentation of *rpart()*, *cp* is a threshold on the proportional improvement in fit. Only splits improving the fit by at least the value of *cp* will be permitted. A large value for the threshold means that acceptable splits must improve the fit a lot.[7]

The three predictors in Fig. 3.5 were selected by the CART procedure from a larger set of 12 predictors.

1. Term: Nominal sentence length in years. (The nominal sentence is the sentence given by the trial judge. Inmates are often released before their nominal sentence is fully served.)

---

[6]Because of confidentiality concerns, the data may not be shared.

[7]The tree diagram is formatted differently from the tree diagram used for the Titanic data to empha-size the terminal nodes.

```
library(rpart) # Load the CART library
library(rpart.plot) # Load the fancy plotting library

# Partition the data
out<-rpart(Fail~AgeArr+Gang+CDC+Jail+Psych+Term,
           data=temp, method="class",
           minbucket=100,cp=.001)
# Plot a tree
prp(out,extra=1,faclen=10,varlen=15,
box.col=c("red","lightblue")[out$frame$yval])
```

Fig. 3.6 R code for a CART analysis of prison misconduct

2. AgeArr: Age at arrival at the prison reception center in years using 16–20, 21–26, 27–35, and 36 or older.
3. Gang: gang membership with Y for "yes" and N for "no."

Terminal nodes are labeled "No Misconduct" if the majority in that node do not engage in misconduct and "Misconduct" if the majority do. The numbers within each terminal node show left to right the counts of misconduct cases and no misconduct cases respectively.[8] There are 4806 observations in the root node. Among these, observations are sent left if the nominal prison term is equal to or greater than 3.5 years and to the right if the nominal prison term is less than 3.5 years. Likewise, at each subsequent split, the observations meeting the condition specified are sent left.

The story is simple. Inmates with nominal prison terms over 14 years, who are under 22 years of age, and who are gang members are more likely than not to be reported for misconduct (i.e., 56 cases v. 45 cases). Inmates with nominal terms of less than 3.5 years are relatively unlikely to be reported for prison misconduct regardless of age, gang membership or any other 9 predictors in the data (i.e., 513 cases v. 2810 cases). In the other three terminal nodes, no-misconduct cases are the majority. One might say that a very long nominal terms puts an observation over the top but by itself is not associated with a preponderance of reported misconduct. Each of the five terminal nodes but the one on the far right are defined by interaction effects.

There are readily available (post hoc) explanations for these results. Judges impose far longer prison terms on individuals who have committed very serious, usually violent, crimes. The data suggest that the judges are on to something. And it is well known that young gang members can be especially difficult especially when housed with members of rival gangs.

At the same time, the partitions are arrived at inductively, and the regression model implied is no doubt badly misspecified. For example, there is no information on the

---

[8]In R, the character variable default order left to right is alphabetical.

security level in which the inmate is placed, and higher security levels are thought to reduce incidents of serious misconduct.[9]

Moreover, a conventional analysis using logistic regression would look very different. It is likely that most of the predictors would have been entered only as main effects, and unlikely that the 4-way interactions on the left branches would have been included. Neither approach is likely to be correct by conventional regression analysis thinking.

Nevertheless, suppose at intake, prison administrators wanted to intervene in a manner that could reduce prison misconduct. Absent other information, it might make sense to distinguish young gang members with very long sentences from other inmates. In effect, the prison administrators would be using the classification tree to make forecasts that would help inform placement and supervision decisions.

Although such thinking can have real merit, there are complications. We will have shifted into a level II analysis if the results are to be used for forecasting. One would need to consider how the data were realized, the impact the CART's extensive data snooping, and out-of-sample performance. In addition, the consequences of failing to identify a very dangerous inmate at intake can be enormously different from the consequences of incorrectly labeling a low-risk inmate as dangerous. The different consequences of can have very different costs. In the first instance, a homicide could result. In the second instance, an inmate might be precluded from participating in prison programs that could be beneficial. It stands to reason, therefore, that the differential costs of forecasting errors should be introduced into the CART algorithm. We turn to that now.

3.5 Classification Errors and Costs

Looking back at the earlier details on how splits are determined, there is little explicit concern about classification errors, but it can be shown that all three impurity functions treat classification errors symmetrically. Incorrectly classifying an A as a B, is treated the same as incorrectly classifying a B as an A. Similar reasoning carries over when the assigned classes are used for forecasting. The class assigned to a terminal node is determined by a majority vote. All observations in a given terminal node get a single vote that has the exact same weight for all. But is that always reasonable?

Consider the second terminal node from the left in Fig. 3.5. The vote is close, but the no misconduct cases win. It follows that the 108 inmates who in fact had reported misconduct are misclassified. But suppose each vote for no misconduct inmates counted as half a vote. The misconduct vote would carry the day, and the terminal node would be assigned to the misconduct class. There would then be 125 classification errors, but because each would count half as much as before, overall

---

[9]The issues are actually tricky and beyond the scope of this discussion. At intake, how an inmate will be placed and supervised are unknown and are, therefore, not relevant predictors. Yet, the training data need to take placement and supervision into account.

Table 3.3 CART confusion table for classifying inmate misconduct (N = 4816)

	Classify as no misconduct	Classify as misconduct	Model error
No misconduct	3762	45	.01
Misconduct	953	56	.95
Use error	.20	.45	Overall error = .21

error would be reduced from 108 to $125 \times .5 = 62.5$ Whereas the original cost ratio was 1 to 1, it is now 2 to 1. In concrete terms, a misclassified misconduct cases is taken to be twice as costly as a misclassified no misconduct case.

As we examine in depth shortly, introducing "asymmetric" costs for classification errors can be a game changer that actually begins with the criteria by which splits are determined and involves far more than re-weighting the votes in terminal nodes. We will see that by altering the prior, the measures of impurity in Eq. 3.8 are replaced by measures of the expected costs of classification errors when a split is determined.[10]

Whether there actually are asymmetric costs resulting from classification errors depends on what is done with the classification tree. If the CART results are just archived in some academic journal, there are probably no costs one way or the other. If the results are used to guide future research, costs can be a real issue. In genomic research, for example, follow-up research would be wasted if a genomic snip is incorrectly identified as important. Conversely, a significant research lead might be missed if an important genomic snip is incorrectly overlooked. These two costs are probably not be the same. In applied research, costs can be very important, as the prison example should make clear. A way is needed to build in the differential costs classification errors.

3.5.1 Default Costs in CART

Without any apparent consideration of costs, the CART algorithm can make classification decisions about the misconduct of inmates. But in fact, costs are built in. To see how, we need to examine Table 3.3, which is constructed from the prison misconduct analysis.

As noted earlier, tables of the form of Table 3.3 are often called confusion tables. They can summarize the classification performance (or as we see later, forecasting performance) of a particular classifier. Here, that classifier is CART. There is a row

---

[10]But as Therneau and Atkinson (2015: Sect. 3.3.2) state,"When altered priors are used, they affect only the choice of split. The ordinary losses and priors are used to compute the risk of the node. The altered priors simply help the impurity rule choose splits that are likely to be good in terms of the risk." For example, the deviance or mean squared error are computed as usual to show how much better the fit has become.

for each actual outcome. There is a column for each classified outcome. Correct classifications are in the main diagonal. Misclassifications are the off-diagonal elements. Thus, we learn that 998 out of 4806 cases were incorrectly classified. But, how good this is depends on the baseline.

Had no predictors been used, classification could have been done from the misconduct marginal distribution alone. Applying the Bayes classifier, all cases could have been classified as having no reported misconduct. Then, 999 out of 4806 of the cases would have been incorrectly classified. Clearly, there is no meaningful improvement by this yardstick.

However, there is lots more going on in the table. The overall fit ignores how well CART does when the two response variable categories separated. Consider first what happens when one conditions on the actual class. In this case, the absence of misconduct can be classified very well — 99 % of the cases are classified correctly. In contrast, instances of misconduct are misclassified about 95 % of the time. The overall error rate masks these important differences. CART performs very well when there is no misconduct and very poorly when there is misconduct.

The columns in Table 3.3 are also instructive. Now the conditioning is with respect to the assigned class, not the actual class. If the no misconduct class is assigned, it is wrong for about 20 % of the observations. If the misconduct class is assigned, it is wrong for about 45 % of the observations. So, mistakes are relatively more common when misconduct is assigned, but we do better with the misconduct class that one might expect. If one is thinking ahead to possible forecasting applications, there may be some hope.

Where are costs in all this? Key information about costs is contained in the two off-diagonal cells. There are 45 no misconduct cases incorrectly classified and 953 misconduct cases incorrectly classified. The former one might call false positives and the latter one might call false negatives. The ratio of the cell counts is $953/45 = 21.2$. There are about 21 false negatives for each false positive. Stated a little differently, one false positive is "worth" about 21 false negatives, and it's cost is, therefore, about 21 times greater. According to the confusion table, it is 21 times more costly to misclassify a case of no misconduct (i.e., a false positive) than to misclassify a case of misconduct (i.e., a false negative).

All of the performance results in the table depend on the 21 to 1 cost ratio produced by default, and one has to wonder if corrections administrators and other stakeholder think that the 21 to 1 cost ratio makes sense. The analysis is shaped by treating false positives as far more costly than false negatives. In practice, prison misconduct false negatives are usually thought to be more costly (Berk 2012), so this analysis may well have it upside down. And if that's right, all of the various measures of classification performance are highly suspect and potentially very misleading.

Important lessons follow. First, the CART algorithm (and every other classification procedure for that matter) *necessarily* introduces the costs of classification errors at least implicitly when classes are assigned. There is no way to circumvent this. Even if the data analyst never considers such costs, they are built in. To not consider the relative costs of misclassifications is to leave the relative cost determinations to the data and the classification algorithm. Second, the way cases are classified will vary depending on the cost ratios. As a result, the entire confusion table can change dramatically depending on the cost ratio. Finally, the classes assigned can serve as forecasts when the predictor values are known and the outcome class is not. But if the assigned classes depend on the false negative to false positive cost ratio, so do the forecasts.

If costs are so important, there is a need to understand how they are incorporated into the CART algorithm. This will set the stage for a data analyst to introduce costs explicitly. In other words, it is desirable — some might say essential — to treat the relative costs of classification/forecasting errors as an *input* to the algorithm. Unless this is done, the results risk being unresponsive to the empirical questions being asked.

3.5.2 Prior Probabilities and Relative Misclassification Costs

The marginal distribution of any categorical response variable will have a proportion of the observations in each response category. In the prison example, .21 of the inmates had a reported incident of misconduct, and .89 of the inmates had not. However, before looking at the data, one might already hold strong beliefs from past research or other information about what those marginal proportions should be. For example, the design through which the data were collected may have over-sampled inmates reported for misconduct in order to have a sufficient number of them in the study. But for many uses of the results, it would make sense to weight the observations back to the actual proportion of inmates who engage in misconduct. For a level II analysis, proportions can be conceptualized as the "prior probabilities" associated with the response variable. The word "prior" comes from Bayesian statistical traditions in which the "prior" refers to the beliefs of the data analyst, before the data are examined, about the probability density or distribution of some parameter.

There has been some work within Bayesian traditions capitalizing on several different kinds of CART priors (Chipman et al. 1998; 1999), including a "pinball prior" for tree size and some features of tree shape (Wu et al. 2007). That is, key features of the tree itself are given a prior probability distribution. The ideas advanced are truly interesting, and have led to some important statistical learning spinoffs (Chipman et al. 2010). But in practice, the technical complications are considerable, and it is not even clear that there will often be credible information available to make such priors more than tuning parameters. Tuning parameters are important and useful, but they are not a feature of probability distributions specified before the data analysis begins. Consequently, for present purposes, we will use the term "prior" only with reference to the marginal probability distribution of the response variable. Consistent with most exposition of CART, we will proceed as if a level II analysis is appropriate, but in broad brush strokes the lessons learned apply as well to level I approaches.

Assume that a credible level II analysis has been undertaken with CART. Drawing heavily on Therneau and Atkinson (2015), suppose the training data has N

observations and C classes for the response variable. The CART algorithm produces K terminal nodes. Define π_i for $i = 1, 2, \ldots$, as the prior probability of being in class i. For the binary cases, i is here represented by 1 or 2. $L(i, j)$ is the loss matrix. The elements in the main diagonal (i.e., $i = j$) are the costs of a correct classification, assumed to be 0.0. The off-diagonal elements (i.e. $i \neq j$) are the costs of classification errors, assumed to be positive.

A is a terminal node, and $\tau(x)$ is the true class for an observation, where x represents the vector of predictor variable values for that observation. We let $\tau(A)$ be the class assigned to node A. N_i and N_A are the number of observations in the sample that are in class i and in node A, respectively, with N_{iA} the number of observations of class i in node A. The following relationships in each terminal node hold.

1. $P(A)$ is the probability of cases appearing in node A, which is equivalent to $\sum_{i=1}^{C} \pi_i P[x \in A | \tau(x) = i]$, where π_i is a prior probability. For each class i, the prior probability of a case being in class i is multiplied by the probability that class i cases will be in node A. This product is summed over classes. $P(A)$ can be estimated by $\sum_{i=1}^{C} \pi_i (N_{iA}/N_i)$. Because prior probabilities figure directly in these calculations, prior probabilities can affect the tree structure.

2. Then, $p(i|A)$ is the conditional probability of class i given that a case is in node A, or $P[\tau(x) = i | x \in A]$. The value of $p(i|A)$ can be estimated by the number of cases of class i in node A, divided by the total number of cases in that node and equals $\pi_i P[x \in A | \tau(x) = i] / P[x \in A]$, which can also be estimated by $\pi_i (N_{iA}/N_i) / \sum_{i=1}^{C} \pi_i (N_{iA}/N_i)$. The conditional probability of a case with true class i landing in A depends in part on the prior probability that a case is class i to begin with.

3. $R(A)$ is the "risk" associated with node A, such that $\sum_{i=1}^{C} p(i|A)L(i, \tau(A))$. In other words, the risk associated with node A is for a binary response the conditional probability of a case of type $i = 1$ falling in that node times costs that follow, plus the conditional probability of a case of type $i = 2$ falling in that node times costs that follow. Risk is a function of both the conditional probabilities and the costs. Because the conditional probabilities depend on the prior probabilities, the prior probabilities affect risks.

4. $R(T)$ is the risk of the entire tree T, which equals $\sum_{j=1}^{K} P(A_j)R(A_j)$, where A_j is for each of the K terminal nodes of the tree. We are now just adding the total risk associated with each terminal node, weighted by the probability of cases falling in that node. This can also be seen as the "expected cost" of the entire tree.

To help make these concepts more concrete, Fig. 3.7 provides a numerical illustration constructed from fictional training data. There are 10,000 high school students in the data. 2000 dropped out (D) and 8000 graduated (G). From these figures one can estimate the "objective" prior as $p(D) = .2$, and $p(G) = .8$. It is called "objective" because it is estimated empirically. We will see later that the objective prior can be altered in useful ways. Shown is a confusion table for terminal node A in which the actual outcome is tabulated by the classified outcome. For example, there are 50 false negatives and 250 false positives. On the margins of the table are the row and column

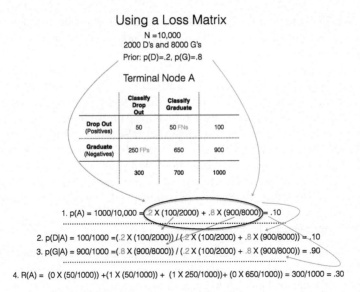

Fig. 3.7   Terminal node A calculations for Dropouts (D) and Graduates (G)

totals, not the usual error rates. With the table in place, one can illustrate how the expressions just described are employed.

What is the estimated probability of a case falling in this terminal node? One can immediately intuit that the probability is $1000/10,000 = .10$. That result can be unpacked as shown in line #1, consistent with the formal expressions above. The key point is that the estimated prior distribution (in red) plays a role.

What is the estimated conditional probability that the case will be a high school drop out, given that a case lands in terminal node A? One can immediately intuit that the estimated conditional probability is $100/1000 = .10$. Line #2 shows how this probability can be unpacked and again the prior is a player, consistent with the formal expression above. Likewise, what is the estimated conditional probability that the case is a high school graduate, given that a case lands in terminal node A? The intuitive answer is $900/1000 = .90$ which is unpacked in line #3. As before, the prior is involved.

Finally, in line #4 we get to the risk associated with terminal node A. The four probabilities come from the four interior entries in the table. These probabilities are affected by the prior through the conditional probabilities on the margins of the table. For the risk calculations, we need to introduce costs. As before, there are no costs associated with correct classifications. For incorrect classifications, we use for now a cost of 1.0. The loss matrix $L(i, j)$ has 0s along the main diagonal and 1s in the off-diagonal cells.

Again building on intuition, the risk for terminal node A is the sum of the estimated conditional probabilities of a case falling in each cell of the table, each multiplied by the cost of falling in that cell, given that the observation has landed in terminal node A to begin with. In effect, risk is an expected cost, and with a value of 1.0 for the cost of misclassifications, the expected risk is nothing more than the proportion of cases misclassified. That value for this example is .30.

For example, there are 1000 cases in the table. The estimated conditional probability of falling in the upper left cell is $50/1000 = .05$. Because this cell only contains correct classifications, the cost is 0.0. It makes no contribution to the risk. For the lower left hand cell, the estimated conditional probability is $250/1000 = .25$. Because this cell contains misclassifications (i.e., false positives), the estimated conditional probability is multiplied by a cost-value of 1.0. The same reasoning applies to the two cells on the right side of the table. When all of the expected costs are summed, the result is .30. When the cost of a false positive or a false negative is equal to 1, it makes sense that the risk for terminal node A is simply the proportion misclassified.

There are four general lessons.

1. The calculations just illustrated apply to each terminal node and, therefore, the full tree. When all misclassifications are given a cost of 1.0, the risk for the tree as a whole is the total number of cases misclassified.
2. The prior's effects cascades down all the way to the final risk calculations. These calculations depend on the estimated probabilities associated with each cell that in turn are influenced by all of the row and column estimated conditional probabilities. If the prior is different, what follows will be different as well. In short, the expected number of classification errors in a terminal node is affected by the priors. Where these are distributed within the confusion table is affected too.
3. Replacing $L(i \neq j) = 1$ with $L(i \neq j) = m$, where m is some constant, just scales up or down the risk by some arbitrary amount and makes no difference to the CART algorithm. It is a bit like measuring a person's height in inches rather than feet. Each misclassification has a cost of 12 rather than 1.
4. In this example, the costs of false positives and false negatives are taken to be the same. That is the usual CART default. Therefore, if one just lets the data determine everything, it is the same as (a) making the costs of all classification errors the same and (b) taking the empirical distribution of the response as the appropriate prior distribution. This is exactly what was done for the results in Fig. 3.5.

But what does one do if as in Table 3.3 the empirical balance of false negatives to false positives is unsatisfactory? It would seem that the most direct response would be to alter the costs in the loss matrix to make them asymmetric. The off-diagonal elements in the loss matrix would not longer be the same. False negatives are then made more (or less) costly relative to false positives. For example, instead of the loss matrix $\begin{bmatrix} 0 & 1 \\ 1 & 0 \end{bmatrix}$, one might use the loss matrix $\begin{bmatrix} 0 & 10 \\ 1 & 0 \end{bmatrix}$.

Because false positives and false negatives are now being weighted differently, one might well expect CART output to be affected. Looking back at second righthand side term in the expression in line #4, imagine that the 1 was replaced by a 10. False negatives are made 10 times more costly. It makes sense that in an effort to minimize

(or at least reduce) risk, the algorithm would aggressively seek ways to reduce the
number of false negatives, even if it meant increasing substantially the number of
false positives. That, in turn, would presumably impact the classification tree and the
confusion table.

One possible approach is to use the loss matrix as an argument in the Gini function (Therneau and Atkinson 2015: Sect. 3.2). As the "generalized" Gini function,
impurity is defined then as

$$G(p) = (1/2) \sum_i \sum_j L(i, j) p_i p_j. \tag{3.9}$$

Unfortunately, this approach does not work in practice (Therneau and Atkinson
2015: 7). $G(p)$ is not necessarily concave, which was a key motivation for each of
the three impurity functions. In addition, calculation of the generalized Gini function
"symmetrizes" the loss matrix. It is as if the loss matrix were added to its transpose.
For the binary case, any cost asymmetry is lost. Both problems apply as well to
categorical response variables with more than two categories, although consequences
for the content of the loss matrix are a bit more complicated.

However, one need not work with the Gini index directly. Recall from the algebraic
treatment several pages back that the probability of class i in node A, $p(i|A)$, can be
estimated by the expression $\pi_i(N_{iA}/N_i)/\sum_{i=1}^C \pi_i(N_{iA}/N_i)$, and its associated risk
is $p(i|A)L(i, \tau(A))$. Therefore, the risk associated with a class in a given node is
scaled by the product of the prior probabilities and the entries in the loss matrix. This
was implicit in expression #4 in Fig. 3.7. To see the consequences, suppose there
exist a new $\tilde{\pi}$ and a new $\tilde{L}$ so that

$$\tilde{\pi}_i \tilde{L}(i, j) = \pi_i L(i, j). \tag{3.10}$$

The risks are identical, and it does not matter what the particular values of $\tilde{\pi}$ and $\tilde{L}$
happen to be as long as the equality holds. This opens the door for lots of possibilities.
If one just thinks of the righthand side as the weight given to the classification errors
for class i in a given node, and if more or less weight is desired, one can alter either
the prior, or the costs, or both. In practice, it is less work to alter one of them, and
the choice can depend on how the software is written. In the binary response case, if
one wanted to alter the weights by altering just the prior distribution to π_i^* from π_i,
one would use

$$\tilde{\pi}_i^* = \frac{\pi_i L_i^*}{\pi_i L_i^* + \pi_j L_j^*}. \tag{3.11}$$

With index for each response class, the values of π_i are the probabilities associated
with the empirical prior distribution. The values of L_i^* are the new costs. Because
of the normalization, all that matters in the loss matrix is relative costs. Thus, one
just has to know, for example, that the cost of one kind of classification error is three
times the cost of another kind of classification error, not their actual values.

Let's try an example of changing the prior so that the reasoning is clear. Suppose for the prison data one were to let the data determine everything. Then, the empirical prior distribution is about .8 for no misconduct and about .2 for misconduct. The cost of a false negative or a false positive is taken to be 1.0.

Suppose we want the cost of a false negative to be twice the cost of a false positive; the 1 to 1 ratio would be 1 to 2. For no misconduct, we let $\pi_1 \times 1.0 = .80 \times 1.0 = .80$. For misconduct, we let $\pi_2 \times 2.0 = .20 \times 2.0 = .40$. These values need to be normalized so that as probabilities they sum to 1.0. Normalizing π_1^*, we compute $(4/5)/(4/5 + 2/5) = .67$. Normalizing π_2^*, we compute $(2/5)/(4/5 + 2/5) = .33$.

Thus, a 1 to 2 cost ratio for a false positive to a false negative can be imposed using for the prior distribution .67 and .33. There is no need to change the values in $L(i, j)$, which in effect, still have off-diagonal cost elements $L(i \neq j) = 1$. Finally, the same results may be obtained by using Eq. 3.11 with $\pi_1 L_1^* = .80 \times 1.0$ and $\pi_2 L_2^* = .20 \times 2.0$.

It would also be handy if analogous procedures were available for categorical response variables with more than two response categories. However, with more than two response categories, there is more than one cost ratio and often, more adjustments are needed than can be properly captured in a revised prior distribution. We will return to this matter in subsequent chapters.

There still is more to the story. Adjusting the prior only affects one feature of the fitting process, and as Fig. 3.7 shows, terminal nodes are also affected by various conditional proportions in the data. If the goal is to have a certain cost ratio in the off-diagonal cells of a *confusion table for the entire tree*, there is absolutely no guarantee that altering the prior by Eq. 3.8 will get the job done.

In practice, therefore, the prior is a tuning parameter used to arrive at desirable off-diagonal cell counts in a confusion table for the entire tree. For example, if the goal is to have in a confusion table a ratio of 5 to 1 for false negatives versus false positives, the prior calculated by Eq. 3.11 may have to be computed with values for L_i^* and L_j^* that are very different from 5 to 1. Some trial and error will be required. Examples are provided later.

Treating the prior (or loss matrix) as a means to arrive at an acceptable cost ratio in a confusion table may seem a bit unprincipled. But this can be fully consistent with Breiman's algorithmic perspective introduced in Chap. 1. As will become more apparent in the pages ahead, statistical learning and machine learning are *procedures* motivated by fitted values that perform well out-of-sample. Getting a responsive cost ratio is part of that performance. Stated only a bit too cavalierly, in this setting, the ends justify the means.

To summarize, when the CART solution is determined solely by the data, the prior distribution is empirically defined, and the costs in the loss matrix are the same for all classification errors. Equal costs are being assigned even if the data analyst makes no conscious decision about them. Should the balance of false negatives to false positives in a confusion table be unsatisfactory, that balance can be changed. The prior distribution can be altered, and with some trial and error, a more satisfactory cost ratio usually can be obtained. An example follows shortly.

3.6 Pruning

With the discussion of costs behind us, we can now return to the problem of overly complex trees and what can be done. Recall that setting a minimum sample size for each terminal node is one strategy. In *rpart()*, the relevant tuning parameter is *minbucket*. Another strategy is to require some minimum reduction in impurity before a new partitioning of the data is undertaken. In *rpart()*, the relevant tuning parameter is *cp*. Still another strategy to constrain the size of the tree is called "pruning." The pruning process removes undesirable branches by combining nodes that do not reduce heterogeneity sufficiently in trade for the extra complexity added. The process starts at the terminal nodes and works back up the tree until all of the remaining nodes are satisfactory. One can think of the tuning parameters *minbucket* and *cp* as serving to "pre-prune" the tree. The material on pruning that follows draws heavily on Therneau and Atkinson (2015, Sect. 4).

Of late, pruning has not gotten a lot of attention. The problem that pruning addresses is very real. But, as CART has become superseded, pruning has become less salient. Consequently, the discussion of pruning here is relatively short. The main objective is to highlight some important issues raised in the previous chapter that figure significantly in the pages ahead.

For a tree T, recall that the overall risk over K terminal nodes is

$$R(T) = \sum_{j=1}^{K} P(A_j)R(A_j). \tag{3.12}$$

This is the sum over all terminal nodes of the risk associated with each node, each risk first multiplied by the probability of a case falling in that node. It might seem that a reasonable pruning strategy would be to directly minimize Eq. 3.12. What could be better than that? Unfortunately, that would leave a saturated tree untouched. CART would construct enough terminal nodes so that all were homogeneous, even if that meant one node for each observation. With all terminal nodes homogeneous, the risk associated with each would be zero. But, the result would be unstable nodes, serious overfitting of the data, and far too much detail to usefully interpret.

The solution is much like what was seen in the previous chapter. A penalty is introduced for complexity, and under the true model perspective in a level II context, the bias–variance tradeoff reappears. For larger trees with a given sample size, there will be fewer classification errors, implying less bias. But larger trees will have terminal nodes with fewer cases in each, which implies greater instability and hence, greater variance. The trick is to find a sensible balance.

To take complexity into account in CART, a popular solution has been to define an objective function for pruning, called "cost complexity," that includes an explicit penalty for complexity. The penalty is not based on the number of parameters, as in conventional regression, or a function of roughness, as in smoothing. For CART, the penalty is a function of the number of terminal nodes. More precisely, one attempts to minimize

$$R_\alpha(T) = R(T) + \alpha|T|. \tag{3.13}$$

$R_\alpha(T)$ has two parts: the total costs of the classification errors for the tree T, and a penalty for complexity. For the latter, $\alpha \geq 0$ is the complexity parameter playing much the same role as λ in smoothing splines. In place of some measure of roughness, $|T|$ is the number of terminal nodes in tree T.

The value of α quantifies the penalty for each additional terminal node. The larger the value of α, the heavier is the penalty for complexity. When $\alpha = 0$, there is no penalty and a saturated tree results. So, α is the means by which the size of the tree can be determined.

Breiman et al. (1984: Sect. 3.3) prove that for any value of the complexity parameter α, there is a unique, smallest subtree of T that minimizes cost complexity. Thus, there cannot be two subtrees of the same size with the same cost complexity. Given α, there is a unique solution.

In many CART implementations, there are ways the software can select a reasonable value for α, or for parameters that play the same role (Zhang and Singer 1999: Sect. 4.2.3). These defaults are often a good place to start, but will commonly lead to results that are unsatisfactory. The tree selected may make a tradeoff between the variance and the bias that is undesirable for the particular analysis being undertaken. For example, there may be far too much detail to be usefully interpreted.

Alternatively, one can specify by trial and error a value of α that leads to terminal nodes, each with a sufficient number of cases, and that can be sensibly interpreted. Interpretation will depend on both the number of terminal nodes and the kinds of cases that fall in each, so a substantial number of different tree models may need to be examined.

More recent thinking on pruning replaces α with cp. Thus,

$$R_{cp}(T) \equiv R(T) + cp * |T| * R(T_1), \tag{3.14}$$

where $R(T_1)$ is the tree with no splits, $|T|$ is now the number of splits for a tree, and R is the risk as before. The value of cp ranges from 0 to 1. When $cp = 0$, one has a saturated tree. When $cp = 1$, there are no splits. A key advantage over α is that cp is unit free and easier to work with. It can be used to pre-prune a tree, much like the minimum bucket size, or can be tuned with procedures such as cross-validation. Sometimes it can be used in both roles for single analysis.

In practice, whether one determines tree complexity by pre-pruning or pruning (or both) seems to make little practical difference. The goal is to construct a useful classification tree. How exactly that is accomplished is less important as long as the steps undertaken and the various results evaluated are recorded so that the work can be replicated.

The major difficulty is that for a level II analysis, a very aggressive model selection exercise is being undertaken. Beyond the data snooping done by CART itself, there is a search over trees. As already noted many times, all statistical inference can be badly compromised. And the best solution, when feasible, is to have training data, evaluation data, and test data that can be used in much the same way they were used for tuning smoothers. Absent such data, a level I analysis may well have to suffice.

3.6.1 Impurity Versus $R_{cp}(T)$

At this point, one might wonder again why CART does not use Eq. 3.14 from the start when a tree is grown instead of some measure of node impurity. $R_{cp}(T)$ would seem to have built in all of the end-user needs very directly.

As mentioned earlier, the rationale for not using a function of classification errors as a fitting criterion is discussed in Breiman et al. (1984: Sect. 4.1). As a technical matter, there can be at any given node, no single best split. But perhaps a more important reason is that less satisfactory trees can result. Consider two splits. For the first, there are two nodes that are about equally heterogeneous. For the second, one node is far more heterogeneous than the other. Suppose the two splits reduce impurity effectively the same amount. Yet, minimizing some function of classification errors could lead to the first split being chosen even though the second split was preferable. For the second split, the less heterogeneous node might serve as a terminal node, or might readily lead to one. The more heterogeneous node would be more subject to further partitioning. For the first split, both nodes would likely be partitioned substantially further. In general, therefore, more complicated tree structures will follow.

There can be good subject matter reasons as well. Thinking back to the prison example, finding a single node that was filled almost completely with misconduct cases would be a very useful result, even if the other terminal nodes were quite heterogeneous. In contrast, having all of the terminal nodes with roughly the same proportions of misconduct and no misconduct cases, would not be very useful. The point of the exercise is find subsets of inmates with different proclivities for misconduct. Using node impurity as a splitting criterion will largely prevent this kind of problem.

3.7 Missing Data

Missing data are a common problem for statistical analyses, and CART is no exception. Broadly stated, missing data creates for CART the same kinds of difficulties created for conventional linear regression. There is the loss of statistical power with the reduction in sample size and a real likelihood of bias insofar as the observations lost are not effectively a random sample of the total. That is, the data are now randomly realized from a new joint probability distribution that does include cases like those that are missing from the data on hand.

There is one and only one ironclad solution to missing data regardless of the form of data analysis: don't have any. The message is that it pays to invest heavily in the data collection so that missing data do not materialize or are very rare. A fallback position is to try to correct the missing data after the data are collected. There are other alternatives to be sure, but all are risky.

Three kinds of missing data mechanisms are commonly considered. For a given variable or sets of variables, there may be no information about certain observations, and that information is "missing completely at random." By "missing completely at random," one means that the mechanism by which the data are lost is equivalent to simple random sampling. A more complicated case is when the information is missing "conditionally at random." By that one means that after conditioning on certain variables, the data are now missing completely at random. For example, the subset of cases that are male may have information about age that is missing completely at random. Finally, the information may be missing systematically. For example, income levels above $100,000 a year may not be recorded regardless of the values of other variables. In a given data set, any combination of these missing data mechanisms may be operating, and the mix shapes what, if any, corrective measures the data analyst employs.

The easiest response to missing data in a multivariate setting is "listwise deletion." If for any case in the data any variable has a missing entry, that case is struck from the data. If the data are missing completely at random, the price is solely a smaller number of observations. A related response in a multivariate setting is "pairwise" deletion. The analysis proceeds with listwise deletion but only for each pair of variables. For example, if for least squares regression some of the predictors have missing values, the cross-product matrix of predictors is assembled for all pairs of predictors based on the number of complete observations for each pair. Many of the computed covariances can be based on different numbers of observations.[11] The most demanding response to missing data is imputation. The basic idea is to replace each missing value with a value that is a useful approximation of what the missing value would have been. There are many different ways this can be done.

Imputation introduces important complications. To begin, one does not ordinarily want to impute values for the response variable. The risk is that artificial relationships between the response and the predictors will be built into the analysis. Consequently, imputation is typically used with predictors only. If there are missing values for the response variable, listwise deletion is usually the prudent choice.

Imputation for predictors alone is hardly problem free. Because the imputed values are rarely the same as what the missing value would have been, measurement error is introduced. Even random measurement error in predictors can bias estimation.[12]

---

[11]In a least squares regression setting, this is generally not a good idea because the covariance matrix may no longer be positive definite.

[12]Consider a conventional regression with a single predictor. Random measurement error (i.e., IID mean 0), will increase the variance of the predictor, which sits in the denominator of slope expression. Asymptotically, $\hat{\beta} = \frac{\beta}{1+\sigma_\epsilon^2/\sigma_x^2}$, where σ_ϵ^2 is the variance of the measurement error and σ_x^2 is the variance of the predictor. The result is a bias toward 0.0. When there is more than one predictor, each with random measurement error, the regression coefficients can be biased toward 0.0 or away from 0.0.

Another difficulty is that an imputed value is typically noisy and that noise should be considered in how the data are analyzed. In practice this can mean imputing missing data several times and taking any random variation into account. Finally, imputed values for a given predictor will often be less variable than the natural variation in that predictor. The reduction in variability can make estimates from the data less precise and invalidate standard errors.

A detailed discussion of missing data is beyond the scope of this book, and excellent treatments are easily found (Little and Rubin 2015). But it is important to consider how missing data can affect CART in particular and what some of the more common responses can be.

3.7.1 Missing Data with CART

Some of the missing data options for CART overlap with conventional practices, and some are special to CART. For the latter, we emphasize the CART options within *rpart( )*. In either case, there are statistical and subject-matter issues that must be considered in the context of *why* there are missing data to begin with. The "why" helps determine what the best response to the missing data should be.

Just as in conventional practice, listwise deletion is always an option, especially when one can make the case that the data are missing completely at random. If the data are missing conditionally at random, and the requisite conditioning variables are in the dataset, it is sometimes possible to build those conditioning variables into the analysis. Then one is back to missing data by, in effect, simple random sampling.

A second set of options is to impute the data outside of CART itself. To take a simple illustration, a predictor with the missing data is regressed on complete data predictors with which it is likely to be related. The resulting regression equation can then be used to impute what the missing values might be.

For example, suppose that for employed individuals there are some missing data for income. But income is strongly related to education, age, and occupation. For the subset of observations with no missing income data, income is regressed on education, age, and occupation. Then, for the observations that have missing income data, values for the three predictors can be inserted into the estimated regression equation. Predicted values follow that can be used to fill in the holes for the income variable. At that point, CART can be applied as usual.

A useful extension of this strategy is to sample randomly from the predictive distribution to obtain several imputed values for each missing value. CART can then be applied to the data several times with different imputations in place. One can at least get a sense of whether the different imputed values make an important difference (He 2006). If they do, there are averaging strategies derived from procedures addressed in the next chapter.

A third option is to address the missing data for predictors within CART itself. There are a number of ways this might be done. We consider here one of the better approaches, and the one available with *rpart()* in R. As before, we only address missing data for predictors.

The first place where missing data will matter is when a split is chosen. Recall that

$$\Delta I(s, A) = I(A) - p(A_L)I(A_L) - p(A_R)I(A_R), \qquad (3.15)$$

where $I(A)$ is the value of the parent impurity, $p(A_R)$ is the probability of a case falling in the right daughter node, $p(A_L)$ is the probability of a case falling in the left daughter node, $I(A_R)$ is the impurity of the right daughter node, and $I(A_L)$ is the impurity of the left daughter node. CART tries to find the predictor and the split for which $\Delta I(s, A)$ is as large as possible.

Consider the leading term on the righthand side. One can calculate its value without any predictors and so, there are no missing values to worry about. However, to construct the two daughter nodes, predictors are required. Each predictor is evaluated as usual, but using only the predictor values that are not missing. That is, $I(A_R)$ and $I(A_L)$ are computed for each optimal split for each predictor using only the data available for the given predictor. The associated probabilities $p(A_R)$ and $p(A_L)$ are re-estimated for each predictor based on the data actually present. This is essentially pairwise deletion.

But determining the split is only half the story. Now, observations have to be assigned to one of the two daughter nodes. How can this be done if the predictor values needed are missing? CART employs a sort of "CART-lite" to impute those missing values by exploiting "surrogate variables."

Suppose there are ten other predictors $x_1 - x_{10}$ that are to be included in the CART analysis, and suppose there are missing observations for x_1 only, which happens to be the predictor chosen to define the split; the split defines two categories for x_1.

The predictor x_1 now becomes a binary response variable with the two classes determined by the split. CART is applied with binary x_1 as the response and $x_2 - x_{10}$ as potential splitting variables. As before pairwise deletion is employed. Only one partitioning is allowed; a full tree is not constructed. The nine predictors are then ranked by the proportion of cases in x_1 that are misclassified. Predictors that do not do substantially better than the marginal distribution of x_1 are dropped from further consideration.

The variable with the lowest classification error for x_1 is used in place of x_1 to assign cases to one of the two daughter nodes when the observations on x_1 are missing. That is, a predicted class for x_1 is used when the actual classes for x_1 are missing. If there are missing data for the highest ranked predictor of x_1, the second highest predictor is used instead. If there are missing data for the second highest ranked predictor of x_1, the third highest ranked predictor is used instead, and so on. If each of the variables $x_2 - x_{10}$ has missing data, the marginal distribution of the x_1 split is used. For example, if the split is defined so that $x_1 < c$ sends observations to the left and $x_1 \geq c$ sends cases to the right, cases with data missing on x_1, which have no surrogate to use instead, are placed along with the majority of cases.

This is a reasonable, but ad hoc, response to missing data. One can think of alternatives that might perform better. But the greatest risk is that if there are lots of missing data and the surrogate variables are used, the correspondence between the results and the data, had they been complete, can become very tenuous. In practice, the data will rarely be missing completely at random or even conditionally at random. Then, if too many observations are manufactured, a new kind of generalization error will be introduced. The irony is that imputation can fail just when it is needed the most. Imputation can be most helpful when there are only a few instances of missing data for single predictors, but the cases with missing data vary over those predictors. Listwise deletion can then decimate the dataset. Imputation may then be a better approach.

But perhaps the best advice is to avoid the use of surrogate variables. The temptations for misuse are great, and there is no clear missing data threshold beyond which imputation is likely to produce misleading results. Imputation of the missing values for the predictors will often be a software option, not a requirement. (But check what the default is.)

Alternatively, one should at least look carefully at the results with and without using surrogates. Results that are substantially different need to be reported to whomever is going to use the findings. There may then be a way to choose on subject matter grounds which results are more sensible. Sometimes neither set will be sensible, which takes us back to where we began. Great efforts should be made to avoid missing data.

3.8 Statistical Inference with CART

As before, there is no statistical inference for a level I analysis. For a level II analysis, one again must make the case that the data are realized from a joint probability distribution of subject-matter interest. Both Y and X are random variables.

Consistent with the discussion in Chap. 1, one should probably give up on the idea of trying to estimate the true tree structure or the true response surface as features of the joint probability distribution responsible for the data. Even if all of the requisite predictors are available in the data, there is no reason to think that the use of step functions coupled with the stagewise fitting procedure will lead to a model that is at least first order correct.

A potentially more viable approach is to estimate an explicit, tree-based, approximation of the true response surface. For reasons already discussed and soon to be elaborated, the partitions themselves, usually displayed as an inverted tree, should be of little interest. Rather, the tree's fitted values can be very important whether those fitted values are the terminal node proportions or the assigned terminal node classes. The estimation target is those fitted values derived from a tree with the same features as the tree grown with the training data.

But there is a new wrinkle. All of the procedures discussed so far do not engage in model selection once the tuning parameters are determined. The defining features of the procedure are then fixed, and the procedure can simply be applied with test data. To take our earliest example, linear least squares with the selected predictors can be used with the test data, and there are no model selection issues.

CART is fundamentally different. To apply CART to new data means that the data partitioning begins again. Even if all tuning parameters are already determined, extensive model selection is undertaken. Test data do not solve this problem because the test data will be subject to the new partitioning.

Probably the best way to proceed is to reformulate the estimation problem. Interest in the CART response surface approximation remains, but CART is not allowed to partition the test data. Rather, the data partitions determined using the training data and the evaluation data are fixed. This means that the tree structure and terminal nodes are fixed as well. The test data are used solely for prediction. Test data predictor values are dropped down the tree and fitted values computed. Those fitted values serve as asymptotically unbiased estimates of the CART approximation of the true response surface. An honest confusion table can follow. Here are the steps.

1. For a set of potential values for tuning parameters, fit classification trees in the *training* data. Key tuning parameters are likely to be values for the prior and the *cp*.
2. Drop the *evaluation* data down each tree, and compute the fitted values. For classification trees, then construct an evaluation data confusion table. From those tables, performance measures can be obtained.
3. Select a "best" classification tree.
4. Using the selected tree, drop the *test* data down the selected tree and compute the fitted values.
5. Cross-tabulate the predicted outcome classes in the test data by the actual test data response classes. Construct a confusion table from that cross-tabulation. That confusion table provides an asymptotically unbiased estimate of the population confusion table approximation if the population realizations were dropped down the selected tree. The overall misclassification rate provides an estimate of generalization error. If misclassification costs are asymmetric, the different classification errors should be weighted by their relative costs should an overall measure of performance be desired.
6. Apply a nonparametric bootstrap to the *test* data to obtain a family of confusion tables and instructive summary statistics. The distribution of those summary statistics can be used to characterize uncertainty in the estimate of generalization error. Consistent with the earlier discussion of generalization error, the training data and tree structure are fixed. We will explain more about the bootstrap in the next chapter. Also, the last exercise for this chapter addresses the bootstrap with code provided.

Compared to the options offered in the last chapter, the level II formulation is more restricted. Results from the fitting procedure are fixed. They are not re-computed with the test data, so an important source of uncertainty has been neglected. We are back within a generalization error framework discussed in Chap. 1. The training data and the results from the training data are a given. One still must make the case that the data are realized from a substantively relevant population, but with that credibly accomplished, a level II analysis can proceed.

There have been some very interesting efforts to think about statistical inference with CART when there is a single dataset. In particular, Horthorn and colleagues (2006) provide a rationale and R library *party* for using permutation procedures to help determine which splits are justified couple with tests of the null hypothesis that there is actually no association between the response and the split selected. However, it is not clear how the permutation tests properly take into account the full set of tests undertaken, the dependence between tests undertaken for a given split, and test results from earlier splits. The impact of tuning also seems to have been overlooked. In addition, the realized values of the predictors are treated as fixed (once realized). It is not apparent how one thinks about forecasting applications when the realized x-values are treated as fixed. What does one do with a new realized case having x-values not represented in the training data?

Options from a Bayesian perspective have also been proposed (Chipman et al. 1998, 1999). A key feature of the Bayesian approach is the use of several different kinds of prior distributions. But, if Bayesian approaches are to be taken seriously as inferential tools, the priors must be taken seriously as well. In practice, the prior distributions typically are used to tune the results and are really not very different from CART tuning parameters like *cp* or *minbuckets*. That's fine, but undermines Bayesian statistical inference.

A reasonable overall assessment is that there are many unsolved problems with CART level II analyses. Lots of interesting work is in progress about post-model selection inference more generally, but at the moment, no fully satisfactory solutions exist. This may well explain why most CART applications are effectively level I analyses.

3.9   From Classification to Forecasting

Forecasting with CART was covered in pieces earlier. Here is the material summarized and in one place.

When a classification tree is used for forecasting, a level II analysis is being undertaken, and the goal is usually to forecast a class. The training data and tree grown from the training data are treated as fixed. There are new cases for which the predictor values are known but the response class is not. New cases are "dropped down" the tree. The class previously assigned to the terminal node in which a case lands, is the forecasted class. Alternatively, the forecasting process can be understood getting fitted values from the regression equation characterizing all of the terminal nodes (e.g., Eq. 3.1).

A key assumption is that the new cases whose outcomes need to be forecasted are realized from the same joint probability distribution as the training data. Unless the joint probability distribution is for a well defined, finite population, and the new cases have be selected by probability sampling, there is no way to know if the assumption is true. In practice, the validity of the assumption is usually a matter of degree that needs to be argued on subject-matter grounds.[13]

In the prison example introduced earlier, the mix of new inmates who are recently admitted must be effectively the same as the mix of inmates in the training data. The prison setting, staffing, and regulations are also unchanged. These issues need to be addressed by individuals who are very familiar with local scene. Sometimes, data may be brought to bear. Is there evidence, for example, of temporal trends in gang affiliations that inmates might bring into the prison? However, the data will usually not have all of the relevant information and whatever the results, it is difficult to know how large changes need to be before the forecasts become insufficiently accurate.

Probably the best strategy is to keep track of forecasting accuracy over time. For each inmate, actual outcomes can be empirically determined for some reasonable amount of elapsed time after intake (e.g., 2 years). Those outcomes can be compared to the forecast at intake. With a sufficient number of inmates, a confusion table can be constructed. Such analyses can be repeated with new inmates over time so that changes in forecasting accuracy are documented. At some point, declines in forecasting accuracy may be sufficient for stakeholders to ask for an update of the classification tree.

In the past, forecasting was an important application for CART. There are now better forecasting tools, for reasons that will soon be apparent. Nevertheless, CART is often a foundation for these better methods and many of the issues resurface.

3.10 Varying the Prior and the Complexity Parameter

Figure 3.8 shows again the tree diagram for the CART analysis of inmate misconduct. Recall that the empirical distribution of the response variable was used as the prior distribution, the costs were assumed to be the same for false negatives and false positives, and the number of terminal nodes was constrained by setting the minimum terminal node sample size.

Recall also the confusion table. It is reproduced here as Table 3.4. One questionable feature of the table was that there were about 21 false negatives for each false positive, implying that false positives were far more costly than false negatives.

Conversations with prison officials indicated that from their point of view, false negatives were worse than false positives. Failing to anticipate inmate misconduct, which could involve fatal violence, was of far greater concern than incorrectly labeling an inmate as high risk. When pushed, a prison official said that the cost of a false negative was at least twice the cost of a false positive. Hence, the earlier analysis got things upside down.

---

[13]If the population is finite, there technically is no joint probability distribution. There is multivariate histogram. This was discussed in Chap. 1.

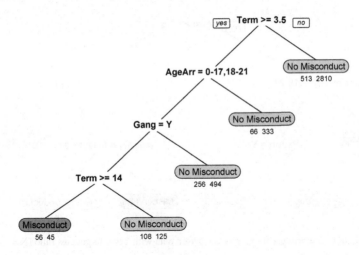

Fig. 3.8 CART recursive partitioning of the prison data with default costs (The *red nodes* represent misconduct, the *blue nodes* represent no misconduct, N = 4806.)

Table 3.4 CART confusion table for classifying inmate misconduct with the default cost ratio (Even with the same data, N's can vary over different analyses because of missing data patterns, N = 4816)

	Classify as no misconduct	Classify as misconduct	Model error
No misconduct	3762	45	.01
Misconduct	953	56	.95
Use error	.20	.45	Overall error = .21

Figure 3.9 shows the tree diagram that results when the target cost ratio of false negatives to false positives in the confusion table is 2 to 1. The code is shown in Fig. 3.10.

Setting appropriate values for *prior* and *cp* is explicit tuning. The process can involve some trial and error and in this illustration, the task was complicated by a tree with relatively few terminal nodes. When there are few terminal nodes, the distribution of fitted classes can be lumpy so that getting the empirical cost ratio right in the confusion table may not be possible. With a specified prior of 52 % misconducts and 48 % no misconducts, the confusion table cost ratio was approximately 2.5 false positives for every false negative. False negatives are about 2.5 times more costly. The results do not change materially with cost ratios between approximately 2 and 3.5.

At first, the terminal nodes in Fig. 3.9 may seem a little odd. There is not a single terminal node in which there are more misconduct cases than no misconduct cases and yet, there are three terminal models with misconduct as the fitted class. The reason is that the counts shown in each terminal node are weighted by the new prior.

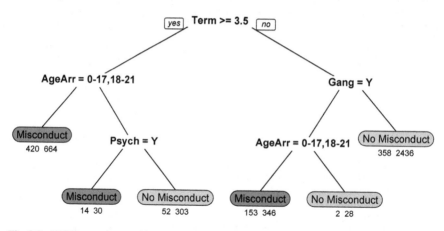

Fig. 3.9 CART recursive partitioning of the prison data with 2 to 1 target cost ratio (N = 4797)

```
# Partition the data
out<-rpart(Fail~AgeArr+Gang+CDC+Jail+Psych+Term,
           data=temp, method="class",
           parms = list(prior = c(.52,.48)),cp=.004)
# Plot a Tree
prp(out,extra=1,faclen=10,varlen=15,under=T
    box.col=c("red","lightblue")[out$frame$yval])
```

Fig. 3.10 R code for the CART analysis of prison misconduct with a 2 to 1 target cost ratio

Misconduct cases constitute about 21 % of the observations but are now treated as if they constitute a little over half. The number of misconduct cases in each terminal node is multiplied by about 2.5 when the fitted class is determined. The ratio of the new prior for misconduct of .52 to the old prior misconduct of .21 is about 2.5.

The partitioning in Fig. 3.9 returns a somewhat different story from the partitioning in Fig. 3.8. Misconduct is the fitted class for young inmates with long nominal terms. Gang membership is not required. For older inmates with long nominal terms, a diagnosed psychological problem leads to a misconduct fitted class. Inmates with shorter nominal terms who are young and gang members are also classified as misconduct cases. All of these results are produced by interaction effects. There are no terminal nodes defined by main effects.

Table 3.5 shows dramatic changes. Increasing relative the costs of false negatives relative to false positives leads to more terminal nodes with misconduct as the assigned class. This is precisely what was intended. As a result, there is a dramatic increase in CART's ability to accurately classify misconduct and in trade, a dramatic reduction in CART's ability to accurately classify no misconduct cases. Overall error is increased a bit, but as already explained, the overall error rate is misleading when the costs of classification errors are asymmetric. The overall error rate treats all clas-

Table 3.5 CART confusion table for classifying inmate misconduct with 2 to 1 target cost ratio (N = 4797)

	Classify as no misconduct	Classify as misconduct	Model error
No misconduct	2767	1040	.27
Misconduct	412	578	.42
Use error	.13	.64	Overall error = .30

sification errors the same. Finally, the use errors have changed as well. When no misconduct is the fitted class, it is incorrect 13 % of the time rather than 20 % of the time. In trade, the use error when misconduct is the fitted class increases from 45 % to 64 %.

The confusion table is constructed from training data only and is no doubt subject to overfitting. For a level I analysis, that comes with the territory. Nevertheless, the changes in use error could have important implications for level II forecasting because the fitted class becomes the forecasted class for new cases when that outcome is not known. By making false negatives more costly, the CART algorithm is, in effect, accepting weaker statistical evidence when misconduct is the fitted class or when misconduct is forecasted; the algorithm is trying harder not to overlook potential misconduct cases. The flip side is that for no misconduct to be the fitted or forecasted class, the algorithm requires stronger statistical evidence. As result, classification and forecasting accuracy (i.e., conditioning on the fitted class) will decline for misconduct outcomes and improve for no misconduct outcomes.

There is nothing mandatory about these results. One might think that there is some sensible way to define an optimal result and a way to produce it. But, even when one has training data, evaluation data and test data, optimality is usually a pipe dream. As a technical matter, several different configurations of tuning parameters values often can lead to very similar results.

The preferred cost ratio complicates matters further. It should be determined by stakeholders, not the data analyst, and depend on decisions that will be informed by the CART tree and confusion table. Such decision-making responsibilities are usually is not included in the job description of a data analyst.

But even with a given cost ratio, how well CART performs is not easily reduced to a single number. For example, some observers might want the tree structure to make subject matter sense. There is no single number by which that can be measured. Other observers may just want a tree structure that is easily interpreted. Again, there is no single number. Still other observers may care little about the tree structure and focus instead on classification accuracy. However, there can be several measures of classification accuracy extracted from a confusion table. In short, there will often be a substantial disconnect between the goals of explanation, classification and forecasting. Even when one dominates, there may well be no single evaluation yardstick to optimize.

There also can be pragmatic complications. In this illustration, prison officials might want to place all inmates forecasted to be problematic in high security settings. But high security incarceration is very expensive (about like Harvard tuition), and if too many misconduct cases are forecasted, the requisite resources will not be available. In effect, there is some threshold above which the number of false positives and true positives breaks the bank. There can be as well legal and political complications if too many false positives are forecasted. Prison officials can be criticized for "over-incarceration."

In short, a reasonable stance is that CART will sometimes provide useful information but rarely definitive guidance. How helpful the information is will depend on the information with which it competes. When decision-makers are operating in an information vacuum, very weak CART results can be valuable. When a lot is already known, strong CART results can be irrelevant. Fortunately, there are much more powerful statistical learning procedures coming.

3.11 An Example with Three Response Categories

In broad brush strokes, there is no formal problem extending CART to three or more response variable categories. But the bookkeeping is much more demanding and getting the cost ratios right is sometimes quite difficult. To see how this happens, we reanalyze the prison data with the three-category response variable: serious and substantial misconduct, some less serious form of misconduct, and no misconduct. About 78 % of the cases have no reported misconduct, about 20 % have minor reported misconduct, and about 2 % have serious and substantial reported misconduct. The 2 % represents very rare cases that ordinarily present a daunting classification challenge. The available predictors are the same as before.

The first hurdle is arriving at sensible cost ratios for classification errors. Prison administrator were concerned about even minor misconduct because it can be a test of staff authority and lead to more serious problems. Still, reported cases of serious and substantial misconduct were of somewhat greater concern. After some back and forth, the following cost ratios were provisionally agreed upon, which can be compared to the results in Table 3.6. The agreement is about as good as one can get without a large number of terminal nodes.

- Misclassifying a "substantial" as a "none" was taken to be about 5 times worse than misclassifying a "none" as a "substantial." In fact, cell 31/cell 13 = 188/31 = 6.1
- Misclassifying a "substantial" as a "some" was taken to be about about 2 times worse than misclassifying a "some" as a "substantial." In fact, cell 23/cell 32 = 117/70 = 1.7
- Misclassifying a "some" as a "none" was taken to be about 2 times worse than misclassifying a "none" as a "some." In fact, cell 12/cell21 = 1181/301 = 2.0

Table 3.6 CART confusion table for classifying inmate misconduct with three outcome classes and target cost ratios ($N = 4736$)

	Classify as none	Classify as some	Classify as substantial	Model error
None	2438	1181	188	.36
Some	301	443	117	.49
Substantial	31	70	37	.73
Use error	.11	.74	.89	Overall error = .39

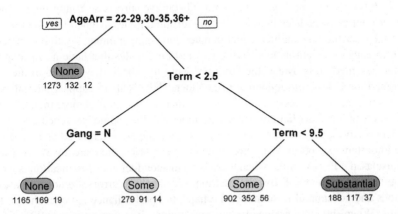

Fig. 3.11 CART recursive partitioning of the prison data with three outcome classes (*Red* terminal nodes represent substantial misconduct, *yellow* terminal nodes represent some misconduct, and *green* terminal nodes represent no misconduct. The order of the numbers below each terminal node is alphabetical: none, some, substantial. $N = 4806$)

```
library(rpart) # Load the CART library
library(rpart.plot) # Load the fancy plotting library
# Partition the data
out<-rpart(Fail3Way~AgeArr+Gang+CDC+Jail+Psych+Term,
           data=temp, method="class",
           parms = list(prior = c(.35,.35,.30)),cp=.01)
#Plot a tree
prp(out,extra=1,faclen=10,varlen=15,under=T
    box.col=c("green","yellow","red")[out$frame$yval])
```

Fig. 3.12 R code for the analysis of prison misconduct

Given reasonable cost ratios in the confusion table (to which we will return), Fig. 3.11 shows the associated classification tree. The R code is provided in Fig. 3.12. With three outcome classes, one reads the classification tree much like before. The main difference is that in each terminal node there is one count for each class arranged in alphabetical order from left to right. As before, the outcome with the largest prior-weighted count determines the class assigned to a terminal node. But here is where the bookkeeping starts to matter. Because the prior has three classes, the weighting is more complicated. Tuning is more intricate. For example, 2 % of the cases in the empirical priors are reported for serious and substantial misconduct, but cost-sensitive prior arrived at assigns a value of 30 %. Such cases are upweighted by a factor of about 15. At the other extreme, the no misconduct cases account for 78 % of the cases in the empirical prior but only 35 % of the tuned cost-sensitive prior. These cases are down weighted by a factor of about .45. In short, all of the votes in each terminal node are given more or less weight than their raw counts indicate.

With the weighting, Fig. 3.11 has no substantive surprises. Young inmates with longer nominal sentences land in the only terminal node assigned the class of substantial or serious misconduct. Older inmates and younger inmates with shorter terms and no gang associations land in the two terminal nodes that have no misconduct as the assigned class. But if the latter are gang members, they placed in the node assigned some, less consequential misconduct. There is also an apparent break point for nominal sentences less than 9.5. years. Inmates with terms of more than 2.5 years but less than 9.5 years land in a terminal node with the "some" assigned class.

The performance measures in the confusion table are interpreted as before with one important exception. With three outcome categories, there are always two ways to misclassify. For example, when there is no misconduct, the classification is wrong about a third of the time. But the vast majority of those errors are not for cases of serious and substantial misconduct. Perhaps, the performance is better than it first seems. When the class assigned is no misconduct, it is correct nearly 90 % of the time. As before, the cost ratios require that there be strong statistical evidence before a case is classified as a no misconduct. Related reasoning can be applied to the other two outcomes.

Outcomes with more than two classes are common and often very desirable. For example, forecasting how an inmate will do on parole has historically been done so that any form of recidivism counts as a failure. The absence of recidivism is a success. Of late and in response to expressed needs to criminal justice stakeholders, more than two outcome classes are increasingly being used (Berk 2012). One might want to distinguish between new arrests for crimes of violence and new arrests for crimes in which there is no violence. There are then three outcome classes: no arrest, an arrest for a crime that is not violent, and an arrest for a violent crime.

Just as with the earlier, two-outcome analysis of prison misconduct, the results are derived solely from training data. Ideally, one would work with training data, evaluation data and test data. In a forecasting setting, the three data sets can be essential because before forecasting with real consequences is undertaken, one must have a classification tree that is tuned well and provides an honest assessment of out-of-sample performance.

3.12   Some Further Cautions in Interpreting CART Results

Just as for any data analysis procedure, the output from CART always demands scrutiny before substantive conclusions are reached. There are commonly three kinds of potential problems: inappropriate response functions, unstable tree structures, and unstable classifications. All can produce results, which if taken at face value, risk serious interpretive errors.

3.12.1   Model Bias

On this point, we can be brief. Should the goal of a CART analysis be to determine the true response surface in the parent joint probability distribution, disappointment will follow. Even if all of the required predictors are included in the data, there is absolutely no guarantee that the correct function will be discovered. Why step functions? Why various high-order interactions? And no claims can be made that the stagewise partitioning will perform as well as a less constrained approach. In short, it is likely that by the standard of truth, the $\hat{f}(\mathbf{X})$ is substantially wrong.

For a level I analysis, these limitations are unfortunate, but useful insights may still follow. For a level II analysis, estimates of an approximate response surface in the joint probability distribution using the training data alone will also be biased in unknown ways. Because of the predictor selection process, all statistical inference (including confidence intervals and statistical tests) is compromised. However, asymptotically unbiased estimates of the tree approximation of the true response surface can be constructed when there is sufficient test data, and one can accept a perspective in which the training data and the CART partitioning are fixed.

3.12.2   Model Variance

Estimation variance is not an issue for a CART level I analysis because the enterprise is descriptive. Estimation variance is a significant problem for CART level II analyses. Indeed, one of the reasons why CART is no longer a popular data analysis procedure is that it can be very unstable.

The most obvious difficulty is the stability in classes assigned to terminal nodes. Each fitted class is determined by a vote within a single terminal node. No estimation strength is borrowed from other nodes. Nor is there any smoothing over nodes. Consequently, when the number of observations in a node is small, the results of the within-node vote could come out very differently in a new realized dataset. The instability can be especially troubling when the within-node votes are close. With very small changes in the composition of node, the assigned class can change. If the assigned classes are unstable, generalization error will be inflated. As noted earlier, however, if small samples within nodes is a concern, the problem can be addressed at least in part with tuning. But as also noted, the risk is an increase in bias with respect to the true response surface.

Instability is even a greater problem in the partitioning process. Just as with the assignment of classes to terminal nodes, very small differences based on very few observations can make a critical difference. Moreover, the stagewise process guarantees that when an unstable splitting decisions is made, its consequences cascade down through all subsequent splits. Recall also that although the "best" split is chosen at each stage, there may very little difference in fitting performance between the best split and the second best split.

Just as with conventional stepwise regression, instability in tree structure is exacerbated with predictors that are strongly correlated. Figure 3.13 provides an illustration. We again have a binary outcome represented by A or B, and X and Z as predictors. The tight ellipse in the figure means that the two predictors have a strong linear relationship.

The first split is shown by the red vertical line. The B outcome dominates to the left, and the A outcome dominates to the right. For the partition to the right, two possible partitions are shown. One partition, shown with the green vertical line, splits on Z a second time. The result would be a more complex step function linking Z and the outcome. The other partition, shown with the horizontal yellow line, splits on X. The result would be an interaction effect between X and Z. The two alternatives imply very different tree structures and subject-matter interpretations.

If the vertical green line is chosen, the partition at the upper left favors As 4 to 1. If the horizontal yellow line is chosen, the partition at the upper left favors As 3 to 1. Clearly the difference in impurity is small, and the result of the single, circled A. With a new data realization, a entirely different split will likely be chosen.

Figure 3.14 addresses the same issues when the two predictors are not as strongly related in a linear fashion. The As and Bs are more spread out on the $X-Z$ plane. After the initial split, the next split is determined by a larger number of observations. The difference in impurity between the horizontal and vertical splits no longer depends

Fig. 3.13 Greater instability in CART partitioning when X and Z are highly correlated (The *red vertical line* is the first split. The *yellow* and *green lines* represent two possible choices for the second split.)

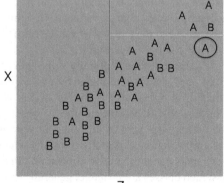

Fig. 3.14 Less instability in CART partitioning when X and Z are not highly correlated

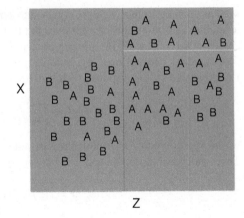

on a single observation. The horizontal split is more homogeneous in A than the vertical split (i.e., 7 out of 10 v. 6 out of 13). Recall that in practice, there are other statistical features of the competing splits to consider, but the point here is with less dependence between X and Z, more stable partitions are likely.

In summary, CART classifications will likely be more stable than the structure of the classification tree. Nevertheless, it is always important to study the distribution of classes within each terminal node. When there are few cases or when the vote is close, the class assigned can be unreliable. Instability in tree structure is more difficult to deal with, but an examination of the sequence of splitting decision can be helpful. (In *rpart()*, that information is easily accessed.) Much as for the terminal nodes, one can consider how many observations determined the split and how much better the winning split was compared to its competitors.

3.13 Regression Trees

The emphasis in this chapter has been on categorical response variables. For reasons that were both pedagogical and practical, classification has been the primary topic. By concentrating on categorical response variables, the full range of fundamental issues surrounding CART are raised.

But CART is certainly not limited to categorical response variables. Quantitative response variables are also fair game. And with the discussion of categorical response variables largely behind us, a transition to quantitative response variables is relatively straightforward. It is possible to be brief.

Perhaps the major operational complication is the kind of regression method to be applied. For example, there are three options in *rpart()* labeled as "anova", "poisson," and "exp." The first is for conventional quantitative response variables such as income. The second is for count response variables such as the number of hurricanes in a given hurricane season. The third is for survival response variables such as the time from release from prison to a new arrest. Code to be written, options available, and output differ a bit over the three. Beneath the hood, the algorithmic details differ a bit too. The splitting criterion is now some variant on the deviance.

Consider a conventional regression application as an illustration. Node impurity is represented by the response within-node sum of squares:

$$i(\tau) = \sum (y_i - \bar{y}(\tau))^2, \tag{3.16}$$

where the summation is over all cases in node τ, and $\bar{y}(\tau)$ is the mean of those cases. Then, much as before, the split s is chosen to maximize

$$\Delta(s, \tau) = i(\tau) - i(\tau_L) - i(\tau_R). \tag{3.17}$$

Recall that for the split decision when the response is categorical, the Gini impurities are weighted by the proportion of cases in each potential daughter node. For the sum of squares impurities, there is no weighting. But because the sum of squares is a sum over observations, the number of cases in each daughter node matters; there is implicit weighting. One can be more direct by reformulating the problem in units of variances. Impurity for the parent node is represented by the variance of its y-values. Likewise, impurity in the derived nodes is represented by each of their variances. Before they are added, the two variances are weighted by the proportion of cases in their respective node. The proportion weights provide the opportunity to employ different weights. Ishwaran (2015) examined three kinds: no weighting, weighting by the node proportions and weighting by the node proportions squared (called "heavy" weighting). Conventional weighting is said to work best for regression trees when predictors are very noisy.

No asymmetric cost weights can be used because there is no reasonable way to consider false positives and false negatives without a categorical response variable. Ideally, one would alter the way impurity is computed. This is easily done for quantile regression applications, but not for least squares applications. There is interesting work in progress on quantile regression trees (Chaudhuri and Loh 2002; Bhat et al. 2011).

To get the impurity for the entire tree, one sums over all terminal nodes to arrive at $R(T)$. In *rpart()*, regression trees can be pruned using the *cp* tuning parameter. Just as with categorical response variables, one can also "pre-prune" using the *cp*.

The summary statistic for each terminal node is usually the node's mean. In principle, a wide variety of summary statistics could be computed (e.g., the median). And just like for conventional regression, one can compute overall measures of fit. Unfortunately, with all of the searching over possible splits and predictors, it is not clear how to adjust for the degrees of freedom used up. There is no summary measure of fit that can account for this form of overfitting. As usual, the best course of action is to use test data to get an honest assessment of fit but as discussed earlier, this is has it own complications.

Just as in parametric regression, the fitted values can be used for forecasting. Each new observation for which the outcome is unknown is dropped down the tree. The fitted value for the terminal node in which an observation lands become the forecast. Typically, that is the conditional mean.

All of the earlier concerns about CART still apply, save for those linked to the classes assigned. Potential bias and instability remain serious problems. Possible remedies, insofar as they exist, are also effectively the same.

3.13.1 A CART Application for the Correlates of a Student's GPA in High School

Figure 3.15 shows a regression tree for applicants to a large public university. Figure 3.16 shows the code. The response variable is a student's GPA in high school. Predictors include the verbal SAT score, the mathematics SAT score, gender, and household income. Grade point average can be as high as 5.0 because the scoring gives performance in advanced placement classes extra weight. The mean GPA in each node is shown along with the number of cases in that node.[14]

Students with Math SAT scores above 695 and verbal SAT scores above 675 have the highest mean grade point average. Their mean is 4.2. Students with verbal SAT scores less than 565 and math SAT scores below 515 have the lowest mean grade point average. Their mean is 3.4. The two terminal nodes are characterized by interaction effects between the verbal and math SATs. All of the other branches suggest rather complicated and not easily explained relationships. For example, students with verbal SAT scores below 565 and math SAT scores above 515, get an extra boost if they are from families with incomes over $77,000. That students from higher income household do a bit better is no surprise. But why that boost only materializes within a certain set of SAT score values is not apparent. The role of gender is even more obscure. Claims are sometimes made that one of CART's assets is the ease with which a classification or regression tree can be interpreted. In practice, splits based on reductions in impurity often do not lead to results with credible subject-matter interpretations.

There are no confusion tables for quantitative response variables. But one can get a sense of fit performance from Fig. 3.17 produced by *rsq.rpart()*.[15] Both plots show the number of splits on the horizontal axis. On the vertical axis for the plot on the left is the usual R^2. The Apparent R^2 (in blue) is computed from the data used to grow the regression tree. The X relative R^2 (in green) is computed using cross-validation in an effort to get a more honest measure of fit. In this case, the two are almost identical and approach .20 as the number of splits increases. The cross-validation R^2 levels out a bit sooner. There is little improvement in the quality of the fit when the

---

[14]These data cannot be shared.

[15]The function defaults to only black and white. If you want color (or something else) you need to get into the source code. It's not a big deal.

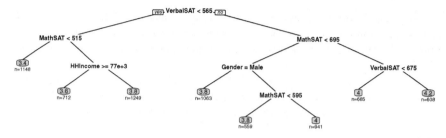

Fig. 3.15 CART recursive partitioning of high school GPA data (The number in each terminal node is the conditional mean. $N = 6965$)

```
# Construct CART Partitions
out<-rpart(GPA~VerbalSAT+MathSAT+HHIncome+Gender,
           data=temp, method="anova", cp=.005)
# Construct a CART tree
prp(out,extra=1,faclen=10,varlen=15,under=T)
# Get Fit Plots
par(mfrow=c(1,1))
rsq.rpart(out)
```

Fig. 3.16 R code for the analysis of the high school GPA data

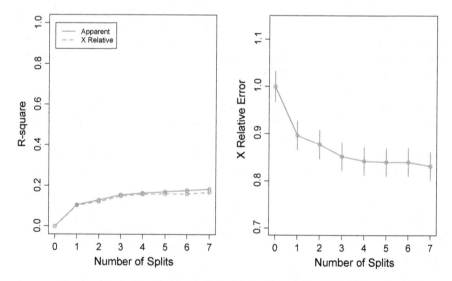

Fig. 3.17 Plots of GPA regression fit. (The *left* figure shows the increase in R^2 with increases in the number of splits. The *solid line* is computed in-sample. The *dashed line* is computed through cross-validation. The *left* figure shows the reduction in relative fitting error with increases in the number of splits. The *vertical lines* are *error bars*.)

number greater than 3. It is also apparent from the similarity of the two lines that the CART search procedures do not seem to have produced problematic overfitting in this instance. This follows from the large number of observations and small number of predictors. Relative to the number of observations, the amount of data snooping is modest. Relatively few degrees have been spent.

The plot on the right side shows the relative improvement in fit. On the vertical axis is the proportional reduction in mean squared error. The vertical lines shows plus and minus one standard error estimated by cross-validation. For this plot, we see that there is little evidence of systematic improvement after the first split, and no evidence of systematic improvement after the 3rd split. The first two errors bars do not overlap at all. Subsequent error bars overlap to varying degrees. The availability of these error bars is helpful, but given all of the problems with CART level II analyses, they should not be taken literally. Moreover, there seems to be no formal justification for using "the 1-SE rule" rather some some other rule (e.g., a 2-SE rule).

For this application, one could probably make a good case for a level II analysis. A relevant joint probability distribution could probably be defined with each observation realized independently. Figure 3.17 suggests that the consequences of data snooping may not be serious. And the number of observations is large enough to make good use of asymptotics. One might want to grow a new regression tree with up to three splits and base any interpretations or applications on that single tree, especially if this were done in test data. The estimation target would be the fitted values from that tree as a feature of the joint probability distribution.

3.14 Multivariate Adaptive Regression Splines (MARS)

Multivariate Adaptive Regression Splines (MARS) can be viewed as another kind of smoother, in the traditions of the last chapter, or as a twist on classification and regression trees. This brief discussion will build on the latter and especially regression trees because MARS assumes that the response variable is quantitative. An excellent and far more extensive exposition of MARS can be found in Hastie et al. (2009: Sect. 9.4).

A key difference between CART and MARS is in the nature of the basis functions used. The MARS formulation is the broadly familiar

$$f(X) = \beta_0 + \sum_{m=1}^{M} \beta_m h_m(X), \tag{3.18}$$

where as before, there are M weighted basis functions $h_m(X)$. But each $h_m(X)$ is a product variable composed of linear piecewise splines. This takes a little explaining.

Just as for CART, the basis functions are determined by searching over all predictors and breakpoints. In CART, this leads to a step function. In MARS, this leads to a V-shaped function composed of two linear piecewise splines, with its minimum value of 0.0 at the breakpoint chosen. The two splines are mirror images of one another; hence the V-shape. Hastie et al. (2009: 322) call the two splines a "reflected pair."

Figure 3.18 is an illustration with a hypothetical breakpoint at 0.5. To the left of breakpoint, the values of the basis function are the positive values of the predictor X subtracted from the breakpoint value. To the right of breakpoint, the values of the basis function are the positive values of the breakpoint subtracted from the predictor X. For CART, the analog to Fig. 3.18 is a step function having a basis function value of 0.0 to the left of the breakpoint and a basis function value of 1.0 to the right. The linear splines formulation does not work for categorical predictors. When there are categorical predictors, MARS goes back to indicator variables just like CART.

Another important difference from CART is that as various breakpoints and predictors are considered, they are *multiplied* by the previous linear piecewise functions already included. The linear basis expansion is undertaken with the sum of products of linear piecewise splines. Exactly how this works need not concern us here. But the use of linear piecewise splines combined with sums of products means that there is no tree representation to inspect.

Like regression trees, each new product is evaluated by the reduction in the error sum of squares. Substantial overfitting can result, so an analogue to pruning is avail-

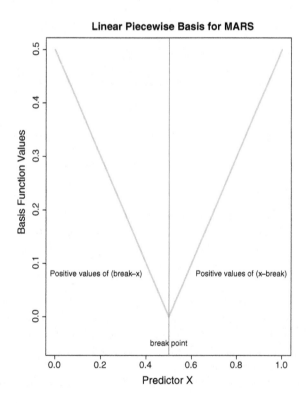

Fig. 3.18 MARS linear basis function with an illustrative break point at 0.5

able. Various tuning parameters are also available to help determine how complex a model is permitted.

MARS output can include the equation actually estimated, and an ANOVA-type partitioning of the explained variance to represent predictor "importance." There are, therefore, parallels to conventional regression. A lot more is said about variable "importance" in the next several chapters.

MARS can be extended to classification tasks. For both classification and regression, it can perform better than CART when step function approximations of $f(\mathbf{X})$ are unsatisfactory. But it has many of the same limitations. MARS has been largely superseded by more recent statistical learning procedures and unlike CART, has not been incorporated into any of these formulations.

3.15 Summary and Conclusions

CART can sometimes be an effective statistical learning tool. It is relatively easy to use, builds directly on familiar regression procedures, does not demand great computing power, and generates output that can be presented in an accessible manner. CART also provides a useful way to introduce the costs of classification errors. However, CART also has some important limitations.

First, if one wants an unbiased estimate of the true $f(\mathbf{X})$, there is no reason to believe that CART's $\hat{f}(X)$ will provide it or that it will even come close. Despite the flexible ways in which CART can respond to data, substantial bias is a real possibility. All fitting procedures are limited by the data available. Key predictors may not be available. But even if the requisite data are available, the use of step functions and the stagewise estimation procedure are significant complications. One can always settle for a level I analysis. A fallback level II strategy is to work with approximate population trees and test data. Asymptotically valid statistical inference, including statistical tests and confidence intervals, can follow.

Second, the splitting decisions can be very unstable. A few observations can in some situations dramatically affect which variables are selected and the precise values used for partitioning the data. Then, all subsequent partitions can be affected. This instability is closely related to overfitting, which can substantially limit the generalizability of the results. The findings from the data examined may not generalize well to other random realizations from the same population (let alone to data from other populations).

Third, for classification, the classes assigned to terminal nodes can be unstable too. When the computed proportions for the terminal node classes are about the same, the movement of just a few cases from one side of a proportion threshold to the other can change the assigned class. It is important to carefully inspect the distribution of proportions in each terminal node to get a sense of how serious the instability problem may be.

Fourth, even moderately elaborate tree diagrams will seriously tax substantive understanding. The problem is not just complexity. CART is trying in a single-minded manner to use associations in the data to maximize the homogeneity of its data partitions. How those associations come to be represented may have nothing remotely to do with subject matter understandings or how subject matter experts think about those associations. High order interaction effects are dramatic illustration.

Exercises

Problem Set 1

The purpose of this exercise is to provide an initial sense of how CART compares to conventional linear regression when the response variable is quantitative.

1. To begin, construct a regression dataset with known properties:

```
x1=rnorm(300)
x2=rnrom(300)
error=2*rnorm(300)
y1=1+(2*x1)+(3*x2)+error
```

Apply conventional linear regression using *lm()*. Then apply *rpart()*, and print the tree using *prp()* from the library *rpart.plot()*. Compare the regression output to the way in which the data were actually generated. Compare the tree diagram to the way in which the data were actually generated. Compare how well linear regression and CART fit the data. For CART, use *rsq.rpart()* from the library *library(rpart.plot)* to consider the fit. What do you conclude about the relative merits of linear regression and CART when the $f(X)$ is actually linear and additive?

2. Now, redefine the two predictors as binary factors and reconstruct the response variable.

```
x11=(x1 > 0)
x22=(x2 > 0)
y=1+(2*x11)+(3*x22)+error
```

Proceed as before comparing linear regression to CART. How do they compare? What do you conclude about the relative merits of linear regression and CART when the $f(X)$ is actually a step function and additive?

3. Under what circumstances is CART likely to perform better than linear regression? Consider separately the matter of how well the fitted values correspond to the observed values and the interpretation of how the predictors are related to the response.

Problem Set 2

The goal of the following exercises is to give you some hands-on experience with CART in comparison to some of the procedures covered in earlier chapters. An initial hurdle is getting R to do what you want. There are lots of examples in the chapter. Also, make generous use of *help()* and I have provided a number of hints along the way. However, I have tried to guide you to results in the least complicated way possible and as a consequence, some of the more subtle features of CART are not explored. Feel free to play with these in addition. You can't break anything.

Load the data set called "frogs" from the DAAG library. The data are from a study of ecological factors that may affect the presence of certain frog populations. The binary response variable is pres.abs. Use the help command to learn about the data. For ease of interpretation, limit yourself to the following predictors: altitude, distance, NoOfPools, NoOfSites, avrain, meanmin and meanmax.

1. Use logistic regression from *glm()* to consider how the predictors are related to whether frogs are present. Which predictors seem to matter? Do their signs make sense?

2. Using the procedure *stepAIC()* from the *MASS* library with the default for stepwise direction, find the model that minimizes the AIC. Which predictors remain? Do their signs make sense?

3. Using *table()*, construct a confusion table for the model arrived at by the stepwise procedure. The observed class is pres.abs. You will need to assign class labels to cases to get the "predicted" class. The procedure *glm()* stores under the name "fitted.values" the estimated conditional probabilities of the presence of frogs. If the probability is greater than .5, assign a 1 to that case. If the probability is equal to or less than .5, assign a 0 to that case. Now cross-tabulate the true class by the assigned class. What fraction of the cases is classified incorrectly? Is classification more accurate for the true presence of frogs or the true absence of frogs? What is a rationale for using .5 as the threshold for class assignment? What is the cost ratio in the table? What are its implications for an overall measure of classification performance? (Hint: some classifications are likely to be relatively more costly than others. This needs to be taken into account for all confusion tables, not just those from CART.)

4. Using your best model from the stepwise procedure, apply the generalized additive model. You can use *gam()* in either the *gam* or *mvcv* library. Use smoothers for each predictor. Let the procedure decide how many degrees of freedom to use for each smooth. Look at the numerical output and the smoothed plots. How do the results compare to those from logistic regression?

5. Construct a confusion table for the model arrived at through GAM. Once again, the observed class is pres.abs. Use the same logic as applied previously to *glm()* to determine the assigned class. What fraction of the cases is classified incorrectly? Is classification more accurate for the true presence of frogs or the true absence of frogs? How do these results compare to the GLM results? (Hint: don't forget to cost-weight the overall measure of classification accuracy.)

6. Going back to using all of the predictors you began with, apply CART to the frog data via the procedure *rpart()* in the library *rpart*. For now, accept all of the default settings. But it is usually a good idea to specify the method (here, method="class") rather than let *rpart()* try to figure it out from your response variable. Use the *print()* command to see some key numerical output. Try to figure out what each piece of information means. Use *rpart.plot()* to construct a tree diagram. What predictors does CART select as important? How do they

compare with your results from GLM and GAM? How do the interpretations of the results compare?

7. Use *predict()* to assign class labels to cases. You will need to use the help command for *predict.rpart()* to figure out how to do this. Then construct a confusion table for the assigned class and the observed class. What fraction of the cases is classified incorrectly? Is classification more accurate for the true presence of frogs or the true absence of frogs? How do these results compare to the GLM and GAM results? If the three differ substantially, explain why you think this has happened. Alternatively, if the three are much the same explain why you think this has happened.

8. Run the CART analysis again with different priors. Take a close look at the information available for *rpart()* using the help command. For example, for a perfectly balanced prior in *rpart()* you would include *parms=list(prior= c(.50,.50))*. Try a prior of .5 for presence and then a prior of .30 for presence. (For this *rpart()* parameter, the prior probability of 0 comes first and the prior probability of 1 comes second.) What happens to the ratio of false negatives to false positives? What happens to the overall amount of cost-weighted classification error compared to the default?

9. Using Eq. 3.11 set the prior so that in the confusion table false negatives are ten times more costly than false positives (with pres.abs = 1 called a "positive" and pres.abs = 0 called a "negative"). Apply CART. Study the output from *print()*, the tree diagram using *rpart.plot()*, and the confusion table. What has changed enough to affect your interpretations of the results? What has not changed enough to affect your interpretations of the results?

10. Construct two random samples with replacement of the same size as the dataset. Use the *sample()* command to select at random the rows of data you need and use those values to define a new sample with R's indexing capability, *x[r,c]*. For the two new samples, apply CART with the default parameters. Construct a tree diagram for each. How do the two trees compare to each other and to your earlier results with default settings? What does this tell you about how stable your CART results are and about potential problems with overfitting.

11. Repeat what you have just done, but now set the minimum terminal node size to 50. You will need the argument *control = rpart.control (minbucket = 50))* in your call to *rpart()*. How do the three trees compare now? What are the implications for overfitting in CART?

Problem Set 3

Here is another opportunity to become familiar with CART, but this time with a quantitative response variable. From the library *car*, load the data set "Freedman." The dataset contains for 100 American cities the crime rate, population size, population density, and percent nonwhite of the population. The goal is to see what is associated with the crime rate.

1. Using the *gam( )* from the library *gam*, regress the crime rate on the smoothed values of the three predictors. Examine the numerical output and the plots. Describe how the crime rate is related to the three predictors.
2. Repeat the analysis using *rpart( )* and the default settings. Describe how the crime rate is related to the three predictors. How do the conclusions differ from those using the generalized additive model?
3. Plot the fitted values from the GAM analysis against the fitted values from the CART analysis. The fitted values for *gam( )* are stored automatically. You will need to construct the fitted values for CART using *predict.rpart( )*. What would the plot look like if the two sets of fitted values corresponded perfectly? What do you see instead? What does the scatterplot tell you about how the two sets of fitted values are related?
4. Overlay on the scatterplot the least squares line for the two sets of fitted values using *abline( )*. If that regression line had a slope of 1.0 and an intercept of 0.0, what would that indicate about the relationship between the two sets of fitted values? What does that overlaid regression line indicate about how the two sets of fitted values are related?
5. Using *scatter.smooth( )*, apply a lowess smoother to the scatterplot of the two sets of fitted values. Try several different spans. What do you conclude about the functional form of the relationship between the two sets of fitted values?
6. For the GAM results and the CART results, use *cor( )* to compute separately the correlations between the fitted values and the observed values for the crime rate. What procedure has fitted values that are more highly correlated with the crime rate? Can you use this to determine which modeling approach fits the data better? If yes, explain why. If no, explain why.

Problem Set 4

1. At a number of places, the bootstrap has been mentioned and applied. The basic idea behind the bootstrap is easy enough in broad brushstrokes. But the details can be challenging even for math-stat types because there are important subtleties and many different bootstrap variants. Fortunately, for many of the applications that have been discussed and that will be discussed, uncertainty in some important features of the output can be usefully addressed with procedures available in R. Currently, *boot( )* is popular because of its great flexibility. But it has a relatively steep learning curve, and some readers may prefer to write their own bootstrap code.

    The code below produces a bootstrap distribution of the proportion of correct classifications in a CART confusion table using the Titanic data and the outcome class of survival. From the empirical distribution, one can consider the sampling distribution for the proportion correctly classified and construct a confidence interval.

    The code is meant to only be illustrative. As already mentioned, it probably makes little sense to consider a level II analysis for the Titanic data. However, code like this will work for test data should a level II analysis be appropriate. The main difference is that there would be no new CART fit for each bootstrap sample.

The rpart step shown in the code would not be included. Rather, the rpart-object would be computed outside of the function and called when *predict()* was used with test data.

Run the code and consider the output. Then try it with another dataset and test data. Interpret the CART confusion table and the distribution of the proportion of cases correctly classified.

```
# Application of nonparametric bootstrap for CART
library(PASWR)
library(boot)
library(rpart)
data("titanic3")
attach(titanic3)
temp<-data.frame(survived,pclass,sex,age) # Select variables
working<-na.omit(temp) # Remove NAs
detach(titanic3)

# Define the function to be bootstraped
confusion<-function(data,i) # i is the index for the bootstrap sample
{
  working2<-working[i,] # names the bootstrap sample for each i
  out<-rpart(survived~sex+age+pclass,data=working2,method="class")
  preds<-predict(out,data=working2)
  conf<-table(preds[,2]>.5,working2$survived) # Confusion table as usual
  fit<-(conf[1,1]+conf[2,2])/dim(working2)[1] # Proportion correct
  return(fit)
}

# Apply the bootstrap and examine the output
fitting<-boot(working,confusion,R=300) # Look at the object
plot(fitting)
quantile(fitting$t,probs=c(.025,.975))
```

Chapter 4
Bagging

4.1 Introduction

In this chapter, we make a major transition. We have thus far focused on statistical procedures that produce a single set of results: regression coefficients, measures of fit, residuals, classifications, and others. There is but one regression equation, one set of smoothed values, or one classification tree. Most statistical procedures operate in a similar fashion.

The discussion now shifts to statistical learning that builds on many sets of outputs aggregated to produce results. Such algorithms make a number of passes over the data. On each pass, inputs are linked to outputs just as before. But the ultimate results of interest are the collection of all the results from all passes over the data.

Bayesian model averaging may be a familiar illustration from another statistical tradition (Madigan et al. 1996; Hoeting et al. 1999). In Bayesian model averaging, there is an assumed $f(X)$; there is a "true model." A number of potentially true models, differing in the predictors selected, are evaluated. The model output is then averaged with weights determined by model uncertainty. Output from models with greater uncertainty are given less weight. From a statistical learning perspective, Bayesian model averaging has a number of complications, including the dependence that is necessarily built in across model results (Xu and Golay 2006). Also, it is not clear why a model with less uncertainty is necessarily closer to the true model. We address shortly how statistical learning procedures relying on multiple results proceed rather differently.

Aggregate results from many passes over the data can have several important benefits. For example, under the right circumstances, averaging over sets of fitted values can increase their stability. The averaging tends to cancel out results shaped by idiosyncratic features of the data. In turn, generalization error is reduced. An increase

---

The original version of this chapter was revised: See the "Chapter Note" section at the end of this chapter for details. The erratum to this chapter is available at https://doi.org/10.1007/978-3-319-44048-4_10.

R.A. Berk, *Statistical Learning from a Regression Perspective*,
Springer Texts in Statistics, DOI 10.1007/978-3-319-44048-4_4

in stability permits the use of more complex functions of the predictors when they are needed.

In this chapter, we focus on bagging, which capitalizes on a particular kind of averaging process that can address complexity and stability. In more traditional terms, bagging can have beneficial consequences for the bias-variance tradeoff. Sometimes you can have your cake and eat it too.

Although bagging can be applied to a wide variety of statistical procedures, we will again concentrate on classifiers. The rationale is largely the same: the exposition is more effective and the step to quantitative responses is easy to make. We begin with a return to the problem of overfitting. Although overfitting has been discussed several times in earlier chapters, it needs to be linked more directly to CART to help set the stage for a full exposition of bagging and subsequent procedures.

4.2   The Bagging Algorithm

The notion of combining fitted values from a number of fitting attempts has been suggested by several authors (LeBlanc and Tibshirani 1996; Mojirsheibani 1997, 1999). In an important sense, the whole becomes more than the sum of its parts. It is a bit like crowd sourcing.

"Bagging," which stands for "Bootstrap Aggregation," is perhaps the earliest procedure to exploit sets of fitted values over random samples of the data. Unlike model averaging, bagging is not a way to arrive at a model. Bagging is an algorithm that can help improve the performance of fitted values from a given statistical procedure. Breiman's remarkable 1996 paper on bagging is well worth a careful read.

For training data having N observations and a binary response variable, bagging takes the following form.

1. Take a random sample of size N *with replacement* from the data. These are sometimes called "bootstrap samples."
2. Construct a classification tree as usual.
3. Assign a class to each terminal node as usual, and store the class attached to each case and the predictor values that define the neighborhood in which in each terminal node resides (e.g., males under 30 years of age with a high school diploma).
4. Repeat Steps 1–3 a large number of times.
5. For each observation in the dataset, count the number of times over trees that it is classified in one category and the number of times over trees it is classified in the other category.
6. Assign each observation to a final class by a majority vote over the set of trees. If the outcome has two classes, and more than 50 % of the time over a large number of trees a given observation is classified as a 1, that becomes its classification. The same reasoning applies to the 0 class. The winning class is determined by a majority vote.

Although there remain important variations and details to consider, these are the key steps to produce "bagged" classification trees. Averaging occurs in the votes over classification trees. The voting results for each case are proportions that can be seen as means for response variables coded as 1 or 0.

The assigned class for each case is used much as it was for CART. Confusion tables are good place to start, especially if imputation or forecasting is in the offing. But there is no longer a single tree to interpret because there are many trees and no such thing as an average tree. Predictor values are linked to fitted classes, but not in a manner that can be substantively interpreted. We have a true blackbox statistical learning procedure. There will be more of them.

The idea of classifying by averaging over the results from a large number of bootstrap samples generalizes easily to a wide variety of classifiers beyond CART. Later we show that bagging can be usefully applied to quantitative responses as well. Nothing fundamentally changes.

4.3 Some Bagging Details

The bagging algorithm may seem straightforward. Bagging is just as way to average out unwanted noise. But there are a number of subtleties that we will need to carry forward in this chapter and later chapters.

4.3.1 Revisiting the CART Instability Problem

One good way to motivate bagging is to consider again the instability of classification trees. That instability can be readily apparent even across bootstrap samples that necessarily share large fractions of the data.

Figure 4.1 shows two such classification trees from the Titanic data. Although, as before, the first split for both is on gender, the two trees subsequently part company. The next two splits are the same for both trees, but the thresholds differ. Then, the splits that follow on the right branch differ in some of the predictors selected as well as thresholds. And the counts in all of the terminal nodes vary as well across the two trees. All of these differences lead to somewhat different classifications. For example, there are 10 boys between 9.5 and 13 years of age who are excluded from the far left terminal node on the top tree but who are not excluded from the far left terminal node on the bottom tree. Overall, about 10 % of the cases common to both trees were classified differently. The bottom tree was far more likely to assign the class of "survived" than the top tree. Again, this is a best case scenario in the sense that about 68 % of the observations in the two analyses are shared, and the overall sample size is relatively large.

A classification tree can be used for level I analyses when all one cares about is characterizing the data on hand. Instability becomes relevant for level II analyses.

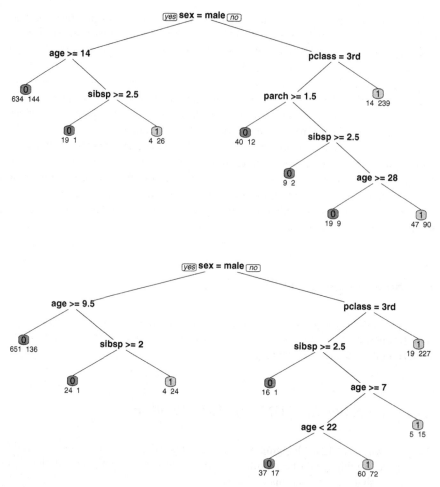

Fig. 4.1 Classification tree analysis of Titanic survival for two bootstrap samples of 1309 observations from the same training data (The *red nodes* are assigned the class of "perished," and the *blue nodes* are assigned the class of "survived")

For example, instability is a concern for generalization error, which speaks to performance in test data, not the data on hand. The same reasoning applies to bagging. Because bagging addresses instability, a level II perspective is required.

4.3.2 Some Background on Resampling

The top bagging priority is to reduce instability, and it all begins with resampling. Over the past two decades, many resampling procedures have been developed that can provide information about the sampling distributions of data-derived estimates. The bootstrap is perhaps the most well known. Other techniques include the jack-

Fig. 4.2 A schematic for
bootstrap sampling

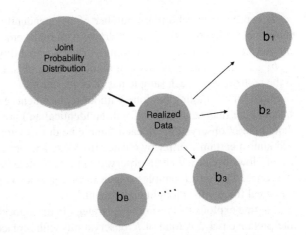

knife (Efron and Tibshirani 1993: Sect. 10.5) and permutation tests (Edgington and
Onghena 2007). Resampling procedures can provide asymptotically valid tests and
confidence intervals making fewer assumptions than conventional methods and can
sometimes be applied when there are no conventional methods at all.[1] For a discussion of bagging, we only need a few ideas from the bootstrap, and in particular,
how one can generate a very large number of random sampling from training data.
There are very good and extensive treatments of the bootstrap provided by Efron and
Tibshirani (1993) and Hall (1997). Code in R to do a CART bootstrap is provided as
part of an exercise at the end of the chapter.

The bootstrap is essentially a simulation of the frequentist thought experiment
and as such, is automatically a level II formulation. For the frequentist, the data
on hand are realized independently from a joint probability distribution or a finite
population. In Fig. 4.2, the process is shown by the thick arrow toward the left side.
The data on hand are seen as a single set of independent realizations from a limitless
number of realized datasets that could be produced. Sample statistics in principle
can be computed from each these realized datasets leading to one or more sampling
distributions. From these, confidence intervals and statistical tests can follow. For
example, if the mean were computed from each of the realized datasets, the result
would be a sampling distribution for the mean. In practice, however, the data analyst
usually gets to see only one realized dataset, and that is what the figure shows.
Depending on the setting, the realized data could be training data, evaluation data,
or test data.

---

[1] Recall that the jackknife can be seen as N-fold cross validation. Permutation tests are essentially
the same as randomization tests and boil down to randomly shuffling some feature of the data
on hand. For example, consider a conventional regression with a single predictor. Under the null
hypothesis that the regression coefficient equals 0.0, one requires the sampling distribution of
the regression coefficient if the null hypothesis is true. It can be effective to simulate that null
distribution by randomly shuffling the response variable over and over, each time computing the
value of the regression coefficient. With this approximation of the null distribution in hand, it is
easy to calculate whether a regression coefficient as big or bigger than the one computed from the
training data appears less the 5 % of the time. A statistical test has been performed with a critical
value of .05. Good (2004) provides a very accessible treatment.

To approximate a limitless number of independently realized datasets, a large number of probability samples are drawn with replacement from the single realized dataset; hence the term "resampling." These probability samples are denoted by $b_1, b_2 \ldots, b_B$, where B is the total number of samples. If there are N observations in the realized data, each sample has N observations.[2]

Should the sampling be done without replacement, each sample of the realized data and the realized data itself will be identical and nothing has been gained. But should the N observations in each sample be drawn *with* replacement, the samples will almost certainly differ by chance from one another and from the realized data. This follows because a given observation in the realized data may be selected more than once. The set of samples drawn in this manner is meant to approximate the canonical frequentist thought experiment.[3]

Bagging exploits this resampling strategy in the algorithm's first step, but with an interpretative twist. A total of N observations with replacement is drawn. Sampling with replacement on the average causes about 37 % of cases to be excluded from a given sample. It follows that a substantial number of cases are selected more than once. From a frequentist perspective, one has the formal sampling properties required, but there is less information in such samples than had all of the observations appeared only once. Some statistical power can be lost, and procedures that are sample-size dependent can suffer.[4]

But, the resampling is not being used to construct an empirical sampling distribution. The resampling is an algorithmic device that allows one to draw a large number of random samples from the training data. Each sample is used to grow a tree whose fitted values are then averaged over trees. There is no estimation. There are also no confidence intervals or statistical tests.

At the same time, the sampling with replacement means that for each tree, a random sample of about 37 % of the observations are excluded from the tree-growing calculations. Each tree, therefore, automatically has "hold-out" observations, often called "out-of-bag" (OOB) observations. OOB observations are an immediate source of test data. Having valid test data as a byproduct of sampling with replacement is huge. Up to this point, test data had to be obtained as part of the data collection process or constructed from split samples.

---

[2] In more complete treatments, there can be more than or less than N observations in each bootstrap sample. Sampling without replacement is also an option as long as the sample size is less than N. However, some statistical procedures such as CART, are sample-size dependent. With more observation one can grow larger trees. It can make good sense, therefore to start with bootstrap samples having the same number of observations as the training data.

[3] There are many different kinds of bootstrap procedures, and it remains an important research area. The resampling just described is sometimes called a "pairs" bootstrap because both Y and X are sampled, or a "nonparametric" bootstrap because there is no model specified through which the realized data were generated.

[4] If one draws random samples *without* replacement with $.50 \times N$ observations, one has on the average a dataset with about the same information content as N observations drawn at random with replacement (Buja and Stuetzle 2006). Still, sampling with replacement is the usual approach.

4.3.3 Votes and Probabilities

For each case in the bootstrap sample, there is a vote over trees. For a binary outcome, the class with the majority vote is the class assigned to that case. For outcomes with more than two classes, the class with a plurality is the class assigned to that case. Because each classifier is grown with a random sample of the training data, the proportion of votes each class musters has the look and feel of probabilities. However, the samples drawn in bagging are not fully independent, which undermines the usual assumption of independent trials, and compromises treating vote proportions are probabilities. But it's worse.

One must be clear about what such probabilities could represent (Breiman 1996: Sect. 4.2). Suppose for a particular set of predictor values the true outcome probability of a 1 is .80. Suppose also that each classification tree votes for 1, given those x-values. Although the true probability of a 1 is .80, the vote "probability" over trees is 1.0. Clearly, two different kinds of outcomes are in play: how a tree votes and the outcome class for a given case. They must not be confused. More will be said about this in the next chapter.

4.3.4 Imputation and Forecasting

Obtaining fitted classes for imputation or forecasting follows directly from the way fitted values from the training data are computed. Recall that for a single classification tree, a new set of predictor values with an unknown outcome are "dropped down" the tree. The assigned class of the terminal node in which the case lands is the imputed or forecasted class. Also recall that this process can be represented in a conventional regression structure where the task is prediction. There is nothing mysterious going on.

When there are K classification trees, the set of predictor values is dropped down each of the K trees. Then as before, a vote is taken. The winning class is the forecast for those x-values. But as just noted, the winning proportion is not an estimate of the probability that the imputation or forecast is correct. This seems to be an all too common error.

4.3.5 Margins

The meaning of "margin" in bagging is somewhat different from the meaning of "margin" in margin maximizing forms of statistical learning (e.g., adaboost, support vector machines). But the statistical goals are the same: to arrive at stable classifications. From a bagging perspective, Bremen (2001a: 7) defines the margin as

$$mg(\mathbf{X}, Y) = av_k I(h_k(\mathbf{X}) = Y) - \max_{j \neq Y} av_k I(h_k(\mathbf{X}) = j), \qquad (4.1)$$

where for randomly realized data and a given case, there is an ensemble of K classifiers denoted by $h_k(\mathbf{X})$, Y is the correct class, j is some other class, and $I(.)$ is the indicator function as before. The K classifiers might be K classification trees. In words, over the K classifiers, there is a proportion of times the case is classified correctly, and a maximum proportion of times the case is classified incorrectly. The difference in the two proportions is the margin for that case.[5] "The larger the margin, the more confidence in the classification" (Breimen 2001: 7).

Suppose that over all of the bagged trees, an observation is correctly classified 75 % of the time and incorrectly classified 25 % of the time. The margin is $.75 - .25 = .50$. A negative margin implies misclassification. If an observation is correctly classified 30 % of the time and incorrectly classified 70 % of the time, the margin is $.30 - .70 = -.40$.

A lopsided vote in favor of the correct class conveys that despite noise introduced by the resampling, most of the time the case is classified correctly. One can say that the correct classification for that case is highly reliable. A lopsided vote in favor of the incorrect class is also highly reliable; reliable and wrong. If the vote is very close, the case is just about as likely to be misclassified as classified correctly. Systematic relationships between the response and the predictors cannot meaningfully overcome the algorithm-generated noise. One can say that the classification, whether correct or incorrect, is unreliable.

One can only know when a classification is correct, if the actual class is known. That will be true in training data, evaluation data, and test data. In that context, margins can be used as diagnostic tools. How reliable are the correct classifications? How reliable are the incorrect classifications? Ideally, the former are very reliable and the latter are not. In new realizations of the data, there is then a good chance that many of the incorrect classifications will be overturned. One might also be able to identify particular types of cases for which misclassifications are likely and/or unreliable.

Forecasting applications differ because the actual outcome is not known. The votes over classifiers still represent reliability, but whether the classification is correct or incorrect is not known. Nevertheless, reliability is important. Suppose for a given case, the vote is close. Because vote is close, bagging the very same data again could easily result in a close vote the other way. The initial forecasted class is not reliable; the forecast could have easily been different. It is usually important for stakeholders who will use the forecast to know the forecast's reliability, even if they do not know whether the forecast is correct. Should the vote be lopsided, the forecasted class is reliable, and even though the true class is not known, the forecast may be given more credibility.

Whatever the level of confidence, it is with respect to the performance of the bagged classifier itself. Was it able to classify particular cases with sufficient reliability? It is not confidence about any larger issues such as whether the fitted values

[5]The average of an indicator variable is a proportion. The "*max*" allows for more than two outcome classes with the proper comparison a worse case scenario.

are good approximations of the true response surface. It is nothing like a model diagnostic or model misspecification test. There is often confusion on this point.

In summary, large margins can be a major asset. For each case, the margin can be a measure of reliability for the class assigned. Larger margins imply greater bagging reliability. Forecasting is different. In the earlier prison inmate instance, housing decisions at intake were based on an inmate's forecasted misconduct class. If the vote for a given inmate is equivocal, prison staff properly might decide to base the housing decision on other information. If the vote is decisive, prison staff properly might base the housing decision primarily on the class assigned.

4.3.6 Using Out-Of-Bag Observations as Test Data

In conventional CART software, a tree is grown with training data, and the training data used to grow the tree are used again to compute the number of classification errors. The training data are dropped down the tree to determine how well the tree performs. The training data are said to be "resubstituted" when tree performance is evaluated.

In some implementations of bagging, out-of-bag observations from each tree can be treated as a test dataset and dropped down the tree. There need be no resubstitution. A record is kept of the class with which each out-of-bag observation is labeled, as well as its values on all of the predictors. Then in the averaging process, only those class labels are used. In other words, the averaging for a given case over trees is done only using the trees for which that case was not used to grow the tree. This leads to still more honest fitted values and more honest confusion tables than with conventional bagging.

4.3.7 Bagging and Bias

Although the major target of bagging is the variance of fitted values, there can be in certain situations a reduction in the bias as well. Figure 4.3 illustrates how bagging can affect the bias. To keep the graph simple, there is a smooth nonlinear $f(X)$ linking a single predictor to a quantitative response Y. The true response function is shown.

Imagine that a regression tree is applied one time to each of three different bootstrap samples of the data. Each time, only one break in the predictor is allowed. (Such trees are sometimes called "stumps.") Three step functions that could result are overlaid as open rectangles. One has a very rough approximation of the $f(X)$. If that function is the estimation target, there is substantial bias.

Suppose now that there are eleven bootstrap samples and eleven stumps. Eleven step functions that could result are shown with the light blue rectangles. Clearly, the approximation is better and bias is reduced. Because in bagging there are often hundreds of trees, there is the possibility of approximating complex functions rather

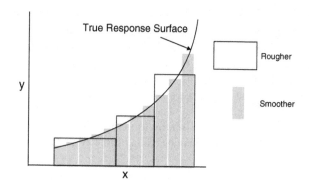

Fig. 4.3 How bagging smooths using a set of step functions to approximate the true response surface

well. The same reasoning applies to categorical outcomes. In short, bagging can reduce bias by what is, in effect, smoothing (Bühlmann and Yu 2002).

In addition, noted earlier was an indirect impact that bagging can have on bias. Because of the averaging in bagging, one can employ more complex functions of the data with less worry about the impact of overfitting on generalization error. For example, bagging gives more license to grow very large trees with few observations in terminal nodes. The larger trees can lead to less bias while bagging increases the stability of fitted values.

4.3.8 Level I and Level II Analyses with Bagging

As always, a level I analysis is justified. For bagging that may mean little more than studying a histogram of the fitted values or examining a confusion table derived from resubstituted data. There might also be interest in the margins. But such analyses go primarily to how well the bagging procedure performs. Because there is no longer a tree to interpret, there is little that can be easily done to describe how the predictors are related to response. In the next chapter, some tools will be introduced that can help.

However, the usual motivation for bagging and the usual interest in margins imply concerns about generalization error. Generalization error is a level II matter. Moreover, bagged output can then be seen as estimates. Assuming that the training data plausibly can be treated as independent random realizations from a relevant joint probability distribution, the level II issues are much the same as discussed for CART. There is an estimation target, which is the population approximation of the true response surface. The details of that approximation depend on the classifier being used. If the classifier is adaptive (i.e., inductive), model selection can be a serious estimation complication. As before, the best hope is to have test data. The training data and bagging results are taken to be fixed. If test data are used to construct fitted values, the observed class and the fitted classes can be tabulated in a confusion table from which various kind of generalization error can be estimated. For example, there can be an overall misclassification proportion weighted by the asymmetric costs of classification errors. There can also be misclassification proportions for either of the two (or more) outcome classes. One can also use the fitted classes from the test data as asymptotically unbiased estimates of the bagging approximation response surface. Imputation and forecasting directly follow.

4.4 Some Limitations of Bagging

In general, bagging is a reasonably safe procedure. But it is hardly a panacea. Sometimes it does not help and on occasion it can make things worse.

4.4.1 Sometimes Bagging Cannot Help

Bagging only returns an average of fitted values that is different from those that could be obtained from one pass over the original data if the fitting procedure is a nonlinear or an adaptive function of the data (Hastie et al. 2009: 282). For example, there is no reason to apply bagging to conventional linear regression. The average of the fitted values over a large number of bootstrap samples would be effectively the same as the fitted values obtained from conventional linear regression applied once to the training data. In contrast, there can be useful differences for smoothing splines when the value of λ is determined empirically. This point helps to underscore an earlier discussion about the bootstrap samples used in bagging: in bagging, the goal is not to approximate a sampling distribution but to allow for many passes over the data.

4.4.2 Sometimes Bagging Can Make the Bias Worse

Look again at Fig. 4.3. Suppose $f(X)$ is really very jagged, much like a step function. Then, the smoothing that bagging accomplishes can increase bias because the smoothing on the average moves the fitted values away from the true response surface. One does not want the sharp corners of the CART estimates "sanded off". Classification can also be adversely affected.

Weak classifiers can also create problems, especially when the distribution of the response is highly unbalanced. Weak classifiers are sometimes defined as those that do not do materially better than the marginal distribution. Suppose the marginal distribution of the response is unbalanced so that it is very difficult for a fitting procedure using the predictors to perform better than the marginal distribution. Under

Fig. 4.4 Good and bad
influence in bagging

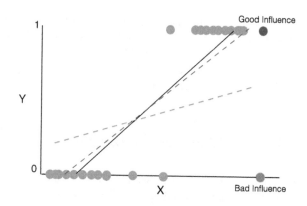

those circumstances the rare class will likely be misclassified most of the time because
votes will be typically won by the class that is far more common.[6]

To illustrate this point, suppose there is a binary response variable, and for the
moment, we are interested in a single observation that actually happens to be a
"success." Over K classification trees, that observation is classified as a success
about two times out of ten. So, the classification for that observation will be wrong
about 80 % of the time. But if one classifies by majority vote, the class assigned would
be a failure and that would be wrong 100 % of the time. Because the K classifiers
do a poor job, the majority vote makes things worse. Stronger classifiers typically
would place that observation in terminal nodes where the major of the cases were
successes. Then the vote over trees would help.

In practice, such problems will be rare if the data analyst pays attention to how
the classifier performs before bagging is applied. If it performs very poorly, bagging
risks making things worse. We show in later chapters that if one has a set of weak
classifiers, alternative procedures may be called for that can help.

4.4.3 Sometimes Bagging Can Make the Variance Worse

Bagging sometimes can also perform poorly with respect to the variance (Grandvalet
2004). Figure 4.4 shows a scatterplot with a binary outcome. The observations are
represented by filled circles. The light blue circles represent the mass of the data.
The dark blue circle and the red circle are high leverage observations because they
are outliers in the x-direction. Consider now their role for the fitted values.

To keep the exposition simple, suppose that within the range of X, true response
surface is a linear function of the X. The solid black line shows the fitted values with
both the blue circle and the red circle excluded from the dataset. Suppose that the blue

---

[6]Moreover, sometimes the procedure will fail because none of the rare cases are included in a given
bootstrap sample.

outlier is not included in the data. The broken red line shows the fitted values with the lower-right outlier included. The lines are rather different, implying that whether that red outlier is included in the analysis alters the response function substantially. Therefore, the outlier is influential. In a bagging application, the fitted values will vary widely depending on whether the red observation happens to be included. Then, averaging over classifiers reduces the variance of the fitted values. Bagging works as it should.

In contrast, suppose that the red outlier is excluded from the data. Whether the blue outlier is included makes a small difference in the fitted values. It happens to fall near the line generated by the other fitted values. The broken blue line shows the result. Deleting the blue outlier does not change the fit a great deal. Therefore, it is not influential. Rather, it helps to stabilize the fitted values. When it is excluded because of bootstrap sampling that added stability is lost. Bagging may increase the variance. In practice, however, such situations are very rare, and the increase in variance is likely to be small.

The problems with bagging just described have their analogues for quantitative responses. Bagging is at its best when the problem to overcome is instability. Bagging when the fitted values are already very stable can make things worse. In practice, it can be useful to inspect several of the K classifiers derived from different bootstrap samples to see how serious the instability may be.

4.5   A Bagging Illustration

In practice, bagging is not used much as a stand-alone procedure. There are far better statistical learning tools. But like classification and regression trees, it can be a key component of more effective approaches and many of the details need to be understood.

Consider now bagging applied to the Titanic data largely to show some R-code. The library in R is *ipred* and bagging procedure itself is *bagging()*.[7] We use the same classification tree specification as before, which assumes symmetric costs for classification errors. Table 4.1 is the confusion table constructed solely from the training data and Fig. 4.5 shows the code responsible. By all of the performance measures shown in the table, the fit is quite good, but the table is constructed from in-sample data. Also, there is no tree to interpret.

---

[7]The package *ipred()* is written by A. Peters, T. Hothorn, B.D. Ripley, T. Therneau, and B. Atkinson. There are number of bagging-related procedures in *ipred()*.

Table 4.1 Bagged classification tree confusion table for survival on the Titanic (N = 1309)

	Classify perished	Classify survived	Model error
Perished	759	50	.05
Survived	100	400	.21
Use error	.12	.10	Overall error = .12

```
## Bagging
library(PASWR) # Where the data are
data("titanic3") # Load data
library(ipred) # Load library

# Bag Classification trees
out1<-bagging(as.factor(survived)~sex+age+pclass+sibsp+parch,
              data=titanic3,coob=T, keepX=T, nbagg=50,
              minsplit=10, cp=.05, xval=0)

fitted<-predict(out1, newdata=titanic3,
                type="class") # fitted class
tab<-table(titanic3$survived,fitted) # confusion table
prop.table(tab,1) # use error
prop.table(tab,2) # model error
```

Fig. 4.5 R code for bagging Titanic data

4.6 Bagging a Quantitative Response Variable

Bagging works by the same principles when the response variable is quantitative. Recall that CART constructs a regression tree by maximizing the reduction in the error sum of squares at each split. Each case is placed in a terminal node with a conditional mean. That mean is the fitted value for all cases of that terminal node.

All of the concerns about CART instability apply, especially given the potential impact that outliers can have on the fitting process when the response variable is quantitative. Because of the sum of squares loss function, a few cases that fall a substantial distance from the mass of the data can produce results that can vary substantially over samples, do not characterize well the mass of the data, and do not generalize well either.

With a numerical response variable, bagging averages over trees in much the same way it averages over trees when the response variable is categorical. For each tree, each observation is placed in a terminal node and assigned the mean of that terminal node. Then, the average of these assigned means over trees is computed for each observation. This average value for each case is the bagged fitted value used. The averaging process will tend to moderate instability. If for each tree, the OOB data that are placed in terminal nodes is used in the averaging, stability can be improved more effectively.

4.7 Summary and Conclusions

Bagging is an important conceptual advance and a useful tool in practice. The conceptual advance is to aggregate fitted values from a large number of bootstrap samples. Ideally, many sets of fitted values, each with low bias but high variance, may be averaged in a manner than can effectively reduce the bite in the bias–variance tradeoff. Thanks to bagging, there can be a way to usefully address this long-standing dilemma in statistics. Moreover, the ways in which bagging aggregates the fitted values is the basis for other statistical learning developments.

In practice, bagging can generate fitted values that often reproduce the data well and forecast with considerable accuracy. Both masters are served without making unrealistic demands on available computing power. Bagging can also be usefully applied to a wide variety of fitting procedures. However, bagging is not much used as a stand-alone procedure because there are statistical learning procedures readily available that import the best features of bagging, add some new wrinkles, and then perform better.

In addition, bagging also suffers from several problems. Perhaps most important, there is no way within the procedure itself to depict how the predictors are related to the response. With test data or OOB data, one can obtain a more honest set of fitted values and a more honest evaluation of how good the fitted values really are. But as an explanatory device, bagging is pretty much a bust. Other tools are needed, which are considered in the next chapter.

A second problem is that because so much of the data are shared from tree to tree, the fitted values are not independent. The common set of available predictors can build in additional dependence. Consequently, the averaging is not as effective as it could be. This too is addressed shortly.

Third, bagging may not help much if the fitting function is consistently and substantially inappropriate. Large and systematic errors in the fitted values are just reproduced a large number of times and do not, therefore, cancel out in the averaging process. For categorical response variables, bagging a very weak classifier can sometimes make things worse.

Fourth, the bootstrap sampling can lead to problems when categorical predictors or outcomes are highly unbalanced. For any given bootstrap sample, the unbalanced variable can become a constant. Depending on the fitting function being bagged, the entire procedure may abort.

Finally, bagging can actually increase instability if there are outliers that help to anchor the fit. Such outliers will be lost to some of the bootstrap samples. It is difficult in practice to know whether this is a problem or not.

Bagging can be extended so that many of these problems are usefully addressed, even if full solutions are not available. We turn to some of these potential solutions in the next chapter. They are found in another form of statistical learning, still farther away from conventional regression analysis.

Exercises

Problem Set 1

The sampling done in bagging must be with replacement. Run the following code and compare the tables. How many duplicate observations are there in s1 compared to s2? Write code to find out. Run the code a second time. Again, how many duplicate observations are there in s1 compared to s2? Write code to find out. What have you learned about the differences between the samples drawn by the two methods?

```
x<-1:100
s1<-sample(x,replace=T)
table(s1)
s2<-sample(x,replace=F)
table(s2)
```

Problem Set 2

The goal of this exercise is to compare the performance of linear regression, CART, and bagging applied to CART. Construct the following data set in which the response is a quadratic function of a single predictor.

```
x1=rnorm(500)
x12=x1^2
y=1+(2*(x12))+(2*rnorm(500))
```

1. Plot the $1 + (2 \times x12)$ against x1. This is the "true" relationship between the response and the predictor without the complication of the disturbances. This is the $f(X)$ you hope to recover from the data.
2. Proceed as if you know that the $f(X)$ is quadratic. Fit a linear model with x12 as the predictor. Then plot the fitted values against x1. You can see how well linear regression does when the functional form is known.
3. Now suppose that you do not know that the $f(X)$ is quadratic. Apply linear regression to the same response variable using x1 (not x12) as the sole predictor. Construct the predicted values and plot the fitted values against x1. How do the fitted values compare to what you know to be the correct $f(X)$? (It is common to assume the functional form is linear when the functional form is unknown.)
4. Apply CART to the same response variable using rpart() and x1 (not x12) as the sole predictor. Use the default settings. Construct the predicted values, using predict(). Then plot the fitted values against x1. How do the CART fitted values compare to what you know to be the correct $f(X)$? How do the CART fitted values compare to the fitted values from the linear regression with x1 as the sole predictor?

5. Apply bagging to the same response variable using *bagging()* from the *ipred()* library, and x1 as the sole predictor. Use the default settings. Construct the predicted values using *predict()*. Then plot the fitted values against x1. How do the bagged fitted values compare to the linear regression fitted values?

6. You know that the relationship between the response and x1 should be a smooth parabola. How do the fitted values from CART compare to the fitted values from bagging? What feature of bagging is highlighted?

Problem Set 3

Load the dataset "Freedman" from the *car* library. For 100 American cities, there are four variables: the crime rate, the population, population density, and proportion nonwhite. As before, the crime rate is the response and the other variables are predictors.

1. Use *rpart()* and its default values to fit a CART model. Compute the root mean square error for the model. One way to do this is to use *predict.rpart()* to obtain the fitted values and with the observed values for the variable "crime," compute the root mean square error in R. Then use *bagging()* from the library *ipred* and the out-of-bag observations to obtain a bagged value for the root mean square error for the same CART model. Compare the two estimates of fit and explain what you see. Keep in mind that at least two things are going on: (1) in-sample v. out-of-sample comparisons, and (2) the averaging that bagging provides.

2. Using *sd()*, compute the standard deviation for the CART fitted values and the bagged fitted values. Compare the two standard deviations and explain what you see.

Problem Set 4

Load the dataset "frogs" from the library *DAAG*. Using "pres.abs" as the response, build a CART model under the default settings.

1. Construct a confusion table with "pres.abs" and the predicted classes from the model. Now, using *bagging()* from the library *ipred*, bag the CART model using the out-of-bag observations. Construct a confusion table with "pres.abs" and the bagged predicted classes from the model. Compare the two confusion tables and explain why they differ. Keep in mind that at least two things are going on: (1) in-sample v. out-of-sample comparisons, and (2) the averaging that bagging provides.

Chapter 5
Random Forests

5.1 Introduction and Overview

Just as in bagging, imagine growing a large number of classification or regression trees with bootstrap samples from training data. But now, as each tree is grown, take a random sample of predictors before each node is split. For example, if there are 20 predictors, choose a random five as candidates for defining the split. Then construct the best split, as usual, but selecting only from the five chosen. Repeat this process for each prospective split. Do not prune. Thus, each tree is produced from a random sample of cases, and at each split a random sample of predictors. Compute the mean or proportion for each tree's terminal nodes just as in bagging. Finally, for each case, average over trees as in bagging, but only when that case is out-of-bag. Breiman calls such as procedure a "random forest" (Breiman 2001a).

The random forest algorithm is very much like the bagging algorithm. Again let N be the number of observations in the training data and assume for now that the response variable is binary.

1. Take a random sample of size N with replacement from the data.
2. Take a random sample *without* replacement of the predictors.
3. Construct the first recursive partition of the data as usual.
4. Repeat Step 2 for each subsequent split until the tree is as large as desired. Often this leads to one observation in each terminal node. Do not prune. Compute each terminal node proportion as usual.
5. Drop the *out-of-bag* (OOB) data down the tree. Store the class assigned to each observation along with each observation's predictor values.
6. Repeat Steps 1–5 a large number of times (e.g., 500).

The original version of this chapter was revised: See the "Chapter Note" section at the end of this chapter for details. The erratum to this chapter is available at https://doi.org/10.1007/978-3-319-44048-4_10.

© Springer International Publishing Switzerland 2016
R.A. Berk, *Statistical Learning from a Regression Perspective*,
Springer Texts in Statistics, DOI 10.1007/978-3-319-44048-4_5

7. Using only the class assigned to each observation when that observation is OOB, count the number of times over trees that the observation is classified in one category and the number of times over trees it is classified in the other category.
8. Assign each case to a category by a majority vote over the set of trees when that case is OOB. Thus, if 51 % of the time over a large number of trees a given case is classified as a 1, that becomes its assigned classification.

The major differences between the bagging algorithm and the random forests algorithm are the sampling of predictors at each potential split of the training data, and using only the out-of-bag data when fitted values or classes are assigned to each case. Both are in the service of making the output from each tree in the random forest more independent, but there are additional benefits addressed below.

The key output from random forests is the fitted values, which if classes, are displayed in a confusion table. Because the fitted values are for out-of-bag observations, the confusion table effectively is constructed from test data. Still, the black box produced is every bit as opaque as the bagging black box. There are other algorithms that can be used in concert with random forests to provide a peek at what may be going on inside the box.

Finally, even when random forests is being used solely to describe associations in the data, there is more going on than a level I analysis. The use of OOB data to obtain honest fitted values implies level II concerns broadly and concerns about generalization error in particular. Most discussions of random forests consider results from a dataset as estimates so that, for example, fitted proportions from a sample are called probabilities even if it is unclear exactly what is being estimated and where that estimand resides. We will return to these issues toward the end of this chapter but many of the level II perspectives from bagging carry over.

5.1.1 Unpacking How Random Forests Works

Just like for CART and bagging, beneath a simple algorithm are a host of important details and subtleties. To begin, random forests uses CART as a key building block but in this new setting, CART can be made far more effective. Large trees can produce fitted values less biased with respect to the true response surface. With large trees necessarily comes a more complex $\hat{f}(\mathbf{X})$. Ordinarily, however, an increase in the number of terminal nodes leads to a smaller number of observations in each. The fitted values are more vulnerable to instability. From a level II perspective, the bias–variance tradeoff remains a serious problem. But by averaging over trees, the fitted values case-by-case are made more stable. Ideally, both the bias and the variance can be reduced.[1]

---

[1]One might think weighting trees by some measure of generalization error would help. Better performing trees would be given more weight in the averaging. So far at least, the gains are at best small (Winham et al. 2013). Because better performing trees tend to have more variation over terminal node fitted values, a form of self-weighting is in play.

Another way to make CART more effective is to sample predictors. One benefit is that the fitted values across trees are more independent. Consequently, the gains from averaging over a large number of trees can be more dramatic. Another benefit is that because only a few predictors are considered for each potential partitioning, there can be overall more predictors than observations; p can be very large and even larger than N. This is a major asset in the era of big data. In principle, having access to a very large number of predictors can help legitimately to improve the fit and any forecasting that might follow.

A third benefit can be understood by revisiting the rationale used by CART to determine whether a particular split is to be made for a given tree. Different sets of predictors are evaluated for different splits so that a wide variety of mean functions are evaluated, each potentially constructed from rather different basis functions. Recall the CART splitting criterion for binary response variables:

$$\Delta I(s, A) = I(A) - p(A_L)I(A_L) - p(A_R)I(A_R), \tag{5.1}$$

where $I(A)$ is the value of the parent impurity, $p(A_R)$ is the probability of a case falling in the right daughter node, $p(A_L)$ is the probability of a case falling in the left daughter node, $I(A_R)$ is the impurity of the right daughter node, and $I(A_L)$ is the impurity of the left daughter node. The CART algorithm tries to find the predictor and the split for which $\Delta I(s, A)$ is as large as possible.[2]

The usefulness of a potential split is a function of the two new impurities and the probability of cases falling into either of the prospective daughter nodes. Suppose there is a predictor that could produce splits in which one of the daughter nodes is very homogeneous but has relatively few observations, whereas the other node is quite heterogeneous but has relatively many observations. Suppose there is another predictor that could generate two nodes of about the same size, each of which is only moderately homogeneous. If these two predictors were competing against each other, the second predictor might well be chosen, and the small, relatively homogeneous, region that the first predictor would exploit be ignored. However, if the second predictor were not in the pool of competitors, the first might be selected instead.

Similar issues arise with predictors that are substantially correlated. There may be little difference empirically between the two so that when they compete to be a splitting variable, one might be chosen almost as readily as the other. But they would not partition the data in exactly the same way. The two partitions that could be defined would largely overlap with each partition having unique content as well. The unique content defined by the predictor not chosen would be excluded.

---

[2]Geurts and his colleagues (2006) have proposed another method for selecting predictors that can decrease dependence across trees and further open up the predictor competition. They do not build each tree from a bootstrap sample of the data. Rather, for each random sample of predictors, they select splits for each predictor at random (with equal probability), subject to some minimum number of observations in the smaller of the two partitions. Then, as in random forests, the predictor that reduces heterogeneity the most is chosen to define the two subsets of observations. They claim that this approach will reduce the overall heterogeneity at least as much as other ensemble procedures without a substantial increase in bias. However, this conclusion would seem to depend on how good the predictors really are.

Moreover, with the shared area now removed from consideration, the chances that the neglected predictor would be selected later for that tree are significantly reduced because its relationship with the response variable has been eroded. But all is not lost. There will be other trees in the forest and other chances to compete. For one or more subsequent trees, the slighted variable will be competing against others, but not the one with which it is strongly correlated.

In practice, the opportunity for weak predictors to contribute is huge. One by one, they may not help much but in the aggregate, their impact can be substantial. Conventional regression models typically exclude such variables by design. The associations with the response one by one are too small to be interesting in subject matter terms. In practice, weak predictors are treated as noise and swept into the disturbance term. But a large number of small associations, when considered as a group, can lead to much better fitted values and much more accurate imputations and forecasts.

5.2   An Initial Random Forests Illustration

Random forests has its roots in CART and bagging. One might expect, therefore, that when random forests is used for classification, a confusion table will be a key output. But for random forests, the confusion table is constructed from the OOB observations so that out-of-sample performance is represented. Such confusion tables can be called "honest."

We revisit the domestic violence example described earlier with an analysis that shows some of the complexities of working with very challenging data. The data are so challenging that some readers may be underwhelmed with how well random forests performs.[3] More definitive performance is illustrated later. The primary goal for the moment is to raise important application issues. The secondary goal is to undercut some of the hype that many associate with the procedures covered in this and the next three chapters. The procedures are very good to be sure. But, compelling results are never guaranteed.

There are a little over 500 observations, and even if just double interactions are considered, there are well over 100 predictors. This time, the goal is not to forecast new calls for service to the police department that likely involve domestic violence, but only those calls in which there is evidence that felony domestic violence has actually occurred. Such incidents represent about 6 % of the cases. They are very small as a fraction of all domestic violence calls for service. As such, they would normally be extremely difficult to forecast with better skill than could be obtained using the marginal distribution of the response alone. One would make only six mistakes in 100 households if one classified all households as not having new incidents of serious domestic violence.

---

[3] All of the other procedures tried performed even more poorly.

Table 5.1 Confusion table for a serious domestic violence incidents using a 10 to 1 target cost ratio (N = 516)

	No serious DV forecasted	Serious DV forecasted	Model error
No serious DV	341	146	.30
Serious DV	15	14	.52
Use error	.04	.91	Total error = .31

Using the response variable as the only source of information would in this case mean never correctly identifying any serious domestic violence households. The policy recommendation might be for the police to assume that the domestic violence incident to which they had been called would be the last serious one for that household. This would almost certainly be an unsatisfactory result, which implies that there are significant costs from false negatives. The default cost ratio of 1 to 1 is not responsive to the policy setting.

With a target cost ratio of 10 to 1 for false negatives to false positives favored by the police department, one obtains the results in Table 5.1.[4] The empirical cost ratio of false positives to false negatives is 146/15. The cost ratio value of 9.7 to 1 means that each false negative is worth nearly 10 times more than each false positive. This is effectively the 10 to 1 cost ratio sought and in practice, it is very difficult to hit the target cost ratio exactly. In practice, moreover, the differences between a confusion table with a 10 to 1 cost ratio and a confusion table with a 9.7 to 1 cost ratio will usually not matter.

Table 5.1 shows that random forests incorrectly classifies households 31 times out of 100 overall. The value of 31 can be interpreted as the overall average cost of a classification error. But noted earlier, the usual overall error gives all errors equal weight. Having decided from policy considerations that the proper cost ratio is 10 to 1, the proper average cost .57 (i.e., $[(10 \times 15) + 146]/516$). But, the overall measure of cost-weighted generalization error neglects some very important features of the table more relevant to real decision-making.

From the model error, one can see that about 30 % of the of the cases with no subsequent DV are classified incorrectly and about 52 % of the cases with subsequent DV are classified incorrectly. That this application of random forests correctly classifies only about half the DV cases may be disappointing, but without using any of the predictors, no DV cases whatsoever would be correctly classified.[5]

If the results from Table 5.1 are to be used to inform real decisions, use error is especially instructive. When a forecast is for no subsequent DV, the assigned class is incorrect only about 4 % of the time. When a forecast is for subsequent DV, the assigned class is incorrect about 91 % of the time. The large difference in forecasting skill results substantially from the 10 to 1 cost ratio. Implicit is a policy preference

---

[4]R code is not provided because it is too early in the exposition. Lots of R code is provided later.

[5]It might seem strange that the classification accuracy of one outcome is not 1 minus the classification accuracy of the other. If a case is not classified as DV, it must be classified as a DV case. But one is conditioning on the actual outcome, and the denominators of the model errors differ. Accuracy depends in part on the base.

to accept a relatively large number of false positives (i.e., 146) so that the number of false negatives is relatively low (i.e., 15). The 146 false positives lead to poor accuracy with the DV class that is predicted.

At the same time, the policy preference means that classification accuracy when no DV is the assigned class is improved compared to the baseline. Recall, that if the marginal distribution of the response is used, all 515 cases are predicted to be arrest-free, and 6 % of the cases are not arrest-free. From Table 5.1, 69 % percent of the cases are predicted to be arrest-free, and 4 % of those cases are not arrest-free. Because the base of 6 % is very small, it is impossible to obtain large improvements in percentage units; even perfect forecasting would only reduce the forecasting errors by 6 percentage points. In such circumstances, it is common to report ratios, and then the forecasting errors is reduced by one-third (2 %/6 %).

In short, the procedure accepts much weaker evidence to assign the serious DV class than to assign the no serious DV class. In this illustration, it takes very strong statistical evidence for a case to be classified as no serious DV. High accuracy follows for forecasts of no serious DV.

Although confusion tables using OOB data are an essential feature of random forests output, there are other kinds of output that can be very helpful. These are derived from additional algorithms that will be discussed shortly. In preparation and to help provide readers with better access to the technical literature, we turn to a few formalities.

5.3   A Few Technical Formalities

With some initial material on random forests behind us, it is useful to take a somewhat more formal look at the procedure. We build on an exposition by Breiman (2001a). The concepts considered make more rigorous some ideas that we have used in the past two chapters, and provide important groundwork for material to come. We also consider whether random forests overfits as the number of trees in the forest increases. As before, we emphasize categorical, and especially binary, response variables.

It will be important to keep straight randomness introduced by the algorithm and randomness introduced by the data. One can undertake a level I analysis despite randomness from algorithm because it has nothing to do with how the data were generated. The moment interest includes generalizing beyond the data on hand, randomness in the data are in play, and a level II analysis must follow. Most formal expositions of random forests emphasize level II issues.

In order to help readers who may wish to read Breiman's treatment of random forests or subsequent work that draws directly from it, Breiman's notation is adopted. Bold type is used for vectors and matrices. Capital letters are used for random variables. The terms "predictor" and "input" are used interchangeably.

5.3.1 What Is a Random Forest?

With categorical response variables, a random forest is an ensemble of classifiers. The classifiers are K classification trees, each based in part on chance mechanisms. Like CART, these classifiers can work with more than two response categories. The goal is to exploit the ensemble of K trees to assign classes to observations using information contained in a set of predictors.

We formally represent a random forest as a collection of K tree-structured classifiers $\{f(\mathbf{x}, \Theta_k), k = 1, \ldots\}$, where $\mathbf{x}$ is an input vector of p input values used to assign a class, and k is an index for a given tree. "Each tree casts a unit vote for the most popular class at input x" (Breiman 2001a: 6). As an ensemble of classifiers, a random forest is also a classifier.

Θ_k is a random vector constructed for the kth tree so that it is independent of past random vectors $\Theta_1, \ldots, \Theta_{k-1}$, and is generated from the same distribution. For bagging, it is the means by which observations are selected at random with replacement from the training data. For random forests, it is also the means by which subsets of predictors are sampled without replacement for each potential split. In both cases, Θ_k is a collection of integers. The integers serve as indices determining which cases and which predictors, respectively, are selected. Integers for both sampling procedures can be denoted by Θ_k.

The paramount output from a random forest is an assigned class for each observation determined at its input values $\mathbf{x}_i$. In CART, for example, the class assigned to an observation is the class associated with the terminal node in which an observation falls. With random forests, the class assigned to each observation is determined by a vote over the set of tree classifiers when OOB data are used. Classes are assigned to observations much as they are in bagging. It is important conceptually to distinguish between the class assigned by the kth tree and the class assigned by a forest. It is also important to appreciate that when used as a classifier, random forests does not produce probabilities for the response variable classes. There is not even an analogy to the fitted values from logistic regression.

5.3.2 Margins and Generalization Error for Classifiers in General

For ease of exposition, consider first any ensemble classifier, not random forests in particular. Suppose there is a training dataset with input values and associated values for a categorical response. As before, each observation in the training dataset is realized at random and independently. The set of inputs and a response are random variables.

There is an ensemble of K classifiers, $f_1(\mathbf{x})$, $f_2(\mathbf{x})$, $\ldots$, $f_K(\mathbf{x})$. For the moment, we do not consider how these different classifiers are constructed. The margin function at *the data point* $\mathbf{X}, Y$ is then defined as

$$mg(\mathbf{X}, Y) = av_k I(f_k(\mathbf{X}) = Y) - \max_{j \neq Y} av_k I(f_k(\mathbf{X}) = j), \qquad (5.2)$$

where $I(.)$ is an indicator function, j is an incorrect class, av_k denotes averaging over the set of classifiers for a single realized data point, and max denotes the largest value. For a given set of x-values and the associated observed class, the margin is the average number of votes over classifiers for the correct observed class minus the maximum average number of votes over classifiers for any other class. The term "data point" for this discussion is for the same a row in the dataset. Because Eq. 5.2 applies to any row, it applies to all rows.

From the definition of the margin function, generalization error is then,

$$g = P_{\mathbf{X}, Y}(mg(\mathbf{X}, Y) < 0), \qquad (5.3)$$

where P means probability. In words, Breiman's generalization error is the probability over realizations of a given row of the data that the vote will be won by an incorrect class: the probability that the margin will be negative. Because Eq. 5.3 applies to any row, it applies to realizations for all rows. There are no test data in this formulation of generalization error, and the training data are not fixed. Recall that when Hastie et al. (2009: 220) define generalization error, the training data are fixed and performance is evaluated over realizations of test data. One is, of course, free to define concepts as one wants, but for both definitions, generalization error should be small.

5.3.3 Generalization Error for Random Forests

Now, suppose for the kth classifier $f_k(\mathbf{X}) = f(\mathbf{X}, \Theta_k)$. There are K tree classifiers that comprise a random forest. Breiman proves (2001a) that as the number of trees increases, the estimated generalization error converges to the true generalization error, which is

$$P_{\mathbf{X}, y}(P_\Theta(f(\mathbf{X}, \Theta) = Y) - \max_{j \neq Y} P_\Theta(f(\mathbf{X}, \theta) = j) < 0). \qquad (5.4)$$

$P_\Theta(f(\mathbf{X}, \Theta) = Y)$ is the probability of a correct classification over trees that differ randomly because of the sampling of the training data with replacement and the sampling of predictors. One can think of this as the proportion of times a classification is correct over a limitless number of trees grown from the same dataset. Parallel reasoning for an incorrect classification applies to $P_\Theta(f(\mathbf{X}, \theta) = j)$. Note that the data are fixed.[6] Then, we are essentially back to Eq. 5.3. As before, $P_{\mathbf{X}, Y}$ is the probability of an incorrect classification over realizations of the data themselves. We

---

[6]The concept of training data gets fuzzy at this point. The training data for a given tree is the random sample drawn with replacement from the dataset on hand. But for the random forest that entire dataset is the training data.

address the uncertainty that is a product of random forests and then the uncertainty that is a product of the random variables. Breiman proves that as the number of trees increase without limit, all of these sources of randomness cancel out leaving the true generalization error shown in Eq. 5.4.

What does one mean in this context by "true" generalization error? No claims are made that the classes assigned by a given forest are "correct." In function estimation language, no claims are made that the true $f(\mathbf{X})$ has been found. Rather, one has once again some approximation of the true response surface, and it is the generalization error of that approximation to which an estimated generalization error converges. It is the "true" generalization error of the approximation.[7]

The importance of the convergence is that demonstrably random forests does not overfit as more trees are grown. One might think that with more trees, one would get an increasingly false sense of how well the results generalize. Breiman proves that this is not true. Given all of the concern about overfitting, this is an important result.

There is some work addressing random forests statistical consistency for what appears to be the true response surface. Even if all of the needed predictors are available, there can be situations in which random forests is not consistent (Biau et al. 2008; Biau and Devroye 2010). However, because this work is somewhat stylized, it is not clear what the implications for practice may be. Work that is more recent and somewhat less stylized proves consistency but among other things, requires sparsity (Biau 2012). This means that only a "very few" of the large set of potential predictors are related to the response (Biau 2012: 1067). We are apparently back to the conventional linear regression formulation in which there are two kinds of predictors: those that matter a lot and those that do not matter at all. A look at the variable importance plots reported later in this chapter shows no evidence of sparsity. There may well be other kinds of data for which sparsity can be plausibly defended (e.g., for genomics research).

Another assumption that all of the recent theoretical work seems to share is that the trees in a random forest are "honest" (Wager 2014: 7). By "honest," one means that the data used to determine the fitted value for each terminal node are not the data used to determined the data partitions. By this definition, the trees in Breiman's random forests are *not* honest so the theoretical work does not directly apply. Moreover, "...the bias of CART trees seems to be subtle enough that it does not affect the performance of random forests in most situations" (Wager 2014: 8). It is probably fair to say that the jury is still out on the formal properties of random forests, but that in practice, there is a consensus that it performs well.

---

[7]Because of random forests' chance components and random forests' dependence on sample size, the approximation response surface in the joint probability distribution is the expected random forest grown with the same number of observations as available in the data.

5.3.4   The Strength of a Random Forest

The margin function for a given realized data point in a random forest (not just any classifier) is defined as

$$mr(\mathbf{X}, Y) = P_\Theta(f(\mathbf{X}, \Theta) = Y) - \max_{j \neq Y} P_\Theta(f(\mathbf{X}, \Theta) = j), \qquad (5.5)$$

where $f(\mathbf{X}, \Theta)$ denotes random forest classifications for a given row that can vary because of the chance mechanisms represented by Θ. Because of the randomness build into the random forest algorithm, the margin function is defined using the probability of a correct vote and an incorrect vote over forests grown from the same dataset. It appropriates a piece of the definition of random forests generalization error.

It is a short step from a random forest margin function to a definition of the "strength" of a random forest. We take the expectation over realizations of the data. That is, the expected value of Eq. 5.5 is:

$$s = E_{\mathbf{X}, y} mr(\mathbf{X}, Y). \qquad (5.6)$$

The strength of a random forest is an expected margin over all possible realizations of the data. And no surprise, strong is good.

5.3.5   Dependence

As previously noted, the effectiveness of averaging over trees using votes depends on the independence of the trees. But, how does one think about that independence in this setting? There is apparently some confusion in the literature (to which I plead guilty). Hastie et al. (2009: 598) stress correctly that "... $\rho(x)$ is the theoretical correlation between a pair of random forest trees evaluated at x, induced by repeatedly making training sample draws $\mathbf{Z}$ from the population, and then drawing randomly a pair of random forest trees." That is, it is the expected value of the correlation between the fitted values from randomly selected pairs of trees over realizations of the data. Ideally, that expected correlation is zero.

5.3.6   Implications

Dependence is important because Breiman shows (Breiman 2001a: 6) that the upper bound for the generalization error is

$$g^* = \frac{\bar{\rho}(1 - s^2)}{s^2}, \qquad (5.7)$$

where $\bar{\rho}$ is the expected correlation over pairs of trees as just described, and s is the strength of the random forest. Ideally, the former is small and the latter is large.

Equation 5.7 implies that both the sizes of margins and that ways in which the random forest algorithm introduces randomness are critical. The random forest algorithm already does a pretty good job reducing the expected correlation. But in practice, random forest sometimes can be tuned to help. For example, sampling fewer inputs at each splitting opportunity can in some situations improve performance, and the random forest software in R emphasized here (i.e., *randomForest( )*) has a default function for determining the number of predictors that seems to work quite well.[8]

5.3.7 Putting It All Together

Why does random forests work so well as a classifier? Although there are not yet any formal proofs, recent work by Wyner and colleagues (2015) provides a conceptual framework coupled with simulations that support some very instructive intuitions. We will see later that their thinking applies to boosting as well.

It has become common practice, and often the default practice, to grow trees as large as the data will allow. Terminal nodes are often perfectly homogeneous. Indeed, sometimes tuning parameters are set so that each terminal node can contain a single observation. Consequently, in the bootstrap sample used to grow each tree, the fit to the data can be perfect; for each observation, the tree assigns the correct class. When this happens, one has an interpolating classifier (Wyner et al. 2015: 9).

Figure 5.1 provides a very simple illustration. We again have a 3-dimensional scatter plot for a realized training dataset. There are two numerical predictors X and Z, and a binary outcome represented as red, blue, or purple. The red and blue outcome classes are noiseless in the sense that no matter what the realization of the data, observations in those locations are always red or blue respectively. In contrast, the purple circles can be either red or blue depending on the realization.

The box in the upper left-hand corner results from a single classification tree terminal node with $X < 2$ and $Z > 12$. The node has one observation and, therefore, is necessarily classified correctly. With sufficiently fine-grained partitioning of X and Z using a sufficiently large tree, each circle in Fig. 5.1 can reside in its own terminal node. Each would be classified correctly, and its terminal nodes would be perfectly homogeneous. One would have what Wyner and his colleagues call an interpolation of the data.

Things are more complicated in the lower right-hand box. For observations with $X > 7$ and $Z < -4$, the outcome class can vary over realizations. It could be a blue outcome for one data realization and a red outcome for another data realization. Suppose in one realization of the training data, it is red and is classified as red. One still has an interpolation of the realized data. But for test data that classification could

---

[8] There are other implementations for random forests in R that are briefly discussed later.

Fig. 5.1 Visualization of
interpolation for a single
classification tree with *blue*
and *red* outcomes having no
noise and *purple* outcomes
having some noise

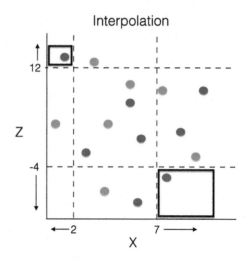

be wrong because the realized value in that location is blue. Generalization error has
been introduced because of overfitting.

However, *because of the interpolation*, one has "local robustness" (Wyner et al.
2015: 9–10). Whatever the error in the fit caused by the purple circle, it is confined to
its own terminal node. That is, all of the classifications for the other circles are made
separately from the noisy circle, so that the damage is very limited. In an important
sense, overfitting has some demonstrable benefits.

But there is still overfitting for a given tree. Enter random forests. Each tree is
grown with a random sample of the training data (with replacement). Whatever the
expected value is for the outcome, sometimes the lower right-hand box will contain
a red outcome and sometimes it will contain a blue outcome. By the Bayes decision
rule, a vote taken over trees for terminal nodes defined just like the lower right-hand
box will classify observations that land in that region as red or blue, depending on
the majority vote. This is the best one can do with respect to generalization error.

Voting is an averaging process that improves on the generalization error from
a single tree. Although each tree will overfit, averaging over trees compensates.
Because for real data most points will be purple, the averaging is essential as a form
of regularization.

There is even more going on. First, the striving to interpolate is helped by the
sampling of predictors. Imagine that in Fig. 5.1 one location has a red circle right on
top of a blue circle. There is no way with X and Z alone to arrive at an interpolation
point at that location.[9] One solution is to come upon a variable, W, that in combination
with X and Z could define two terminal nodes, one with the blue circle and one with
the red circle. But, looking back to Eq. 5.1, suppose that for a given prospective
partitioning of the data, W does not make a sufficient contribution to homogeneity
to be selected as the next partitioning variable. Even if it is strongly related to the

---

[9]As discussed in Chap. 1, there might be a solution is some linear basis expansion of X and Z.

response, it is also too strongly related to X. An opportunity to distinguish between a red circle and a blue circle is lost. This problem can be solved by sampling predictors. Suppose, there is a predictor U that, like X, is strongly related to the response, but unlike X is only moderately related to Z. If for some split, X is not available as a potential partitioning variable but U is, U, W, and Z can participate sequentially in the partitioning process.[10]

Second, the random sampling helps in the situation just described. Over trees, the covariances among the variables will vary. Consequently, there will be variation in how strongly X and W are related to the response and to each other. This provides an opportunity in some samples for W to be less competitive with X. For example, in some samples, there can be prospective partitions for which W reduces heterogeneity sufficiently, even if X is an earlier partitioning variable. The result will be some different terminal nodes that, in turn, will affect the vote over trees.

Finally, a larger number of training observations can really help. With larger samples, one can grow larger trees. With larger trees, interpolation can better approximated. With a better approximation of interpolation, coupled with averaging over trees, generalization error can be reduced.

Although all of the mechanisms just described are always in play, challenges from real data are substantial. In practice, all of the class labels are noisy so that the circles in Fig. 5.1 would all be purple. A perfect fit in the training data will not lead to a perfect fit in the test data. Moreover, a perfect fit is certainly no guarantee of obtaining unbiased estimates of the true response surface. There will typically be omitted predictors, and the classification trees are still limited by the ways splits are determined and the greedy nature of the tree algorithm. It remains true, however, that "Random forests has gained tremendous popularity due to robust performance across a wide range of data sets. The algorithm is often capable of achieving best-in-class performance with respect to generalization error and is not highly sensitive to choice of tuning parameters, making it an ideal off-the-shelf tool of choice for many applications" (Wyner et al. 2015: 9).

5.4 Random Forests and Adaptive Nearest Neighbor Methods

A conceptual link was made earlier between CART and adaptive nearest neighbor methods. Not surprisingly, similar links can be made between random forests and adaptive nearest neighbor methods. But for random forests, there are a number of more subtle issues (Meinshausen 2006; Lin and Jeon 2006). These are important not just for a deeper understanding of random forests, but for recent theoretical treatments (Biau 2013; Wager 2014; Wager et al. 2014; Wager and Walther 2015).

---

[10] Also, W might be selected farther down in the tree even if it is chosen along with X, depending on the other predictors chosen. They are both in a competition with several other candidate splitting variables.

Recall that in CART, each terminal node represented a region of nearest neighbors. The boundaries of the neighborhood were constructed adaptively when the best predictors and their best splits were determined. With the neighborhood defined, all of the observations inside were used to compute a mean or proportion. This value became the measure of central tendency for the response within that neighborhood. In short, each terminal node and the neighborhood represented had its own conditional mean or conditional proportion.

Consider the case in which equal costs are assumed. This makes for a much easier exposition, and no key points are lost. The calculations that take place within each terminal node implicitly rely on a weight given to each value of the response variable. For a given terminal node, all observations not in that node play no role when the mean or proportion is computed. Consequently, each such observation has a weight of zero. For a given terminal node, all of its observations are used when the mean or proportion is computed. Consequently, each value of the response variable in that node has a weight equal to $1/n_\tau$, where n is the number of observations in terminal node τ. Once the mean or proportion for a terminal node is computed, that mean or proportion can serve as a fitted value for all cases that fall in that terminal node.

Figure 5.2 shows a toy rendering. The tree has a single partitioning of the data. There happen to be three values of the response variable in each terminal node. Consider terminal node A. The mean for terminal node A is 2.33, computed with weights of 1/3 for the values in that node and weights of 0 otherwise; the values of the response variable in terminal node B play no role when the mean of node A is computed. Each of the three observations landing in terminal node A are assigned a value of 2.33 as their fitted value. If the response variable had been binary, the numbers in the two terminal nodes would have been replaced by 1s and 0s. Then a conditional proportion for terminal node A would be the outcome of the weighted

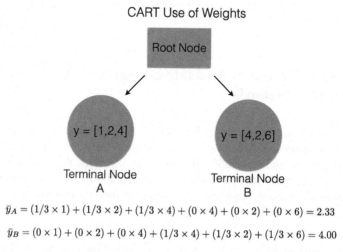

CART Use of Weights

$$\bar{y}_A = (1/3 \times 1) + (1/3 \times 2) + (1/3 \times 4) + (0 \times 4) + (0 \times 2) + (0 \times 6) = 2.33$$

$$\bar{y}_B = (0 \times 1) + (0 \times 2) + (0 \times 4) + (1/3 \times 4) + (1/3 \times 2) + (1/3 \times 6) = 4.00$$

Fig. 5.2 CART weighting used to assign a mean or proportion to a terminal node A or B

averaging. And from this, an assigned class could be determined as usual. The same reasoning applies to terminal node B.

A bit more formally, a conditional mean or proportion for any terminal node τ is

$$\bar{y}_\tau | x = \sum_{i=1}^{N} w_{(i,\tau)} y_i, \tag{5.8}$$

where the sum is taken over the *entire* training dataset, and w_i is the weight for each y_i. The sum of the weights over all observations is 1.0. In practice, most of the weights for the calculations in any terminal will be zero because they are not associated with the terminal node τ. This is no different from the manner in which nearest neighbor methods can work when summary measures of a response variable are computed.

There are two important features of the weighting terminal node by terminal node. First, each terminal node defines a neighborhood. The x-values for each observation determine in which neighborhood the observation belongs. It will often turn out that observations with somewhat different sets of x-values land in the same neighborhood. For example, a partition may be defined by a threshold of 25 years of age. All ages less than 25 sent to one neighborhood and all ages 25 and above are sent to another.

Second, for any given tree, each of the N observations will have a single, nonzero weight because each observation must land in one (and only one) of the terminal nodes. It is in that node that the single weight is determined as the reciprocal of the number of observations. In our toy example, each of the six observations happen to have a weight of 1/3 because both terminal nodes have three observations.

Now imagine that the tree is grown as an element of a random forest. The form of the calculations shown for terminal nodes A and B still apply with the fitted values, in this instance, a conditional mean. However, there are now a large number of such trees. For each observation, random forests average the weights obtained from each tree (Lin and Jeon 2006: 579–580). Consequently, the ith fitted value from a random forest is a weighted average of N values of the response, much like in Fig. 5.2, but using average weights.[11] That is,

$$\hat{y}_i = \sum_{i=1}^{N} \bar{w}_i y_i, \tag{5.9}$$

where $\bar{w}_i$ is the average weight.

The weights can serve another important purpose. Suppose for a given neighborhood defined by x_0, there are 10 observations and, therefore, 10 values for a quantitative response. There are also 10 average weights as just described. If one orders the response values from low to high, the weights conceptualized as

---

[11] For example, if there is a tiny random forest of 3 trees (more like very small stand), and the ith observation has 3 weights of .2, .3, and .1, the average weight over the 3 trees is .2.

Table 5.2 Weights and cumulative weights for a target value x_0

Average weight	Response value	Cumulative weight
.10	66	.10
.11	71	.21
.12	74	.33
.08	78	.41
.09	82	.50
.10	85	.60
.13	87	.73
.07	90	.80
.11	98	.91
.09	99	1.0

probabilities can be used to compute other summary measures than the mean. Table 5.2 can be used to illustrate.

From left to right, there are ten average weights that sum to 1.0, ten response values available for x_0, listed in order, and then cumulative weights. The mean is computed by multiplying each response value by its average weight and adding the products. In this case, the mean is 83. Quantiles are also available. The 10th percentile is 66. The 50th percentile (the median) is 82. The 90th percentile is a little less than 98. In short, one is not limited to the mean of each x_0.

Suppose one has a random forest and a variety of predictor profiles of x-values. When the response is quantitative, there routinely is interest in determining the fitted conditional mean for each profile. But sometimes, there will be interest in fitted conditional medians to "robustify" random forest results or to consider a central tendency measure unaffected by the tails of the distribution. Sometimes, there is subject matter interest in learning about a conditional quantile such as the 25th percentile or the 90th percentile.

For example, in today's world of school accountability based on standardized tests, perhaps students who score especially poorly on standardized tests respond better to smaller classroom sizes than students who excel on standardized tests. The performance distribution on standardized tests, conditioning on classroom size, differs for good versus poor performers. Building on work of Lin and Jeon just discussed, Meinshausen (2006) alters the random forests algorithm so that conditional quantiles can be provided as fitted values. An application is provided later in this chapter using *quantregForest( )* in R.[12]

But there are caveats. In particular, each tree is still grown with a conventional impurity measure, which for a quantitative response is the error sum of squares (Meinshausen 2006: Sect. 3). If one is worried about the impact of a highly skewed response variable distribution, there may well be good reason to worry about the splitting criterion too. For example, one might prefer to minimize the sum of the

---

[12]The package *quantregForest( )* is authored by Nicolai Meinshausen and Lukas Schiesser.

absolute values of the residuals (i.e., L_1 loss) rather than the sum of squared residuals (i.e., L_2 loss) as an impurity measure. This was originally proposed by Breiman and his colleagues in 1984 (Chap. 8), and there have been interesting efforts to build on their ideas (Chaudhuri and Loh 2002; Loh 2014). But L_1 loss does not seem to have yet been incorporated into random forests. We will see later that L_1 loss has been implemented in stochastic gradient boosting.

5.5 Introducing Misclassification Costs

Just as in CART, there is a need when random forests is used as a classifier to consider the relative costs of false negatives and false positives. Otherwise, for each tree, one again has to live with results that depend on the default of equal costs and a prior distribution for the response variable that is the same as its marginal distribution in the data.

Perhaps the most conceptually direct method would be to allow for a cost matrix just as CART does. To date, this option is not available in random forest software, and there is evidence that it might not work effectively if it were.

There are four approaches that have been seriously considered for the binary class case. They differ by whether costs are imposed on the data before each tree is grown, as each tree is grown, or at the end when classes are assigned. Although binary outcomes will be emphasized, the lessons for response variables with more than two categories will be covered as well.

1. Just as in CART, one can use a prior distribution to capture costs as each tree is grown. This has the clear advantages of being based on the mechanics of CART and capitalizing on a straightforward way to translate costs into an appropriate prior.
2. After all of the trees are grown, one can differentially weight the classification votes over trees. For example, one vote for classification in the less common category might count the same as two votes for classification in the more common category. This has the advantage of being easily understood.
3. After all of the trees are grown, one can abandon the majority vote rule and use thresholds that reflect the relative costs of false negatives and false positives. For instance, rather than classifying as 1 all observations when the vote is larger than 50 %, one might classify all observations as 1 when the vote is larger than 33 %. This too is easy to understand.
3. When each bootstrap sample is drawn before a tree is grown, one can oversample cases from one class relative to cases from the other class, in much the same spirit as disproportional stratified sampling used for data collection (Thompson 2002: Chap. 11). Before a tree is grown, one oversamples the cases for which forecasting errors are relatively more costly. Conceptually, this is a lot like altering the prior distribution.

All four approaches share the problem that the actual ratio of false negatives to false positives in the confusion table probably will not sufficiently correspond to the target cost ratio. In practice, this means that whatever method is used to introduce relative costs, that method is simply considered a way to "tune" the results. With some trial and error, an appropriate ratio of false negatives to false positives can usually be achieved. All four also share the problem mentioned earlier that when there are more than two response categories, none of the methods introduce enough new information to directly control all of the relevant cost ratios. But also as before, with some trial and error it is usually possible to approximate well enough the target cost in the confusion table.

Although experience suggests that in general all four methods can tune the results as needed, there may be some preference for tuning by the prior or by stratified bootstrap sampling. Both of these methods will affect the confusion table through the trees themselves. The structure of the trees themselves responds to the costs introduced. Changing the way votes are counted or the thresholds used only affects the classes assigned, and leaves the trees unchanged. The defaults of equal costs and the empirical prior remain in effect. By allowing the trees to respond directly to cost considerations, more responsive forecasts should be produced. Moreover, any output beyond a confusion table will reflect properly the desired costs. More is said about such output shortly.

There is one very important situation in which the stratified sampling approach is likely to be demonstrably superior to the other three approaches. If the response variable is highly unbalanced (e.g., a 95–5 split), any given bootstrap sample may fail to include enough observations for the rare category. Then, a useful tree will be difficult to grow. As observed earlier, it will often be difficult under these circumstances for CART to move beyond the marginal distribution of the response. Oversampling rare cases when the bootstrap sample is drawn will generally eliminate this problem. Using a prior that makes the rare observations less rare can also help, but that help applies in general and will not be sufficient if a given bootstrap sample makes the rare cases even more rare.

We consider some applications in depth shortly. But a very brief illustration is provided now to prime the pump.

5.5.1   A Brief Illustration Using Asymmetric Costs

Table 5.3 was constructed using data from the prison misconduct study described earlier. In this example, the response is incidents of very serious misconduct, not the garden variety kind. As noted previously, such misconduct is relatively rare. Less than about 3 % of the inmates had such reported incidents. So, just as for the domestic violence data shown in Table 5.1, it is extremely difficult to do better than the marginal distribution under the usual CART defaults. In addition, there is simply not a lot of misconduct cases from which the algorithm can learn. Trees in the forest will be unable to partition the rare cases as often as might be desirable; tree depth

Table 5.3 Confusion table for forecasts of serious prison misconduct with a 20 to 1 target cost ratio (N = 4806)

	Forecast no misconduct	Forecast misconduct	Model error
No misconduct	3311	1357	.29
Misconduct	58	80	.42
Use error	.02	.94	Overall error = .29

may be insufficient. In short, when a response distribution is highly unbalanced, very large samples can sometimes help too.

Suppose that the costs of forecasting errors for the rare cases were substantially higher than the costs of forecasting errors for the common cases. These relative costs can be introduced effectively by drawing a stratified bootstrap sample, oversampling the rare cases. And by making the rare cases less rare, problems that might follow from the highly unbalanced response variable can sometimes be overcome.

For Table 5.3, the bootstrap samples for each of the two response categories was set to equal 100.[13] The "50–50" bootstrap distribution was selected by trial and error to produce an empirical cost ratio of false negatives to false positives of about 20 to 1 (actually 23 to 1 here). The cost ratio may be too high for real policy purposes, but it is still within the range considered reasonable by prison officials.

Why 100 cases each? Experience suggests that the sample size for the less common response category should equal about two-thirds of the number of cases in that class. If a larger fraction of the less common cases is sampled, the out-of-bag sample size for that class may be too small. The OOB observations may not be able to provide the quality of test data needed.

With the number of bootstrap observations for the less common category determined to be 100, the 50–50 constraint leads to 100 cases being sampled for the more common response category. In practice, one determines the sample size for the less common outcome and then adjusts the sample size of the more common outcome as needed.

Table 5.3 can be interpreted just as any of the earlier confusion tables. For example, the overall proportion of cases incorrectly identified is 0.29, but that fails to take the target costs of false negatives to false positives (i.e., 20 to 1) into account. Random forests classify 42 % of the incidents of misconduct incorrectly and 29 % of the no misconduct cases incorrectly. Should prison officials use these results for forecasting,

---

[13]Using the procedure *randomForest()* in R written by Leo Breiman and Ann Culter, and later ported to R by Andy Liaw and Matthew Wiener, the stratified sampling argument was *sampsize=c(100,100)*. The order of the two sample sizes depends on the order of the response variable categories. They are ordered alphabetical or numerically low to high depending on how the variable is coded. For classification procedures in R, it is a good idea to always construct the outcome variable as a factor. The procedure *randomForest()* will automatically know that the task is classification. If a binary response variable is defined as numeric with a value of 0 and a value of 1, and if the type of procedure within *randomForest()* is not identified as classification, *randomForest()* will proceed with regression. This is a common error.

a forecast of no serious misconduct would be wrong only 2 times out of 100, and a forecast of serious misconduct would be wrong 94 times out of 100. The very large number of false positives results substantially from the target 20 to 1 cost ratio. But, for very serious inmate misconduct, having about 1 true positive for about 17 false positives (1357/80) may be an acceptable trade-off. The misconduct represented can include homicide, assault, sexual assault, and narcotics trafficking. If not, the cost ratio could be made more symmetric.

To summarize, random forests provides several ways to take the costs of false negatives and false positives into account. Introducing stratified bootstrap sampling seems to work well in practice. Ignoring the relative costs of classification errors does not mean that costs are not affecting the results. The default is equal costs and using the marginal distribution of the response variable as the empirical prior.

5.6 Determining the Importance of the Predictors

Just as for bagging, random forests leaves behind so many trees that collectively they are useless for interpretation. Yet, a goal of statistical learning can be to explore how inputs are related to outputs. Exactly how best to do this is currently unresolved, but there are several useful options available. We begin with a discussion of "variable importance."

5.6.1 Contributions to the Fit

One approach to predictor importance is to record the decrease in the fitting measure (e.g., Gini index, mean square error) each time a given variable is used to define a split. The sum of these reductions for a given tree is a measure of importance for that variable when that tree is grown. For random forests, one can average this measure of importance over the set of trees.

As with conventional variance partitions, however, reductions in the fitting criterion ignore the prediction skill of a model, which many statisticians treat as the gold standard. Fit measures are computed with the data used to build the classifier (i.e., in-sample). They are not computed from test data (i.e., out-of-sample).

Moreover, it can be difficult to translate contributions to a fit statistic into practical terms. Simply asserting that a percentage contribution to a fit statistic is a measure of importance is circular. Importance must be defined outside of the procedure used to measure it. And what is it about contributions to a measure of fit that makes a predictor more or less important? Even if an external definition is provided, is a predictor important if it can account for, say, 10% of the reduction in impurity?

One also must be fully clear that contributions to the fit by themselves are silent on what would happen if in the real world a predictor is manipulated. Causality can only be established by how the data were generated, and causal interpretations depend on there being a real intervention altering one or more predictors (Berk 2003).

5.6.2 Contributions to Prediction

Breiman (2001a) has suggested another form of randomization to assess the role of each predictor. This method is implemented in *randomForest()*. It is based on the reduction in what Breiman calls prediction accuracy when a predictor is shuffled so that the predictor cannot make a systematic contribution to a prediction. For categorical response variables, it is the reduction in *classification* accuracy with OOB data. One conditions on the actual outcome to determine the proportion of times the wrong class is assigned. As such it has a very grounded interpretation that can be directly linked to the rows of a confusion table. For numeric response variables, the standard approach is to use the increase in mean squared error for the OOB data. One is again conditioning on the actual value of Y. The term "prediction", can be a little misleading, but to be consistent with Breiman, we will stick with it here.

Breiman's approach has much in common with the concept of Granger causality (Granger and Newbold 1986: Sect. 7.3). Imagine two times series, Y_t and X_t. If the future conditional distribution of Y given current and past values of Y is the same as the future conditional distribution of Y given current and past values of Y and X, X does not Granger-cause Y.[14] If the two future conditional distributions differ, X is a Granger-cause of Y.

These ideas generalize so that for the baseline conditional distribution, one can condition not just on current and past values of Y but on current and past values of other predictors (but not X). Then X Granger-causes Y, conditional on the other predictors, if including X as a predictor changes the future conditional distribution of Y. In short, the idea of using forecasting performance as a way to characterize the performance of predictors has been advanced in both the statistical and econometrics literature.

Breiman's importance measure of prediction accuracy differs perhaps most significantly from Granger cause in that Breiman does not require time series data and randomly shuffles the values of predictors rather than dropping (or adding) predictors from a procedure. The latter has some important implications discussed shortly.

For Breiman's approach with a categorical response variable, the following algorithm is used to compute each predictor's importance.

1. Construct a measure prediction error ν for each tree as usual by dropping the out-of-bag (OOB) data down the tree. Note that this is out-of-sample because data not used to grow the tree are used to evaluate its predictive skill.
2. If there are p predictors, repeat Step 1 p times, but each time with the values of a given predictor randomly shuffled. The shuffling makes that predictor on the average unrelated to the response and all other predictors. For each shuffled predictor j, compute new measure of prediction error, ν_j.
3. For each of the p predictors, average over trees the difference between the prediction error with no shuffling and the prediction error with the jth predictor shuffled.

---

[14]Sometimes Granger-cause is called predictive cause.

The average increase in prediction error when a given predictor j is shuffled represents the importance of that predictor. That is,

$$I_j = \sum_{k=i}^{K} \left[\frac{1}{K}(\nu_j - \nu) \right], \quad j = 1, \ldots, p, \tag{5.10}$$

where there are K trees, ν_j is the prediction error with predictor j shuffled, and ν is the prediction error with none of the predictors shuffled. It is sometimes possible for prediction accuracy to improve slightly when a variable is shuffled because of the randomness introduced. A negative measure of predictor importance follows. Negative predictor importance can be treated as no decline in accuracy or simply can be ignored.

As written, Eq. 5.10 is somewhat open-ended. The measures of prediction error (ν and ν_j) are not defined. As just noted, for a quantitative response variable, the MSE is an obvious choice. There are more options for categorical response variables: the deviance, percentage of cases classified incorrectly, average change in the margins, or some other measure. Currently, the preferred measure is the proportion (or percentage) of cases misclassified. This has the advantage of allowing direct comparisons between the increases in misclassification and all of the row summaries in a confusion table. In addition, all of the other measures considered to date have been found less satisfactory for one reason or another. For example, some measures are misleadingly sensitive; small changes in the number of classification errors can lead to large changes in the importance measure.

When used with categorical response variables, a significant complication is that Eq. 5.10 will almost always produce different importance measures for given predictors for different categories of the response. That is, there will be for any given predictor a measure of importance for each response class, and the measures will not generally be the same. For example, if there are three response classes, there will be three measures of importance for each predictor that will generally differ. Moreover, this can lead to different rankings of predictors depending on which response category is being considered. Although this may seem odd, it follows directly from the fact that the number of observations in each response class and the margins for each class will typically differ. Consequently, a given increase in the number of misclassifications can have different percentage impacts. A detailed illustration is presented shortly.

Partly in response to such complications, one can standardize the declines in performance. The standard deviation of $(\nu_j - \nu)$ over trees can be computed. In effect, one has a bootstrap estimate over trees of the standard error associated with the increase in classification error, which can be used as a descriptive measure of stability. Larger values imply less stability.

Then, one can divide Eq. 5.10 by this value. The result can be interpreted as a z-score so that importance measures are now all on the same scale. And with a bit of a stretch, confidence intervals can be computed and conventional hypothesis tests performed. It is a stretch because the sampling distribution of the predictor importance measure is usually not known. Perhaps more important, the descriptive gains from standardization are modest at best, as the illustrations that follow make clear.

One of the drawbacks of the shuffling approach to variable importance is that only one variable is shuffled at a time. There is no role for joint importance over several predictors. This can be an issue when predictors are correlated. There will be a contribution to prediction accuracy that is uniquely linked to each predictor and joint contributions shared between two or more predictors. This can also be an issue when a single categorical predictor is represented by a set of indicator variables. The importance of the set is not captured.

There is currently no option in the random forest software to shuffle more than one variable at a time. However, it is relatively easy to apply the prediction procedure in random forests using as input the original dataset with two or more of the predictors shuffled. Then, Eq. 5.10 can be employed as before, where j would now be joined by other predictor subscripts. The main problem is that the number of potential joint contributions can be very large. In practice, some subset selection procedure is likely to be needed, perhaps based on substantive considerations.

It might seem that Granger's approach of examining forecasting skill with and without a given predictor included is effectively the same as Breiman's shuffling approach. And if so, one might consider, for instance, dropping sets of predictors to document their joint contribution. But actually, the two strategies are somewhat different. In Granger's approach, dropping or adding predictors to the model means that the model itself will be reestimated each time. So, the comparisons Granger favors are the result of different predictors being included *and different models*. The impact of neutralizing a predictor and changing the model are confounded. Under Breiman's approach, the model is not reconstructed. The shuffling is undertaken as an additional procedure with the model fixed.

In summary, for many scientists the ability to predict accurately in Brieman's sense is an essential measure of a model's worth. If one cannot predict well, it means that the model cannot usefully reproduce the empirical world. It follows that such a model has little value. And as now stressed a number of times, a model that fits the data well will not necessarily predict well. Put another way, out-of-sample performance is far more compelling than in-sample performance. The take-home message is simple: if prediction skill is the gold standard (or even just a very important criterion by which to evaluate a model), then a predictor's contribution to that skill is surely one reasonable measure of that predictor's importance.

5.6.2.1 Some Examples of Importance Plots with Extensions

Consider now a random forests analysis of data from an educational and job training program for homeless individuals. Because providing such services to homeless individuals was expensive, administrators wanted to know in advance which individuals referred to the program would not likely be helped. For example, they may have had more fundamental needs such as treatment for drug dependence. At the same time, they wanted to make a special effort to identify individuals with promise and were prepared to accept a substantial number of individuals who would not find a steady job when predicted to do so. A provisional cost ratio of 4 to 1 was determined. It was 4 times worse to overlook a promising individual than to mistakenly decide that an individual was promising.

Random forests was applied to training data on a little less than 7000 individuals who had gone through their program. One of the primary outcomes was whether after finishing the program steady employment followed. It did for about 27 % of the graduates of the program. The response variable is still unbalanced, not nearly so seriously as in the past two examples.

Table 5.4 shows the confusion table that resulted. Consistent with stakeholder preferences, there are about 4 false positives for every false negative (i.e., 2626/606). 68 % of those who would find employment were accurately identified in advance. However, because of the imposed 4 to 1 cost ratio, a prediction of success on the job market would be wrong 67 % of the time.

However, we are focusing now on the variable importance plots shown in Fig. 5.3. Reduction in prediction accuracy is shown on the horizontal axis. The code for the random forest analysis and the subsequent importance plots is shown in Fig. 5.4. Keep in mind that although we are using Breiman's term "prediction accuracy," we are actually considering classification accuracy in OOB data.

The upper left figure shows unstandardized reductions in prediction accuracy for employment when each predictor is in turn randomly shuffled. The age at which an individual enters the program is the most important input. When that variable is shuffled, prediction accuracy declines about 2.5 percentage points (i.e., from 68 % to 65.5 %). The importance of all of the other predictors can be interpreted in the same fashion. The bottom four predictors make no contribution to predictive accuracy. Recall that contributions less than 0.0 result from the noise built into the random forests algorithm and in practice are taken to be equal to 0.0.

Predictor importance does not show *how* an input is related to the response. The functional form is not revealed, nor are any of the likely interaction effects with other inputs. Going back to our bread baking metaphor, each input is but an ingredient in a recipe. We can learn how important an input is for prediction, but nothing more.

Table 5.4 Confusion table for employment after training with a 4 to 1 target cost ratio (N = 6723)

	Forecast not employed	Forecast employed	Model error
Not employed	2213	2626	.54
Employed	606	1278	.32
Use error	.21	.67	Overall error = .48

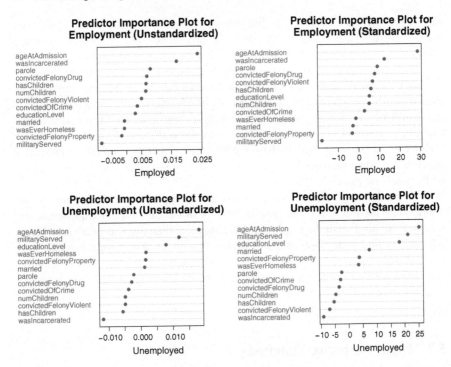

Fig. 5.3 Variable importance plots for employment outcome with a 4 to 1 target cost ratio (N = 6723)

Also not shown is prediction accuracy that is shared among inputs. Consequently, the sum of the individual contributions can be substantially less than 68 %.

The upper right figure shows the standardized contributions to employment prediction accuracy in standard deviation units.

The ordering of the inputs in the upper right figure has changed a bit because of the standardization, and as a descriptive summary, it is not clear what has been gained. It may be tempting to use each input's standard deviation, which can be easily extracted from the output, to construct confidence intervals. But, for a variety of technical reasons, this is not a good idea (Wager et al. 2014).

The bottom two figures repeat the same analyses, but using unemployment as the outcome. One might think that the figures in the bottom row would be very similar to the figures in the top row. Somewhat counterintuitively, they are not. But, recall how classification is accomplished in random forests. For a binary outcome, the class is assigned by majority vote. Two important features of those votes are in play here: the voting margin and the number of actual class members.

Consider a simple example in which there are 500 trees in the random forest. Suppose a given individual receives a vote of 251 to 249 to be assigned to the employment class category. The margin of victory is very small. Suppose that in fact that individual does find a job; the forecast is correct. Now a predictor is shuffled.

The vote might be very different. But suppose it is now just 249 to 251. Only two votes over tress have changed. Yet, the individual is now placed incorrectly in the unemployed class. This increases the prediction error by one individual.

Is that one individual increase in misclassifications enough to matter? Probably not given the usual sample sizes. But if a substantial number of the votes over trees is close, a substantial increase in the number of classification errors could result. And if the sample size is relatively small, the accuracy decline in units of percentage points could be relatively large. Such results are potentiated if the votes in terminal nodes within trees are close as well. Perhaps the key point is that these processes can differ depending on the outcome class, which explains why predictor importance can vary by the outcome class.

In Fig. 5.3, the prediction contributions are generally larger for the upper two figures than for the lower two figures. This is substantially a consequence of the marginal distribution of the response. There are more than twice as many individuals who do not find work compared to individuals who do. As a result, it would take many more classification changes after shuffling for the smaller prediction accuracy declines shown in the lower figures to approximate the larger predictor accuracy declines shown in the upper figures.

5.7 Input Response Functions

Predictor importance is only part of the story. In addition to knowing the importance of each input, it can be very useful to have a description of how each predictor is related to the response. The set of response functions needs to be described.

One useful solution based on an earlier suggestion by Breiman and his colleagues (1984) is "partial dependence plots" (Friedman 2001; Hastie et al. 2009: Sect. 10.13.2). For tree-based approaches, one proceeds as follows.

1. Grow a forest.
2. Suppose x_1 is the initial predictor of interest, and it has v distinct values in the training data. Construct v datasets as follows.

   a. For each of the v distinct values of x_1, make up a new dataset where x_1 only takes on that value, leaving all other variables untouched.
   b. For each of the v datasets, predict the response for each tree in the random forest. There will be for each tree a single value averaged over all observations. For numeric response variables, the predicted value is a mean. For categorical response variables, the predicted value is a proportion.

c. Average each of these predictions over the trees. The result is either an average mean or an average proportion over trees.

d. Plot the average prediction for each value for each of the v datasets against the v values of x_1

3. Go back to Step 2 and repeat for each predictor.

There is a lot going on in this algorithm that may not be immediately apparent. Partial dependence plots show the average relationship between a given input and the response within the fixed, joint distribution of the other inputs. For each of the v values, the values of all other inputs are always the same. Therefore, variation in these other inputs cannot explain away an empirically determined response function for those v values.

Perhaps here is a way to think about it. Suppose the selected input is age. One asks what would the average outcome be if everyone were 21 and nothing else changed? Then one asks, what would the average outcome be if everyone were 22 and nothing else changed? The same question is asked for age 23, age 24 and so on. All that changes is the single age assigned to each case: 21, 22, 23, 24 . . . .

Now in more detail, suppose the response is binary and initially everyone is assigned the age of 20. Much as one would do in conventional regression, the outcome for each case is predicted using all of the other inputs as well. Those fitted values can then be averaged. For a binary outcome, an average class is computed. That average is a proportion.[15] Next, everyone is assigned the age of 21, and the same operations are undertaken. For each age in turn, the identical procedure is applied. One can then see how the outcome class proportions change with age alone because as age changes, none of the other variables do. Should the response be quantitative, each fitted average is a conditional mean. One can then see how the conditional mean changes with age alone.

Commonly, the partial dependence is plotted. Unlike the plots of fitted values constructed from smoothers (e.g., from the generalized additive model), partial dependence plots usually impose no smoothness constraints, and the underlying tree structure tends to produce somewhat bumpy results. In practice, one usually overlays an "eyeball" smoother when the plot is interpreted. Alternatively, it is often possible to overlay a smoother if the software stores the requisite output. In R, *randomForest()* does.

For quantitative response variables, the units on the vertical axis usually are the natural units of the response, whatever they happen to be. For categorical response variables, the units of the response on the vertical axis are centered logits. Consider first the binary case.

Recall that logistic regression equation commonly is written as

$$\log\left(\frac{p}{1-p}\right) = \mathbf{X}\beta, \tag{5.11}$$

---

[15] For example, if getting a job is coded 1 and not getting a job is coded 0, the mean of the 1s and 0s is the proportion who got a job.

where p is the probability of a success. The term on the left-hand side is the log of the odds of a success, often called the "logit". The change in the response for a unit change in a predictor, all other predictors held constant, is in "logits".

For the multinomial case, the most common approach is to build up from the familiar binary formulation. If there are K response categories, there are $K - 1$ equations, each of the same general form as Eq. 5.11. One equation of the K possible equations is redundant because the response categories are exhaustive and mutually exclusive. Thus, if an observation does not fall in categories $1, \ldots, K - 1$, it must fall in the Kth category. This implies that a single category can be chosen as the reference category, just as in the binomial case (i.e., there are two possible outcomes and one equation). Then, for each of the $K - 1$ equations, the logit is the log of the odds for a given category compared to the reference category.

Suppose there are four response categories, and the fourth is chosen as the reference category. There would then be three equations with three different responses, one for $\log(p_1/p_4)$, one for $\log(p_2/p_4)$, and one for $\log(p_3/p_4)$. The predictors would be the same for each equation, but each equation would have its own set of regression coefficients differing in values across equations.

One might think that partial dependence plots would follow a similar convention. But they do not. The choice of the reference category determines which logits will be used, and the logits used affect the regression coefficients that result. Although the overall fit is the same no matter what the reference category, and although one can compute from the set of estimated regression coefficients what the regression coefficients would be were another reference category used, the regression coefficients reported are still different when different reference categories are used.

There is usually no statistical justification for choosing one reference category or another. The choice is usually made on subject matter grounds to make interpretations easier, and the choice can easily vary from data analyst to data analyst. So, the need for a reference category can complicate interpretations of the results and means that a user of the results has to undertake additional work if regression coefficients using another reference category are desired.

Partly in response to these complications, partial dependence plots are based on a somewhat different approach. There are K, rather than $K - 1$, response functions, one for each response variable class. For the logistic model and class k, these take the form of

$$p_k(X) = \frac{e^{f_k(X)}}{\sum_{k=1}^{K} e^{f_k(X)}}. \tag{5.12}$$

There is still a redundancy problem to solve. The solution employed by partial dependence plots is the constraint $\sum_{k=1}^{K} f_k(X) = 0$. This leads to the multinomial deviance loss function and the use of a rather different kind of baseline.

Instead of using a given category as the reference, the unweighted mean of the proportions in the K categories is used as the reference. In much the same spirit as analysis of variance, the response variable units are then in deviations from a mean. More specifically, we let

$$f_k(X) = \log[p_k(X)] - \frac{1}{K} \sum_{k=1}^{K} \log[p_k(X)].$$ (5.13)

Thus, the response is the difference between the logged proportion for category k and the average of the logged proportions for all K categories. The units are essentially logits but with the mean over the K classes as the reference. Consequently, each response category can have its own equation and, therefore, its own partial dependence plot. This approach is applied even when there are only two response categories, and the conventional logit formulation might not present interpretive problems.

To illustrate, consider once again the employment data. Suppose age in years is the predictor whose relationship with the binary employment response variable is of interest. And suppose for an age of say, 25 years, the proportion of individuals finding a job is .20 (computed using the partial dependence algorithm). The logit is $\log(.2) - [\log(.2) + \log(.8)]/2 = -0.693$ (using natural logarithms). This is the value that would be plotted on the vertical axis corresponding to 25 years of age on the horizontal axis. It is the log of the odds with mean proportion over the K categories as the reference.

The same approach can be used for the proportion of 25 year old individuals who do not find a job. That proportion is necessarily .80, so that value plotted is $\log(.8) - [\log(.2) + \log(.8)]/2 = 0.693$. In the binary case, essentially the same information is obtained no matter which response class is examined.

As required, $0.693 - 0.693 = 0$. This implies that one response function is the mirror image of the other. Thus, one partial dependence plot is the mirror image of the other partial dependence plot, and only one of the two is required for interpretation.

It is easy to get from the centered log odds to more familiar units. The values produced by Eq. 5.13 are half the usual log of the odds. From that, one can easily compute the corresponding proportions. For example, multiplying $-.693$ by 2 and exponentiating yields an odds of .25. Then, solving for the numerator proportion results in a value of .20. We are back where we started.[16]

Equation 5.13 would be applied for each year of age. Thus, for 26 years, the proportion of individuals finding a job might be .25. Then the value plotted on the horizontal axis would be 26, and the value on the vertical axis would be $\log(.25) - [\log(.25) + \log(.75)]/2 = -.549$.

The value of $-.549$ is in a region where the response function has been increasing. With one additional year of age, the proportion who find work increases from 0.20 to 0.25, which becomes log odds of -0.693 and -0.549 respectively. All other values produced for different ages can be interpreted in a similar way. Consequently, one can get a sense of how the response variable changes with variation in a given predictor, all other predictors held constant.

---

[16] $e^{[2(-.693)]}/(1 + (e^{[2(-.693)]})) = .20$.

5.7.1   Partial Dependence Plot Examples

Figure 5.5 shows two partial dependence plots constructed from the employment
data with code that can be found toward the bottom of Fig. 5.4. The upper plot shows
the relationship between the input age and the centered log odds of employment.[17]
Age is quantitative. Employment prospects increase nearly linearly with age until
about age 50 at which time they begin to gradually decline. The lower plot shows the
relationship between the input education and the centered log odds of employment.
Education is a factor. The employment prospects are best for individuals who have
a high school or GED certificate. They are worst for individuals who have no high
school degree or GED. Individuals with at least some college fall in between.[18]
Program administrators explained the outcome for those with at least some college
as a result of the job market in which they were seeking work. The jobs were for
largely unskilled labor. There were not many appealing jobs for individuals with
college credits.

In order to get a practical sense of whether employment varies with either input,
it can be useful to transform the logits back to proportions. Suppose that one were
interested in the largest gap in the prospects for employment. From the upper plot,
the largest logit is about 0.39, and the smallest logit is about -0.42. These become
proportions of 0.69 and 0.30 respectively. The proportion who find work nearly
doubles. Age seems to be strongly associated with employment.

It is important not to forget that the response functions displayed in partial dependence plots reflect the relationship between a given predictor and the response, conditioning on all other predictors. All other predictors are being "held constant" in
the manner discussed above. The code in Fig. 5.4 shows that there are a substantial
number of such predictors.

When the response has more than three outcome categories, there are no longer the
symmetries across plots that are found for binary outcomes. For a binary response
variable, it does not matter which of the two categories is used when the partial
dependence plot is constructed. One plot is the mirror image of the other. Figure 5.6
shows what can happen with three outcome categories.

The three employment outcomes in Fig. 5.6 are "no salary," "hourly salary,"
"yearly salary." The first category means that no job was found. For those who
found a job, a yearly salary is for these individuals associated with higher status
positions compared to positions offering an hourly salary. The plot at the top, for
the yearly salary outcome, looks rather like the plot for finding any job. Prospects
are bleak for those under 20, peak around 50 and then gradually taper off. The plot
in the middle, for the hourly salary outcome, has the same general shape, but peaks
around 40 and then falls of far more abruptly. The plot at the bottom, for no salary,
looks much like the top plot, but with a sign reversal. No plot is the mirror image
of another because if the outcome in question is does not occur, *one of two* other

---

[17]The term "centered" is used because mean of the K proportions is the reference.

[18]The bars use the value of zero as the base and move away from 0.0 upwards or downwards.

```
library(randomForest)
# random forests
rf1<-randomForest(Employed~ageAtAdmission+
convictedOfCrime+convictedFelonyViolent+
convictedFelonyProperty+convictedFelonyDrug+
wasIncarcerated+numChildren+parole
married+hasChildren+educationLevel+
wasEverHomeless+militaryServed,
data=TestData,importance=T,sampsize=c(1200,1100))

par(mfrow=c(2,2))

# Variable Importance Plots
varImpPlot(rf1,type=1,scale=F,class="Employed",
main="Forecasting Importance Plot for Employment
(Unstandardized)",col="blue",cex=1,pch=19)

varImpPlot(rf1,type=1,scale=T,class="Employed",
main="Forecasting Importance Plot for Employment
(Standardized)", col="blue",cex=1,pch=19)

varImpPlot(rf1,type=1,scale=F,class="Unemployed",
main="Forecasting Importance Plot for Unemployment
(Unstandardized)", col="blue",cex=1,pch=19)

varImpPlot(rf1,type=1,scale=T,class="Unemployed",
main="Forecasting Importance Plot for Unemployment
(Standardized)", col="blue",cex=1,pch=19)

# Partial Dependence Plots
part1<-partialPlot(rf1,pred.data=TestData,x.var=ageAtAdmission,
rug=T,which.class="Employed")

par(mfrow=c(2,1))

scatter.smooth(part1$x,part1$y,span=1/3,xlab="Age at Admission",
ylab="Centered Log Odds of Employment", main="Partial
Dependence Plot for Employment on Age",col="blue",pch=19)

part2<-partialPlot(rf1,pred.data=TestData,x.var=educationLevel,
rug=T,which.class="Employed", main="Partial Dependence
Plot for Employment on Education", xlab="Educational Level,
ylab="Centered Log Odds of Employment"),ylim=c(-.05,.25))
```

Fig. 5.4 R code for random forests analysis of an employment outcome

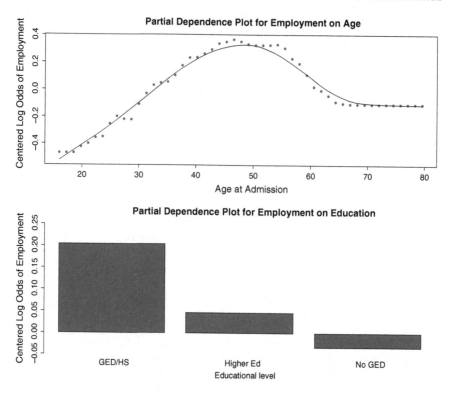

Fig. 5.5 Partial response plots for employment on age and education (N = 6723)

categories will. Moreover, the two other categories change depending on the single outcome whose centered logits are plotted.

In practice, each plot can have a story to tell. For example, comparing the top two plots, being over 50 years old is associated with a small decline in prospects for higher status jobs, In contrast, being over 50 years old is associated with a dramatic decline in prospects for lower status jobs. Part of the explanation can probably be found in the nature of the job. Hourly jobs will often require more physical capacity, which can decrease dramatically starting around age 50.

When there are more than two classes, working with units other than logits is more limited. Suppose the respective proportions at age 30 for the three classes represented in Fig. 5.5 are 0.15, 0.35, and 0.50 respectively. The three centered logits computed for the three response categories are respectively −0.68, 0.16, .52. As before, the sum of the values is 0.0. But there is no mirror image, and one cannot easily get from a single partial dependence plot back to underlying proportions. But one can work with odds.

For example, the largest logit in the top figure is about 0.19. The odds are 1.21. The smallest logit in the top figure is about −.61. The odds are 0.54. For individuals around 50 years old, their odds of getting a job with a yearly salary are about 1.2

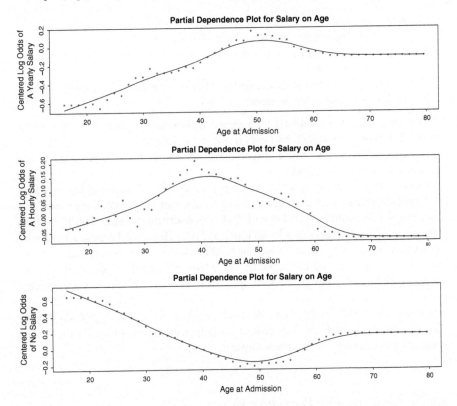

Fig. 5.6 Partial response plots for employment of yearly salary, weekly salary, or no salary on age (N = 6723)

odds units better than average. For individuals around 20 years of age, the odds of getting a job with a yearly salary are about 1.85 odds units worse than average (i.e., 1/.54). Once again, age at the extremes seems to matter substantially.

Finally, just as with variable importance plots, one does not really know *how* each input is linked to the outcome. In particular, variation in an input may well be partitioned between a large number of interaction effects. In econometric language, something akin to reduced form relationships are being represented.[19]

5.8 Classification and the Proximity Matrix

It can be interesting to determine the degree to which individual observations tend to be classified alike. In random forests, this information is contained in the "proximity matrix." The proximity matrix is constructed as follows.

---

[19]They are not literally reduced forms results because there is no structural model.

1. Grow tree as usual.
2. Drop all the training data (in-bag and out-of-bag) down the tree.
3. For all possible pairs of cases, if a pair lands in the same terminal node, increase their proximity by one.
4. Repeat Steps 1–4 until the designated number of trees has been grown.
5. Normalize by dividing by the number of trees.

The result is an $N \times N$ matrix with each cell showing the proportion of trees for which each pair of observations lands in the same terminal node. The higher that proportion, the more alike those observations are in how the trees place them, and the more "proximate" they are.

As noted earlier, working with a very large number observation can improve how well random forests performs because large trees can be grown. Large trees can reduce bias. For example, working with 100,000 observations rather than 10,000 can improve classification accuracy by as much as 50 %. However, because a proximity matrix is $N \times N$, storage can be a serious bottleneck. Storage problems can be partly addressed by only storing the upper or lower triangle, and there are other storage-saving procedures that have been developed. But large datasets still pose a significant problem.

Little subject matter sense can be made of an $N \times N$ matrix of even modest size. Consequently, additional procedures usually need to be applied. We turn to one popular option: multidimensional scaling.

5.8.1 Clustering by Proximity Values

The proportions in a proximity matrix can be seen as measures of similarly, and the matrix is symmetric with 1s along the main diagonal. Consequently, a proximity matrix can be treated as a similarity matrix in much the same spirit as some kernel matrices discussed earlier. As such, it is subject to a variety of clustering procedures with multidimensional scaling (MDS) the one offered by *randomForests()*. The results can be shown in a 2-dimensional plot. The two axes are the first and second principal components (i.e., with the two largest eigenvalues) derived from the proximity matrix. Observations closer in their Euclidian distances are more alike.[20]

Figure 5.7 shows an MDS plot from the proximity matrix constructed for the employment analysis. The results for the first two principle components of the proximity matrix are shown and clearly, there are discernible pattens. The red dots are for individuals who found employment, and the blue dots are for individuals who did

---

[20]The calculations are done by *cmdscale()*, and the plotting is done by *MDSplot()*. The latter automatically calls the former. However, with more than several hundred observations, there is so much overplotting that making sense of the results is very difficult. Labeling the points could help, but not with so much overplotting. Finally, the computational challenges are substantial. For the employment data (N = 6723), doing the MDS using *cmdscale()* on an iMac with an 3.4 GHz intel Core i7 and 32 GB of memory using took about 30 min.

Fig. 5.7 Multidimensional scaling plot of the proximity matrix from the employment analysis: *red dots* for employed and *blue dots* for unemployed

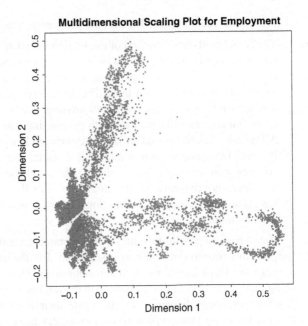

not. Ideally, the individuals who found employment would tend to be alike, and the individuals who did not find employment would tend to be alike. That is, there would be lots of terminal nodes dominated by either employed individuals or unemployed individuals so that they would tend to fall in similar neighborhoods. However, it is difficult to extract much from the figure because of the overplotting. Working with a small random sample of cases would allow for a plot that could be more easily understood, but there would be a substantial risk that important patterns might be overlooked.

In short, better ways need to be found to visualize the proximity matrix. Multidimensional scale has promise, but can be very difficult to interpret with current graphical procedures and large Ns.[21]

5.8.1.1 Using Proximity Values to Impute Missing Data

There are two ways in which random forests can impute missing data. The first and quick method relies on a measure of location. If a predictor is quantitative, the median of the available values is used. If the predictor is categorical, the modal category from the available data is used. Should there be small amounts of missing data, this method may be satisfactory, especially given the computational demands of the second method.

---

[21] This is not to say that MDS is inappropriate in principle or that it will not work well for other kinds of applications.

The second method capitalizes on the proximity matrix in the following manner.

1. The "quick and dirty" method of imputation is first applied to the training data, a random forest is grown, and the proximity values computed.
2. If a missing value is from a quantitative variable, a weighted average of the values for the non-missing cases is used. The proximity values between the case with a missing value and all cases with non-missing values are used as the weights. So, cases that are more like the case with the missing value are given greater weight. All missing values for that variable are imputed in the same fashion.
3. If a missing value is from a categorical value, the imputed value is the most common non-missing value for the variable, with the category counts weighted, as before, by proximity. Again, cases more like the case with the missing value are given greater weight. All missing values for that variable are imputed in the same fashion.

The step using proximity values is then iterated several times. Experience to date suggests that four to six iterations is sufficient. But the use of imputed values tends to make the OOB measures of fit too optimistic. There is really less information being brought to bear in the analysis than the random forest algorithm knows about. The computational demands are also quite daunting and may be impractical for many datasets until more efficient ways to handle the proximities are found. Finally, imputing a single weighted value for each missing observation papers over chance variation in the imputation. How much this matters depends on whether a level II analysis is being undertaken. More will be said about that later.[22]

5.8.1.2   Using Proximities to Detect Outliers

The proximity matrix can be used to spot outliers in the space defined by the predictors. The basic idea is that outliers are observations whose proximities to all other observations in the data are small. The procedures in *randomForest( )* to detect outliers are not implemented for quantitative response variables. For categorical response variables, outliers are defined within categories of the response variable. Within each observed outcome class, each observation is given a value for its "outlyingness" computed as follows.

1. For a given observation, compute the sum of the squares of the proximities with all of the other observations in the same outcome class. Then take the inverse. A large value will indicate that on the average the proximities are small for that observation; the observation is not much like other observations. Do the same for all other observations in that class. One can think of these values as unstandardized.
2. Within each class, compute the median and mean absolute deviation around the median of the unstandardized values.

---

[22]The assumed missing data mechanism is much like missing conditionally at random because of the proximity weighting.

3. Subtract the median from each of the unstandardized values and divide by the mean absolute deviation. In this fashion, the unstandardized values are standardized.
4. Values less than zero are set to 0.0.

These steps are then repeated for each class of the response variable. Observations with values larger than 10 can be considered outliers. Note that an observation does not become suspect because of a single atypical x-value. An outlier is defined by *how it is classified*, which is a function of all of its x-values. It typically lands in terminal nodes where it has little company.

Figure 5.8 is an index plot of outlier values for the employment data, with employed cases represented by red spikes and unemployed cases represented as blue spikes. The R code is shown in Fig. 5.9.

For this analysis, there are perhaps 4 to 6 observations of possible concern, but the outlier measures are close to 10 and with over 9000 observations overall, they would make no material difference in the results if dropped. It might be different if the outlier measures were in the high teens, and there were only a few hundred observations in total.

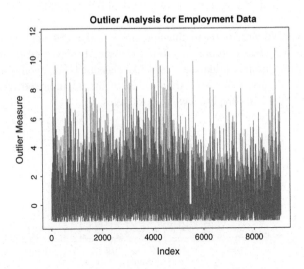

Fig. 5.8 Index plot of outlier measures for employment data with values greater than 10 candidates for deletion (*Red spike* are for employed and *blue spikes* are for unemployed)

```
plot(outlier(rf1),type="h", ylab="Outlier Measure",
    main="Outlier Analysis for Employment Data",
    col=c("red","blue")[as.numeric(TestData$Employed)])
```

Fig. 5.9 R code for index plot of outlier measures

When the data analyst considers dropping one or more outlying cases, a useful diagnostic tool can be a cross tabulation of the classes assigned for the set of observations that two random forest analyses have in common: one with all of the data and one with the outliers removed. If the common observations are, by and large, classified in the same way in both analyses, the outliers do not make an important difference to the classification process.

5.9 Empirical Margins

Recall Breiman's definition of a margin: the difference between the proportion of times over trees that an observation is correctly classified minus the largest proportion of times over trees that an observation is incorrectly classified. That definition can be used for each observation in a dataset. Positive values represent correct classifications, and negative values represent incorrect classifications.

Figure 5.10 shows histograms for two empirical margins. The upper plot is for individuals who were employed. The lower plot is for individuals who are not employed. We are conditioning on the actual response class much as we do for rows of a confusion table. For both histograms, the red, vertical line is located at a margin value of 0.0.

For employed individuals, the median margin is .18 (i.e., .59–.41), which translates into a solid majority vote or more for half of the correctly classified cases. Moreover, 68% of the employed individuals are correctly classified. For unemployed individuals, the median margin is −.07. About 55% of the unemployed individuals are incorrectly classified, although many by close votes.

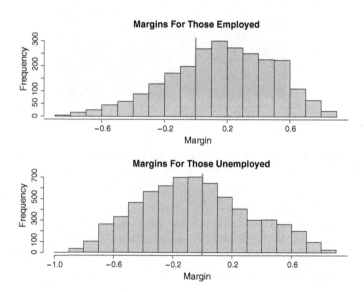

Fig. 5.10 Distribution of margins for employed and unemployed individuals (The *red vertical line* is located at a margin value of 0.0)

The margins can serve an additional performance diagnostic to supplement the rows of a confusion table. In addition to classification accuracy computed from each row, one can learn how definitive both the correct and incorrect classifications are. Ideally, the votes are decisive for the correctly classified cases and razor thin for the incorrectly classified cases. The results in Fig. 5.10 have some of this pattern, but only weakly so. Perhaps the major use of margins is to compare the stability of results from different datasets. One might have results from two datasets that classify with about the same accuracy, but for one of those, the classifications are more stable. The results from that dataset should be preferred because they are less likely to be a result of a random forest luck of the draw.

The stability is with respect to the random forest algorithm itself because margins are derived from votes over trees. The data are fixed. If a new random forest were grown with the same data, the classes assigned to all cases would not likely be the same. The uncertainty captured is created by the random forest algorithm itself. As such, it represents the in-sample reliability of the algorithm and says nothing about accuracy. Indeed, it is possible to have results that are reliably wrong.

There can be no margins in forecasting settings because the outcomes are not yet known. But the votes are easily retrieved by *randomForest()*, and can be very instructive. More decisive votes imply more reliable forecasts. For example, a school administrator may be trying to project whether a particular student will drop out of high school. If so, there may be good reason to intervene with services such as tutoring. The case for intervening should be seen as more credible if the drop out forecast is coupled with high reliability.

There is no clear threshold beyond which reliability is automatically high enough. That will be a judgment call for decision-makers. Moreover, that line may be especially hard to draw when there are more than two outcome classes. Suppose the vote proportions are 0.25, 0.30, and 0.45. The class with 45 % of the votes wins by a substantial plurality. But the majority of votes is cast against that class.

For real world settings in which forecasts from a random forest are made, the best advice may be to use the votes to help determine how much weight should be given to the forecast compared to the weight given to other information. In the school drop out example, an overwhelming vote projecting a drop out may mean discounting a student's apparent show of contrition and promises to do better. If the vote is effectively too close to call, the show of contrition and promises to do better may quite properly carry the day.

5.10 Quantitative Response Variables

There is not very much new that needs to be said about quantitative response variables once one appreciates that random forests handles quantitative response variables much as CART does. Even through for each tree there are still binary partitions of the data, there are no response variable classes and no response class proportions from which to define impurity. Traditionally, impurity is defined as the within-node error sum of squares. A new partition of the data is determined by the split that would most reduce the sum, over the two prospective subsets, of the within-partition error sums of squares. Predicted values are the mean of the response variable in each of the terminal nodes. For each OOB observation, the mean of its terminal node is the fitted value assigned.

For regression trees, therefore, there are no classification errors, only residuals. Concerns about false negatives and positives and their costs are no longer relevant. There are no confusion tables and no measures of importance based on classification errors. To turn a regression tree into a fully operational random forest, the following steps are required.

1. Just as in the classification case, each tree is grown from a random sample (with replacement) of the training data.
2. Just as in the classification case, for each potential partitioning of the data, a random sample (without replacement) of predictors is used.
3. The value assigned to each terminal node is the mean of the response variable values that land in that terminal node.
4. For each tree in the random forest, the fitted value for each OOB case is the mean previously assigned to the terminal node in which it lands.
5. As before, random forest averages over trees. For a given observation, the average of the tree-by-tree fitted values is computed using only the fitted values from trees in which that observation was not used to grow the tree. This is the fitted value that random forest returns.
6. Deviations between these averaged, fitted values and the response variable observed values are used to construct the mean square error reported for the collection of trees that constitutes a random forest. The value of the mean square error can be used to compute a "pseudo" R^2 as $(1 - \text{MSE})/\text{Var}(Y)$.
7. Construction of partial dependence plots is done in the same manner as for classification trees, but now the fitted response is the set of conditional means for different predictor values, not a set of transformed fitted proportions.
8. Input variable importance is computed using the shuffling approach as before. And as before there is a "resubstitution" (in-sample) measure and a OOB (out-of-sample) measure. For the resubstitution measure, each time a given variable is used to define a partitioning of the data for a given tree, the reduction in the within-node error sum of squares is recorded. When the tree is complete, the reductions are summed. The result is a reduction in the error sum of squares that can be attributed to each predictor. These totals, one for each predictor, are then averaged over trees.

   The out-of sample importance measure is also an average over trees. For a given tree, the OOB observations are used to compute each terminal node's error sum of squares. From these, the mean squared error for that tree is computed. Then a designated predictor is shuffled, and mean square error for that tree is computed again. An increase in this mean square error is a decrease in accuracy. The same steps are applied to each tree, and the accuracy decreases are averaged over trees to get an average decrease in accuracy for that predictor. The standard deviation of these decreases over trees can be used to standardize the average decrease, if that is desirable. The same process is employed for each predictor.

Despite the tight connection between regression trees and random forests, there are features found in some implementations of regression trees that have yet to be introduced into random forests, at least within R. But change is underway. Extensions to Poisson regression seem imminent (Mathlourthi et al. 2015), and Ishwaran and colleagues (2008) provide in R a procedure to do survival analysis (and lots more) with random forests using *randomForestSRC()*. Both alter the way splits within each tree are determined so that the reformulation is fundamental. For example, *randomForestSRC()* can pick the predictor and split that maximizes the survival difference in the two offspring nodes. There is also the option to do the analysis with competing risks (Ishwaran et al. 2014) and various weighting options that can be applied to the splitting rule (Ishwaran 2015).

Alternatively, *quantregForest()* only changes how values in each terminal node are used. The intent is to compute quantiles. Instead of storing only the mean of each terminal node as trees are grown, the entire distribution is stored. Recall the earlier discussion surrounding Table 5.2. Once the user decides which quantiles are of interest, they can be easily computed.

If one is worried about the impact of within-node outliers on the conditional mean, the conditional median can be used instead. If for substantive reasons there is interest in, say, the first or third quartile, those can be used. Perhaps most importantly, the quantile option provides a way to take the costs of forecasting errors into account. For example, if the 75th quantile is chosen, the consequences of underestimates are three times more costly than the consequences of overestimates (i.e., $75/25 = 3$).

However, such calculations only affect what is done with the information contained in the terminal nodes across trees. They do not require that the trees themselves be grown again with a linear loss function, let alone a loss function with asymmetric costs. In other words, the trees grown under quadratic loss are not changed. If there are concerns about quadratic loss, they do not apply to each of the splits. Moreover, all of the usual random forests outputs (e.g., variable importance plots) are still a product of a quadratic loss function.

5.11 A Random Forest Illustration Using a Quantitative Response Variable

Several years ago, an effort was made to count the number of homeless in Los Angeles County (Berk et al. 2008). There are over 2000 census tracts in the county, and enumerators were sent to a sample of a little over 500. Their job was to count "unsheltered" homeless who were not to be found in shelters or other temporary housing. Shelter counts were readily available. The details of the sampling need not trouble us here, and in the end, the overall county total was estimated to be about 90,000. We focus here on the street counts only.

Fig. 5.11 For Los Angeles
county census tracts a plot of
actual homeless street counts
against the random forest
fitted homeless street counts
(Least squares line is in *red*,
the 1-to-1 line in *green*, N =
504)

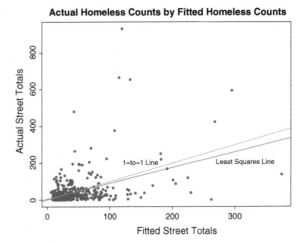

In addition to countywide totals, there was a need to have estimated counts for
tracts not visited. Various stakeholders might wish to have estimates at the tract level
for areas to which enumerators were not sent. Random forests was used with tract-
level predictors to impute the homeless street counts for these tracts. Here, we focus
on the random forests procedure itself, not the imputation. About 21 % of the variance
in the homeless street counts was accounted for by the random forests application
with the follow inputs.[23]

1. MedianInc – median household income
2. PropVacant – proportion of vacant dwellings
3. PropMinority – proportion minority
4. PerCommercial – percentage of land used for commercial purposes
5. PerIndustrial – percentage of the land used for industrial purposes
6. PerResidential – percentage of the land used for residential purposes.

Figure 5.11 is a plot of the actual street totals against the fitted street totals in the
data. One can see that there are a number of outliers that make any fitting exercise
challenging. In Los Angeles county, the homeless are sprinkled over most census
tracts, but a few tracts have very large homeless populations. The green 1-to-1 line
summarizes what a good fit would look like. Ideally the fitted street counts and the
actual street counts should be much the same. The red line summarizes with a least
squares line the quality of the fit actually obtained. Were the horizontal axis extended
to allow for fitted counts with the same large values as the actual counts, the two
lines would diverge dramatically.

The counts in the highly populated census tracts are often badly underestimated.
For example, the largest fitted count is around 400. There are 5 census tracts with

---

[23] As is often the case with quantitative response variables, the defaults in *randomForest()* worked
well.

actual street counts over 400, one of those with a count of approximately 900. From a policy point of view this really matters. The census tracts most in need of services are not accurately characterized by random forests.

Figure 5.12 shows two variable importance plots. On the left, the percentage increase in average OOB mean squared error for each predictor is plotted. On the right, the increase in the average in-sample node impurity for each predictor is plotted. For example, when the percentage of land that is commercial is shuffled, the OOB mean squared error increases by about 7 %, and the proportion of the residential population that is minority has no predictive impact whatsoever. When household median income is shuffled, average node impurity increases by 7e+05, and all of the predictors have some impact on the fit. The ranking of the variables changes depending on the importance measure, but for the reasons discussed earlier, the out-of-sample measures is preferable, especially if forecasting is an important goal.

Figure 5.13 is a partial dependence plot showing a positive association between the percentage of the residential dwellings that are vacant and the number of homeless counted. When vacancy is near zero, the average number of homeless is about 20 per tract. When the vacancy percent is above approximately 10 %, the average count increases to between 60 and 70 (with a spike right around 10 %). The change is very rapid. Beyond 10 % the relationship is essentially flat. At that point, perhaps the needs of squatters are met.

In response to the poor fit for the few census tracts with a very large number of homeless individuals, it is worth giving *quantregForest()* a try. As already noted, a random forest is grown as usual, but the distributions in the terminal nodes of each

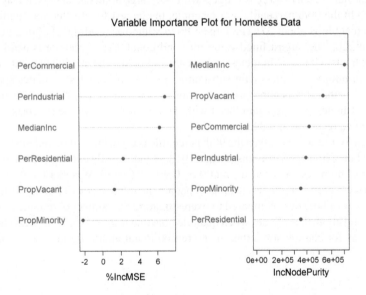

Fig. 5.12 Variable importance plots for street counts (On the *left* is the percent increase in the OOB mean squared error, and on the *right* is the in-sample increase in node impurity. N = 504)

Fig. 5.13 The partial
response plot for street
counts on the proportion of
vacant dwellings in a census
tract (N = 504)

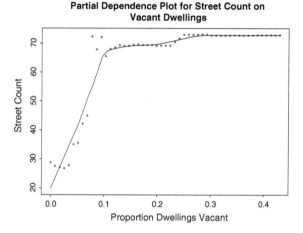

tree are retained for analysis. We will consider the impact of using three different
quantiles: 0.10, 0.50, and 0.90. For these data, quantiles substantially larger than .50
would in practice usually be the focus. The code used in the analyses to follow is
shown in Fig. 5.16.[24]

Figure 5.14 shows three plots laid out just like Fig. 5.11, for the conditional quantiles of 0.10, 0.50 and 0.90. All three fit the data about equally well if the adjusted R^2
is the measure because the outliers are very few. But should there be special concerns
about the half dozen or so census tracts with very large homeless counts, it may make
sense to fit the 90th percentile. For example, the largest fitted value for conditional
10th percentile is about 37. The largest fitted value for conditional 50th percentile
is about 220. The largest fitted value for conditional 90th percentile is nearly 700.
Several tracts with large homeless counts are still badly underestimated, but clearly,
the small number of tracts with substantial number of homeless is better approximated. Whether this is appropriate depends on the relative costs of underestimates
to overestimates. We are again faced with the prospect of asymmetric costs, but for
quantitative response variables.

When for the homeless data the 90th percentile is used, the cost of underestimating
the number of homeless in a census tract is 9 times more costly than overestimating the
number of homeless in a census tract (i.e., $0.90/0.10 = 9$). Whether the 9-to-1 cost
ratio makes sense is a policy decision. What are the relative costs of underestimating
the number of homeless compared to overestimating the number of homeless? More
will be said about these issues when quantile boosting is discussed in the next chapter.
But just as for classification, there is no reason to automatically impose symmetric
costs.

---

[24]The authors are Nicolai Meinshausen and Lukas Schiesser. The version used for these analyses
(version 1.1) seems to have some bugs in the plotting routines, which is why the code shown in
Fig. 5.16 is so lengthy and inelegant. The plots had to be constructed from more basic procedures.

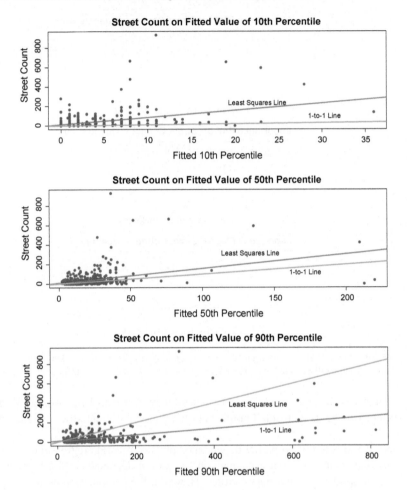

Fig. 5.14 Plot of quantile random forest fitted values against the actual values (Least squares line in *red* and 1-to-1 line in *green*. Quantiles = 0.05, 0.50, 0.90. N = 504)

Figure 5.15 shows three variable importance plots, one for each of the three quantiles being used: 0.10, 0.50, 0.90. The percentage point increase in quantile (linear) out-of-sample loss is the measure of importance. For example, for the conditional 90th percentile, the most important input is the proportion of vacant dwellings, which when shuffled increased the out-of-sample L_1 loss by about 16 percentage points. As before, negative values are treated as 0.0.

Perhaps the most important message is that by this measure of importance, the order of the variables can vary by the conditional quantile estimated. Inputs that are most important for out-of-sample performance when the 90th percentile is the fitted value may not be the most important for out-of-sample performance when the 10th percentile is the fitted value. That is, predictors that help to distinguish between

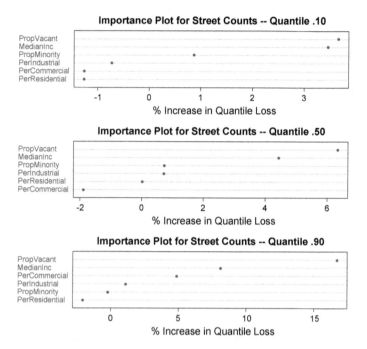

Fig. 5.15 Street count variable importance plots for quantiles of 0.10, 0.50, and 0.90 (Importance is measured by the OOB percentage point increase in the quantile loss after shuffling. N = 504)

census tracts with large numbers of homeless may be of no help distinguishing between census tracts with small numbers of homeless. Different processes may be involved.

There are apparently no partial dependence plots of quantile regression forests. It seems that relatively modest changes in the partial dependence plot algorithm could accommodate conditional quantiles. However, the computation burdens may be substantially increased.

Quantile random forests has some nice features and in particular, the ability to introduce asymmetric costs when the response variable is quantitative. However, the random forest is grown as usual with each split based on quadratic loss. Were one truly committed to linear loss, it would make sense to revise the splitting criterion accordingly. An R library called yarp(), by Adam Kapelner, is under development that among other features will allow for a wide variety of split loss functions. Quantile random forests is a strange hybrid and so far at least, does not seem to be widely used.

5.12   Statistical Inference with Random Forests

As long as users of random forests are content to describe relationships in the data on hand, random forests is a level I procedure. But the use of OOB data to get honest performance assessments and measures of predictor performance speaks to level II

```
library(quantregForest)
X<-as.matrix(HData[,2:7]) # predictors as matrix
Y<-as.numeric(as.matrix(HData[,1])) # response as vector

# Quantile Random Forests
out2<-quantregForest(x=X,y=Y,nodesize=10,importance=T,
                     quantiles = c(.10))
preds<-predict(out2) # Fitted OOB values

# Fitted value plots
par(mfrow=c(3,1))
plot(preds[,1],Y,col="blue",pch=19,
     xlab="Fitted 10th Percentile",
     ylab="Street Count",
     main="Street Count on Fitted Value of 10th Percentile")
abline(lsfit(preds[,1],Y),col="red",lwd=2)
abline(0.0,1.0,lwd=2,col="green")
text(22,220,"Least Squares Line",cex=1)
text(30,90,"1-to-1 Line",cex=1)

plot(preds[,2],Y,col="blue",pch=19,
     xlab="Fitted 50th Percentile",
     ylab="Street Count",
     main="Street Count on Fitted Value of 50th Percentile")
abline(lsfit(preds[,2],Y),col="red",lwd=2)
abline(0.0,1.0,lwd=2,col="green")
text(130,300,"Least Squares Line",cex=1)
text(170,110,"1-to-1 Line",cex=1)

plot(preds[,3],Y,col="blue",pch=19,
     xlab="Fitted 90th Percentile",
     ylab="Street Count",
     main="Street Count on Fitted Value of 90th Percentile")
abline(lsfit(preds[,3],Y),col="red",lwd=2)
abline(0.0,1.0,lwd=2,col="green")
text(500,370,"Least Squares Line",cex=1)
text(550,110,"1-to-1 Line",cex=1)

# Importance Plots
par(mfrow=c(3,1))
imp10<-sort(out2$importance[,1])
dotchart(imp10,col="blue",pch=19,xlab="% Increase
         in Quantile Loss",
         main="Importance Plot for Street Counts -- Quantile .10")
imp50<-sort(out2$importance[,2])
dotchart(imp50,col="blue",pch=19,xlab="% Increase
         in Quantile Loss",
         main="Importance Plot for Street Counts -- Quantile .50")
imp90<-sort(out2$importance[,3])
dotchart(imp90,col="blue",pch=19,xlab="% Increase
         in Quantile Loss",
         main="Importance Plot for Street Counts -- Quantile .90")
```

Fig. 5.16 R code for quantile random forests

concerns and generalization error in particular. If the forecasting is an explicit goal, a level II analysis is being undertaken.

Taking level II analyses a step farther, there have been some recent efforts to provide a rationale and computational procedures for random forests statistical inference (Wager 2014; Wager et al. 2014; Wager and Walther 2015; Mentch and Hooker 2015). The issues are beyond the scope of our discussion in part because the work is at this point still very much in progress. Key complications are the inductive nature of random forests, tree depth dependence on sample size, the sampling of predictors, and summary values for terminal nodes computed from the same data used to grow the trees.

However, if one has test data, one can proceed in the same spirit as in CART. The estimation target is the fitted values from the very same random forest grown with the training data. The test data can be used to estimate generalization error or other features of a confusion table. One can then apply the pairwise (nonparametric) bootstrap to the test data in the fashion discussed in earlier chapters.

5.13   Software and Tuning Parameters

In this chapter, all empirical work has been done with the R procedure *randomForest()*, which works well even for large datasets. But there are some disciplines in which the datasets are extremely large (e.g., 1,000,000 observations, and 5000 predictors) and working with subsets of the data can be counterproductive. For example, in genomics research there may be thousands of predictors.

Over the past few years, new implementations of random forests have been written for R, and some are remarkably fast (Ziegler and König 2014). A recent review by Wright and Ziegler (2015:1) confirms that *randomForest()* is "feature rich and widely used." But the code has not been optimized for high dimensional data.

Wright and Ziegler describe their own random forests implementation, *ranger()*, in some depth. It is indeed very fast, but lacks a number of features that can be very important in practice. All of the other implementations considered are either no more optimized than *randomForest()*, or run faster but lack important features (e.g., partial dependence plots). No doubt, at least some of these packages will add useful features over time. One possible candidate in R is *Rborist()* (Seligman 2015). The programs *rforest()* (Zhang et al. 2009) and *rjungle()* (Schwartz et al. 2010) are also candidates, but neither is currently available in R.[25] There are, in addition, efforts to reconsider random forests more fundamentally for very high dimensional data. For example, Xu and colleagues (2012) try to reduce the number of input dimensions by taking into account information much like that assembled in the *randomForest()* proximity matrix. Readers intending to use random forests should try to stay informed about these developments. Here, we will continue with *randomForest()*.

---

[25]*Rborist* wins the award for the most clever name.

Despite the complexity of the random forest algorithm and the large number of potential tuning parameters, most of the usual defaults work well in practice. However, if one tunes from information contained in the OOB confusion table, the OOB data will slowly become tainted. For example, if for policy or subject matter reasons one needs to tune to approximate a target asymmetric cost ratio in a confusion table, model selection is in play once again. Still, when compared to the results from true test data, the OOB results usually hold up well if the number of cost ratios estimated is modest (e.g., <10) and the sample size is not too small (e.g., >1000). The same holds if on occasion some of the following tuning parameters have to be tweaked.

1. *Node Size* — Unlike in CART, the number of observations in the terminal nodes of each tree can be very small. The goal is to grow trees with as little bias as possible. The high variance that would result can be tolerated because of the averaging over a large number of trees. In the R implementation of random forests, the default sample sizes for the terminal nodes are one for classification and five for regression. These seem to work well. But, if one is interested in estimating a quantile, such as in quantile random forests, then terminal node sizes at least twice as large will often be necessary for regression. If there are only five observations in a terminal node, for instance, it will be difficult to get a good read on, say, the 90th percentile.

2. *Number of Trees* — The number of trees used to constitute a forest needs to be at least several hundred and probably no more that several thousand. In practice, 500 trees is often a good compromise. It sometimes makes sense to do most of the initial development (see below) with about 500 trees and then confirm the results with a run using about 3000 trees. But, the cost is primarily computational time and only if the number of inputs and number of observations are large, do computational burdens become an issue. For example, if there are 100 inputs and 100,000 observations, the number of trees grown becomes an important tuning parameter.

3. *Number of Predictors Sampled* — The number of predictors sampled at each split would seem to be a key tuning parameter that should affect how well random forests performs. Although it may be somewhat surprising, very few predictors need to be randomly sampled at each split, and within sensible bounds on the number sampled, it does not seem to matter much for the OOB error estimates. With a large number of trees, each predictor will have an ample opportunity to contribute, even if very few are drawn for each split. For example, if the average tree in a random forest has ten terminal splits, and if there are 500 trees in the random forest, there will be 5000 chances for predictors to weigh in. Sampling two or three each time should then be adequate unless the number of predictors is quite large (e.g., > 100).
   But a lot depends on the number of predictors and how strongly they are related. If the correlations are substantial, it can be useful to reduce the number of predictors sampled for each partitioning decision. In the original manual for the FORTRAN version of random forests, Breiman recommends starting with the

number of predictors sampled equal to the square root of the number of predictors available. Then, trying a few more or a few less as well can be instructive.

The feature of random forests that will usually make the biggest difference in the results is how the costs of false negatives and false positives are handled, or for quantile random forests, the quantile used. Even through asymmetric costs are introduced by altering one or more of the arguments in *randomForest()*, one should not think of the target cost ratio as a tuning parameter. It is a key factor in the fitting process determined in advance from substantive and policy considerations. However, to arrive at a good approximation of the target cost ratio, some tuning of one or more arguments will usually be necessary (e.g., *sampsize()*).

Computational burdens can be an issue when the training data have a very larger number of observations (e.g., $>100,000$), when the number of inputs is large (e.g., >100), and when a substantial number of inputs are categorical with many classes.[26] It is difficult to tune one's way out of letting the algorithm grind for hours in part because with each new set of tuning values, the algorithm has to run again. Sometimes a better strategy is to work with a random, modest sized subset of training data for tuning, saving the bulk of the data for results that will be used. Doing some initial screening of the predictors to be used can also help, as long as one is aware of the risks. Combining some of the categories for factors with many levels is worth a try. Finally, many of the computational steps in random forests are easily parallelized and will run well on computers with multiple processors. Soon, software with these capabilities and others that increase processing speed will be routinely available and be richly endowed with desirable features.

Also, a cautionary note. Random forests is not designed to be a variable selection procedure. Nevertheless, it can be temping to use the variable importance plots to discard weak predictors. There are at least four problems with this approach. First, there is rarely any need to reduce the number of predictors. The way in which splits are determined for each tree in the forest is a kind of provisional, variable selection method that performs well. In other words, there is almost never a need to drop the unimportant variables and rerun random forests. Second, some argue that if multicolinearity is a serious problem, random forests results can be unstable. But that concern refers primarily to estimates of variable importance. Should that form of instability become an issue, any dimension reduction in the set of predictors is probably best done before the random forests analysis begins. However, one is back in the model selection game. Third, if the goal is to use variable importance to determine the predictors to be introduced into some other procedure, performance in prediction may not be what is needed. For example, prediction importance may be unrelated to causal importance. Finally, as discussed earlier, there are lots of worthy procedures designed for variable/model selection as long as one is prepared to address the damage usually done to level II analyses.

---

[26]Currently, up to 53 classes are allowed for any given categorical input in *randomForest()*.

5.14 Summary and Conclusions

There is substantial evidence that random forests is a very powerful statistical learning tool. If forecasting accuracy is one's main performance criterion, there are no other general purpose tools that have been shown to consistently perform any better. Moreover, random forests comes with a rich menu of post-processing procedures and simple means with which to introduce asymmetric costs. We consider a chief competitor in the next chapter.

But a lot depends on the data analysis task. We will later briefly address deep learning, which for specialized applications has enormous promise with very high dimensional data when great precision in the fitted values is needed. But one must be prepared to invest substantial time (e.g., weeks) in tuning, even when there is access to a very large number of CPUs and GPUs. As some advertisements warn, "don't try this at home." The most powerful desktop and laptop computers can be overmatched by deep learning.

Random forests seems to get its leverage from five features of the algorithm:

1. growing large, low bias trees;
2. using bootstrap samples as training data when each tree is grown;
3. using random samples of predictors for each partitioning of the data;
4. constructing fitted values and output summary statistics from the out-of-bag data; and
5. averaging over trees.

At the same time, very few of random forests' formal properties have been proven. At a deeper level, the precise reasons why random forests performs so well are not understood. There is some hard work ahead for theoretical statisticians. Nevertheless, random forests is gaining in popularity because it seems to work well in practice, provides lots of flexibility, and in R at least, comes packaged with a number of supplementary algorithms that provide a range of useful output.

Exercises

Problem Set 1

The goal of this first exercise is to compare the performance of linear regression, CART, and random forests. Construct the following dataset in which the response is a quadratic function of a single predictor.

```
x1=rnorm(500)
x12=x1^2
y=1+(-5*x12)+(5*rnorm(500))
```

1. Plot the $1 + (-5 \times x12)$ against x1. This is the "true" relationship between the response and the predictor without the complication of the disturbances. This is the $f(X)$ you hope to recover from the data.
2. Proceed as if you know that the relationship between the response and the predictor is quadratic. Fit a linear model with x12 as the predictor. Then plot the fitted values

against x1. The results show how the linear model can perform when you know the correct function form.

3. Now suppose you do not know that the relationship between the response and the predictor is quadratic. Apply CART to the same response variable using rpart() and x1 as the sole predictor. Use the default settings. Construct the predicted values, using predict(). Then plot the fitted values against x1. How do the CART fitted values compare to the linear regression fitted values? How well does CART seem to capture the true $f(X)$?

4. Apply random forests to the same response variable using randomForests() and x1 as the sole predictor. Use the default settings. Construct the predicted values using predict(). Then plot the fitted values against x1. How do the random forest fitted values compare to the linear regression fitted values? How well does random forests seem to capture the true $f(X)$?

5. How do the fitted values from CART compare to the fitted values from random forests? What feature of random forests is highlighted?

6. Construct a partial dependence plot with x1 as the predictor. How well does the plot seem to capture the true $f(X)$?

7. Why in this case does the plot of the random forest fitted values and the partial dependence plot look so similar?

5.14.1   Problem Set 2

Load the dataset SLID from the *car* library. Learn about the data set using the help() command. Treat the variable "wages" as the response and all other variables as predictors. The data have some missing values you will want to remove. Try using na.omit().

1. Using the default settings, apply random forests and examine the fit quality.

2. Set the argument *mtry* at 4. Apply random forests again and examine fit quality. What if anything of importance has changed?

3. Now set ntrees at 100 and then at 1000 applying random forests both times. What if anything of importance has changed?

4. Going back to the default settings, apply random forests and examine the variable importance plots with no scaling for each predictor's standard deviation. Explain what is being measured on the horizontal axis on both plots when no scaling for the standard deviation is being used. Interpret both plots. If they do not rank the variables in the same way, why might that be? Now scale the permutation-based measure and reconstruct that plot. Interpret the results. If the ranks of the variables differ from the unscaled plot, why might that be? Focusing on the permutation-based measures (scaled and unscaled) when might it be better to use one rather than the other?

5. Construct partial dependence plots for each predictor and interpret them.

5.14.2   Problem Set 3

Load the *MASS* library and the dataset called Pima.tr. Read about the data using help().

1. Apply random forests to the data using the diagnosis of diabetes as the response. Use all of the predictors and random forest default settings. Study the confusion table.

   a. How accurately does the random forests procedure forecast overall?
   b. How accurately does the random forests procedure forecast each of the two outcomes separately (i.e., *given* each outcome)? (Hint: you get this from the rows of the confusion table.)
   c. If the results were used to forecast either outcome (i.e., *given* the forecast), what proportions of the time would each of the forecasts be incorrect? (Hint: you get this from the columns of the confusion table.)

2. Construct variable importance plots for each of the two outcomes. Use the unscaled plots of forecasting accuracy. Compare the two plots.

   a. Which predictors are the three most important in forecasts of the presence of diabetes compared to forecasts of the absence of diabetes? Why might they not be the same?

3. Construct and interpret partial dependence plots of each predictor.
4. Suppose now that medical experts believe that the costs of failing to identify future cases of diabetes are four times larger than the costs of falsely identifying future cases of diabetes. For example, if the medical treatment is to get overweight individuals to lose weight, that would likely be beneficial even if the individuals were not at high risk for diabetes. But failing to prescribe a weight loss program for an overweight individual might be an error with very serious consequences. Repeat the analysis just completed but now taking the costs into account by using the stratified bootstrap sampling option in random forests.

   a. How has the confusion table changed?
   b. How have the two variable importance plots changed?
   c. How have the partial dependence plots changed?

5. Plot the margins to consider the reliability of the random forests classifications. You will need at least *margin()* followed by the *plot()*. Are the two classes correctly classified with about the same reliability? If so, why might a physician want to know that? If not, why might a physician want to know that?
6. The votes are stored as part of the random forests object. Construct a histogram of the votes separately for each of the two outcome classes. How do votes differ from margins?

7. Now imagine that a physician did not have the results of the diabetes test but wanted to start treatment immediately, if appropriate. Each of the predictors are known for that patient but not the diagnosis. Using the predictor values for that patient, a random forests forecast is made. What should the physician use to measure the reliability of that forecast? Given some examples of high and low reliability.

Chapter 6
Boosting

6.1 Introduction

As already discussed, one of the reasons why random forests is so effective for a complex $f(\mathbf{X})$ is that it capitalizes interpolation. As a result, it can respond to highly local features of the data in a robust manner. Such flexibility is desirable because it can substantially reduce the bias in fitted values. But the flexibility usually comes at a price: the risk of overfitting. Random forests consciously addresses overfitting using OOB observations to construct the fitted values and measures of fit, and by averaging over trees. The former provides ready-made test data while the latter is a form of regularization. Experience to date suggests that this two-part strategy can be highly effective.

But the two-part strategy, broadly conceived, can be implemented in other ways. Some argue that an alternative method to accommodate highly local features of the data is to give the observations responsible for the local variation more weight in the fitting process. If in the binary case, for example, a fitting function misclassifies those observations, that function can be applied again, but with extra weight given to the observations misclassified. Then, after a large number of fitting attempts, each with difficult-to-classify observations given relatively more weight, overfitting can be reduced if the fitted values from the different fitting attempts are averaged in a sensible fashion. Ideas such as these lead to very powerful statistical learning procedures that can compete with random forests. These procedures are called "boosting."

Boosting as originally conceived gets its name from its ability to take a "weak learning algorithm," which performs just a bit better than random guessing, and "boosting" it into an arbitrarily "strong" learning algorithm (Schapire 1999: 1). It "combines the outputs from many "weak" classifiers to produce a powerful "committee" (Hastie et al. 2009: 337). So, boosting has some of the same look and feel as random forests.

The original version of this chapter was revised: See the "Chapter Note" section at the end of this chapter for details. The erratum to this chapter is available at https://doi.org/10.1007/978-3-319-44048-4_10.

© Springer International Publishing Switzerland 2016
R.A. Berk, *Statistical Learning from a Regression Perspective*,
Springer Texts in Statistics, DOI 10.1007/978-3-319-44048-4_6

But, boosting as initially formulated differs from random forests in at least five
important ways. First, in traditional boosting, there are no chance elements built
in. At each iteration, boosting works with the full training sample and all of the
predictors. Some more recent developments in boosting exploit random samples from
the training data, but these developments are enhancements that are not fundamental
to the usual boosting algorithms. Second, with each iteration, the observations that
are misclassified, or otherwise poorly fitted, are given more relative weight. No such
weighting is used in random forests. Third, the ultimate fitted values are a linear
combination over a large set of earlier fitting attempts. But the combination is not a
simple average as in random forests. The fitted values are weighted in a manner to
be described shortly. Fourth, the fitted values and measures of fit quality are usually
constructed from the data in-sample. There are no out-of-bag observations, although
some recent developments make that an option. Finally, although small trees can be
used as weak learners, boosting is not limited to an ensemble of classification and
regression trees.

To appreciate how these pieces can fit together, we turn to Adaboost.M1 (Freund
and Schapire 1996; 1997), which is perhaps the earliest and the most widely known
boosting procedure. For reasons we soon examine, the "ada" in Adaboost stands for
"adaptive" (Schapire 1999: 2). Adaboost illustrates well boosting's key features and
despite a host of more recent boosting procedures, is still among the best classifiers
available (Mease and Wyner 2008).

6.2 Adaboost

We will treat Adaboost.M1 as the poster child for boosting in part because it provides
such a useful introduction to the method. It was designed originally for classification
problems, which once again are discussed first.

Consider a binary response coded as 1 or -1. Adaboost.M1 then has the following
general structure. The pseudocode that follows is basically a reproduction of what
Hastie et al. (2009) show on their page 339.

1. Initialize the observation weights $w_i = 1/N, i = 1, 2, \ldots, N$ observations.
2. For $m = 1$ to M passes over the data:

   (a) Fit a classifier $G_m(x)$ to the training data using the weights w_i.
   (b) Compute: $err_m = \frac{\sum_{i=1}^{N} w_i I(y_i \neq G_m(x_i))}{\sum_{i=1}^{n} w_i}$.
   (c) Compute $\alpha_m = \log[(1 - err_m)/err_m]$.
   (d) Set $w_i \leftarrow w_i \cdot \exp[\alpha_m \cdot I(y_i \neq G_m(x_i))], i = 1, 2, \ldots, N$.

3. Output $G(x) = \text{sign} \left[\sum_{m=1}^{M} \alpha_m G_m(x) \right]$.

There are N cases and M iterations. $G_m(x)$ is a classifier for pass m over the data
x. It is the source of the fitted values used in the algorithm. Any number of procedures
might be used to build a classifier, but highly truncated trees (called "stumps") are
common. The operator I is an indicator variable equal to 1 if the logical relationship

is true, and 0 otherwise. The binary response is coded 1 and -1 so that the sign defines the outcome.

Classification error for pass m over the data is denoted by err_m; it is essentially the proportion of cases misclassified. In the next step, err_m is in the denominator and $(1 - err_m)$ is in the numerator before the log is taken. A larger value of α_m means a better fit.

The new weights, one for each case, are then computed, The value of w_i is unchanged if the ith case is correctly classified. If the ith case is incorrectly classified, it is "up-weighted" by e^{α_m}. Adaboost.M1 will pay relatively more attention in the next iteration to the cases that were misclassified. In some expositions of Adaboost (Freund and Schapire 1999), α_m is defined as $\frac{1}{2}\log(1-err_m/err_m)$. Then, incorrectly classified cases are up-weighted by e^{α_m} and correctly classified cases are down-weighted by $e^{-\alpha_m}$.

In the final step, classification is determined by a sum of fitted values over the M classifiers G_m, with each set of fitted values weighted by α_m. This is in much the same spirit as the last step in the random forest algorithm, but for adaboost, the contributions from classifiers that fit the data are better and are given more weight, and the class assigned depends on the sign of the sum.

To summarize, Adaboost combines a large number of fitting attempts of the data. Each fitting attempt is undertaken by a classifier using weighted observations. The observation weights are a function of how poorly an observation was fitted in the previous iteration. The fitted values from each iteration are then combined as a weighted sum. There is one weight for each fitting attempt, applied to all of the fitted values, which is a function of the overall classification error of that fitting attempt. The observation weights and the iteration weights both are a function of the classification error, but their forms and purposes are quite different.

6.2.1 A Toy Numerical Example of Adaboost.M1

To help fix these ideas, it is useful to go through a numerical illustration with very simple data. There are five observations with response variable values for $i = 1, 2, 3, 4, 5$ of $1, 1, 1, -1, -1$, respectively.

1. Initialize the observations with each weight $w_i = 1/5$.
2. For the first iteration using the equal weights, suppose the fitted values from some classifier for observations $i = 1, 2, 3, 4, 5$ are $1, 1, 1, 1, 1$. The first three are correct and the last two are incorrect. Therefore, the error for this first iteration is

$$err_1 = \frac{(.20 \times 0) + (.20 \times 0) + (.20 \times 0) + (.20 \times 1) + (.20 \times 1)}{1} = .40.$$

3. The weight to be given to this iteration is then

$$\alpha_1 = \log\frac{(1 - .40)}{.40} = \log(.60/.40) = \log(1.5) = .41.$$

4. The new weights are

$$w_1 = .20 \times e^{(.41 \times 0)} = .20$$

$$w_2 = .20 \times e^{(.41 \times 0)} = .20$$

$$w_3 = .20 \times e^{(.41 \times 0)} = .20$$

$$w_4 = .20 \times e^{(.41 \times 1)} = .30$$

$$w_5 = .20 \times e^{(.41 \times 1)} = .30$$

5. Now we begin the second iteration. We fit the classifier again and for $i = 1, 2, 3, 4, 5$ get 1, 1, 1, 1, −1. The first three and the fifth are correct. The fourth is incorrect. The error for the second iteration is

$$err_2 = \frac{[(.20 \times 0) + (.20 \times 0) + (.20 \times 0) + (.30 \times 1) + (.30 \times 0)]}{1.2} = .25$$

6. The weight to be given to this iteration is

$$\alpha_2 = \log\frac{(1-25)}{.25} = \log(.75/.25) = 1.1.$$

7. We would normally keep iterating, beginning with the calculation of a third set of weights. But suppose we are done. The classes assigned are

$$\hat{y}_1 = \text{sign}[(1 \times .41) + (1 \times 1.1)] > 0 \Rightarrow 1$$
$$\hat{y}_2 = \text{sign}[(1 \times .41) + (1 \times 1.1)] > 0 \Rightarrow 1$$
$$\hat{y}_3 = \text{sign}[(1 \times .41) + (1 \times 1.1)] > 0 \Rightarrow 1$$
$$\hat{y}_4 = \text{sign}[(1 \times .41) + (1 \times 1.1)] > 0 \Rightarrow 1$$
$$\hat{y}_5 = \text{sign}[(1 \times .41) + (-1 \times 1.1)] < 0 \Rightarrow -1.$$

One can see in this toy example how in the second iteration, the misclassified observations are given relatively more weight. One can also see that the class assigned (i.e., +1 or −1) is just a weighted sum of the classes assigned at each iteration. The second iteration had fewer wrong (one out of five rather than two out of five) and so was given more weight in the ultimate averaging. These principles would apply even for very large datasets and thousands of iterations. The key point, however, is that operationally, there is nothing very mysterious going on.

6.2.2 Why Does Boosting Work so Well for Classification?

Despite the operational simplicity of boosting, there is no consensus on why it works so well. At present, there seem to be three complementary perspectives. All three are truly interesting, and each has some useful implications for practice.

6.2.2.1 Boosting as a Margin Maximizer

The first perspective comes from computer science and the boosting pioneers. The basic idea is that boosting is a margin maximizer (Schapire et al. 1998; Schapire and Freund 2012). From AdaBoost, the margin for any given case i is defined as

$$mg^* = \sum_{y=G_m} \alpha_m - \sum_{y \neq G_m} \alpha_m, \tag{6.1}$$

where the sums are over the number of passes through the data for correct classifications or incorrect classifications respectively. This expression is different from Breiman's margin (mr) but in the same spirit. In words, for any given case i, the margin is the difference between the sum of the iteration weights when the classification is correct and the sum of the iteration weights when the classification is incorrect.[1]

Looking back at the toy example, the classifier is two for two for the first three observations, one for two for the last observation, and zero for two for the fourth observation. In practice, there would be hundreds of passes (or more) over the data, but one can nevertheless appreciate that the classifications are most convincing for the first three observations and least convincing for the fourth observation. The fifth observation is in between. Equation 6.1 is just an extension of this idea. The sum of the correct or incorrect classifications becomes the sum of the weights when the classification is correct or the sum of the weights when the classification is incorrect, with the weights equal to α_m. For the first three cases in the toy example, the margin $(.41 + 1.1) - 0 = 1.51$. The margin for the fourth case is $0 - (.41 + 1.1) = -1.51$. The margin for the fifth case is $1.1 - .41 = .69$. The evidence for the first three cases is the highest. The evidence for the fourth case is the lowest, and the evidence for the fifth case is in between.

And now the punch line. "Boosting is particularly good at finding classifiers with large margins in that it concentrates on those examples whose margins are small (or negative) and forces the base learning algorithm to generate good classifications for those examples" (Schapire et al. 1998: 1656).[2] Indeed, as the number of passes through the data increase, the margins over observations generally increase, although

---

[1] A more general definition is provided by Schapire and his colleagues (2008: 1697). A wonderfully rich and more recent discussion about the central role of margins in boosting can be found in Schapire and Freund (2012). The book is a remarkable mix from a computer science perspective of the formal mathematics and very accessible discussions of what the mathematics means.

[2] In computer science parlance, an "example" is an observation or case.

whether they are maximized depends on the base classifier. For instance, the margins are generally not maximized for stump classification trees but are maximized for large classification trees. This should sound familiar. A closely related point was made for random forests.

Improvements in the margin over passes through the data reformulates the overfitting problem. It is possible in principle to fit the training data perfectly. One would ordinarily halt the boosting well before that point because of concerns about overfitting. But with a perfect fit of the data, generalization error in test data can be surprisingly good because the weighed averaging works in a manner much like the averaging in bagging or random forests. (Look again at the final step in the Adaboost.M1 algorithm.) Moreover, boosting *past* a perfect fit of the data can further reduce generalization error because the margins are getting larger. In short, concerns about overfitting for boosting seem to have been overstated.

There is one exception in which overfitting has actually been understated. When a classifier is also used to compute the probabilities associated with each class, boosting to minimize generalization error pushes the conditional proportions/probabilities for each observation toward 0.0 or 1.0 (Mease et al. 2007; Buja et al. 2008). This follows from the margin maximizing property of boosting. We will have more to say about this shortly.

In summary, one reason why boosting works so well as a classifier is that it proceeds as a margin maximizer. An important implication for using classifiers such as Adaboost.M1 is that overfitting can in practice not be a serious problem. One can even boost past the point at which the fit in the training data is perfect. Another important implication for practice is that if classification trees are used as the classifier, large trees are desirable. And if large trees are desirable, so are large samples.

6.2.2.2   Boosting as a Statistical Optimizer

The second perspective sees Adaboost as a stagewise additive model using basis functions in much the same spirit as CART and random forests. Consider again the final step in the algorithm for Adaboost.M1

$$G(x) = \text{sign} \left[\sum_{m=1}^{M} \alpha_m G_m(x) \right]. \tag{6.2}$$

Each pass through the data involves the application of a classifier $G_m(x)$, the culmination of which is a stage. The results of M stages are combined in an additive fashion with the M values of α_m as the computed weights. This means that each $G_m(x)$ relies on a linear basis expansion of X, much as discussed in Chap. 1.

If boosting can be formulated as a stagewise additive model, an important question is what loss function is being used. From Friedman and his colleagues (2000), Adaboost.M1 iterations are implicitly targeting

$$f(X) = \frac{1}{2}\log\frac{P(Y=1|X)}{P(Y=-1|X)}. \tag{6.3}$$

This is just one-half of the usual log-odds (logit) function for $P(Y=1|X)$. The $1/2$ results from using the sign to determine the class. This is the "population minimizer" for an exponential loss function $e^{-yf(x)}$. More formally,

$$\arg\min_{f(x)} E_{Y|x}(e^{-Yf(x)}) = \frac{1}{2}(\log)\frac{P(Y=1|x)}{P(Y=-1|x)} \tag{6.4}$$

Adaboost.M1 is attempting to minimize exponential loss with the observed class and the predicted class as its arguments. The focus on exponential loss raises at least two important issues for practice.

First, emphasizing the mathematical relationship between the exponential loss function and conditional probabilities can paper over a key point in practice. Although at each stage, the true conditional probability is indeed the minimizer, over stages there can be gross overfitting of the estimated probabilities. In other words, the margin maximizing feature of boosting can trump the loss function optimizing feature of boosting.

Second, a focus on the exponential loss function naturally raises the question of whether there are other loss functions that might perform better. Hastie and his colleagues (2009: 345–346) show that minimizing the negative binomial log likelihood (i.e., the deviance) is also (as in Adaboost) in service of finding the true conditional probabilities, or the within-sample conditional proportions (i.e., a level II or level I analysis respectively). Might this loss function, implemented as "Logitboost," be preferred? On the matter of overfitting conditional probabilities, the answer is no. The same overfitting problems surface (Mease et al. 2007).

With respect to estimating class membership, the answer is maybe. Hastie et al. (2009: 346–349) show that the Logitboost loss function is somewhat more robust to outliers than the Adaboost loss function. They argue that, therefore, Logitboost may be preferred if a significant number of the observed classes of the response variable are likely to be systematically wrong or noisy. There are other boosting options as well (Friedman et al. 2000). But, it is not clear how the various competitors fare in practice and for our purposes at the moment, that is beside the point. The loss function optimization explanation, whatever the proposed loss function, is at best a partial explanation for the success of boosting.

6.2.2.3 Boosting as an Interpolator

The third perspective has already been introduced. One key to the success of random forests is that it is an interpolator that is then locally robust. Another key is the averaging over a large number of trees. Although the details certainly differ, these attributes also apply to boosting (Wyner et al. 2015). As the margins are increased, the fitted values better approximate an interpolation of the data. Then, the weighted average of fitted values provides much the same stability as the vote over trees provides for random forests; "...the additional iterations in boosting way beyond the point at which perfect classification in the training data (i.e., interpolation) has occurred has the effect of smoothing out the effects of noise rather than leading to more and more overfitting" (Wyner et al. 2105: 24).

All three perspectives help explain why boosting performs so well as a classifier. From a statistical perspective, boosting is a stagewise optimizer targeting the same kinds of conditional probabilities that are the target for logistic regression. One of several different loss functions can be used depending on the details of the data. This framework places boosting squarely within statistical traditions. But boosting is far more than a round-about way to do logistic regression. The margin maximization perspective helps to explain why and dramatically reduces concerns about overfitting, at least for classification. When the classifiers are trees, large trees perform better, which suggests that in general, complex base classifiers are to be preferred. Finally, the interpolation perspective links boosting to random forests and shows that boosting classifiers have many of the same beneficial properties. In so doing, there is a deeper understanding about why maximizing margins can be so helpful, although it is not nearly the whole story. In the end, interpolation may be the key.

The implications for classification in practice are fourfold

1. complex base learners (e.g., large classification trees) help;
2. boosting beyond a perfect fit in the training data can help;
3. a large number of observations can help; and
4. a rich set of predictors can help (subject to the usual caveats such as very high multicollinearity).

6.3   Stochastic Gradient Boosting

At present, there are many different kinds of boosting that all but boosting mavens will find overwhelming. Moreover, there is very little guidance about which form of boosting should be used in which circumstances. For practitioners, therefore, stochastic gradient boosting is a major advance (Friedman 2001; 2002). It is not quite a one-size-fits-all boosting procedure, but within a single statistical framework provides a rich menu of options. As such, it follows directly from the statistical perspective on boosting.

Here is a rough summary of the procedure for classification. Suppose that the response variable in the training data is binary and coded as 1 or 0. The procedure is initialized with some constant such as the overall proportion of 1s. This constant serves as the fitted values from which residuals are obtained by subtraction in the usual way. The residuals are then appended to the training data as a new variable. Next, a random sample of the data is drawn without replacement. One might, for example, sample half the data. A regression tree, not a classification tree, is applied to the sample with the residuals as the response. Another set of fitted values is obtained.

From these, a new set of residuals is obtained and appended. Another random sample is taken from the training data and the fitting process is repeated. The entire cycle is repeated many times: (1) fitted values, (2) residuals, (3) sampling, (4) a regression tree. In the end, the fitted values from each pass through the data are combined in a linear fashion. For classification, these can be interpreted as proportions or probabilities depending on whether the analysis is at level I or level II respectively. Commonly, observations with $\hat{y}_i > 0.5$ are assigned a 1, and observations with $\hat{y}_i \leq 0.5$ are assigned a 0.

The weighting so central to boosting occurs implicitly through the residuals from each pass. Larger positive or negative residuals imply that for those observations, the fitted values are less successful. As the regression tree attempts to maximize the quality of the fit overall, it responds more to the observations with larger positive or negative residuals.

Consider now somewhat more formally the sources of the term "gradient" in stochastic gradient boosting. Either numerical or categorical response variables are allowed along with a variety of loss functions. As with random forests, trees are a key component of the algorithm. The discussion that follows on boosting trees draws heavily on Ridgeway (1999) and on Hastie et al. (2009: Sects. 10.9–4.10).

A *given* tree can be represented as

$$T(x; \Theta) = \sum_{j=1}^{J} \gamma_j I(x \in R_j), \tag{6.5}$$

with, as before, the tree parameters $\Theta = \{R_j, \gamma_j\}$, where j is an index of the terminal node, $j, \ldots, J$, R_j a predictor-space region defined by the jth terminal node, and γ_j is the value assigned to each observation in the jth terminal node. The goal is to construct values for the unknown parameters Θ so that the loss function is minimized. At this point, no particular loss L is specified, and we seek

$$\hat{\Theta} = \arg\min_{\Theta} \sum_{j=1}^{J} \sum_{x_i \in R_j} L(y_i, \gamma_j). \tag{6.6}$$

As noted earlier, minimizing the loss function for a single tree is challenging. For stochastic gradient boosting, the challenge is even greater because we seek to minimize the loss over a set of trees. As a rough-and-ready approximation, we once again proceed in a stagewise fashion so that at iteration m, we need to find

$$\hat{\Theta}_m = \arg\min_{\Theta_m} \sum_{i=1}^{N} L(y_i, f_{m-1}(x_i) + T(x_i; \Theta_m)), \tag{6.7}$$

where $f_{m-1}(x_i)$ are the results of the previous tree. Given the results from the previous tree, the intent is to reduce the loss as much as possible using the fitted values from the next tree. This can be accomplished through an astute determination of

$\hat{\Theta}_m = [R_{jm}, \gamma_{jm}]$ for $j = 1, 2, \ldots, J_m$. Thus, Eq. 6.7 expresses the aspiration of updating the fitted values in an optimal manner.

Equation 6.7 can be reformulated as a numerical optimization task. In this framework, g_{im} is the gradient for the ith observation on iteration m, defined as the partial derivative of the loss with respect to the fitting function. Thus,

$$g_{im} = -\left[\frac{\partial L(y_i, f(x_i))}{\partial f(x_i)}\right]_{f(x_i)=f_{m-1}(x_i)}. \qquad (6.8)$$

Equation 6.8 represents for each observation i the potential reduction in the loss as the fitting function $f(x_i)$ is altered. The larger the absolute value of g_{im}, the greater is the change in the loss as $f(x_i)$ changes. So, an effective fitting function would respond more to the larger absolute values of g_{im} than small ones.

The g_{im} will generally vary across observations. A way must be found to exploit the g_{im} so that over all of the observations, the loss is reduced the most it can be. One approach is to use a numerical method called "steepest descent," in which a "step length" ρ_m is found so that

$$\rho_m = \arg\min_{\rho} L(\mathbf{f}_{m-1} - \rho\mathbf{g}_m). \qquad (6.9)$$

In other words, a scalar ρ_m is determined for iteration m so that when it multiplies the vector of gradients, the loss function from the previous iteration is reduced the most it can be.

Figure 6.1 illustrates the basics of the process when there are two predictors, X_1 and X_2. There is a single location, represented by the red filled circle, where the smallest loss can be found. The algorithm starts at some arbitrary point and proceeds in steps determined by the direction and step length for which the loss is reduced the most, subject to a constraint on the length of the step. Often the step lengths are reduced in flatter regions of the function so that the minimum is not overshot. Typically there will be many more predictors, but the ideas represented in Fig. 6.1 generalize.

The link between the method of steepest descent and gradient boosting is g_{im}. Consider the disparities between tree-generated fitted values and the actual values of the response. Those disparities are a critical input to the loss function. The size of the loss depends on all of the N disparities, but larger disparities make greater contributions to the loss than smaller disparities. Thus, a fitting function will reduce the loss more substantially if it does an especially good job at reducing the larger disparities between its fitted values and the actual values. There is a greater payoff in concentrating on the larger disparities. Disparities resulting from the fitting process play much the same role as the gradients in the method of steepest descent.

And now the payoff. Friedman (2002) shows that if one uses certain transformations of the disparities as the gradients (details soon), there is a least squares solution to finding effective parameter values for the fitting function. That is,

Fig. 6.1 An illustration of steepest descent looking down into a convex loss function (The predictors are X_1 and X_2. Loss is represented on the vertical axis.)

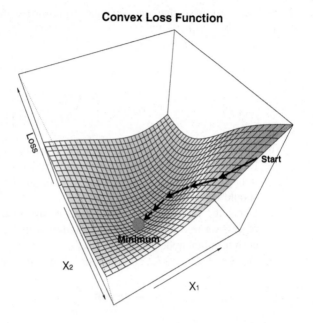

$$\tilde{\Theta}_m = \arg\min_{\Theta} \sum_{i=1}^{N} (-g_{im} - T(x_i; \Theta))^2. \qquad (6.10)$$

What this means in practice is that if one fits successive regression trees by least squares, each time using as the "response variable" a certain transformation of the disparities produced by the previous regression tree, one can obtain a useful approximation of the required parameters. For a binary outcome, the classifier that results, based on a large number of combined regression trees, can be much like Adaboost or Adaboost itself. Moreover, by recasting the boosting process in gradient terms, many useful variants follow including the boosting of fitting procedures for quantitative response variables.

We turn, then, to stochastic gradient boosting, implemented in R as *gbm()*, that is a generalization of Friedman's original gradient boosting. Among the differences are the use of sampling in the spirit of bagging and a form of shrinkage.[3]

Consider a training dataset with N observations and p variables, including the response y and the predictors x.

---

[3]For very large datasets, there is a scalable version of tree boosting called *XGBoost()* (Chen and Guestrin 2016) that can provide remarkable speed improvements but has yet to include the range of useful loss functions found in *gbm()*. More will be said about *XGBoost()* when "deep learning" is briefly considered in Chap. 8.

1. Initialize $f_0(x)$ so that the constant κ minimizes the loss function: $f_0(x) = \arg\min_\kappa \sum_{i=1}^{N} L(y_i, \kappa)$.[4]
2. For m in $1, \ldots, M$, do steps a–e.

   (a) For $i = 1, 2, \ldots, N$ compute the negative gradient as the working response

   $$r_{im} = -\left[\frac{\partial L(y_i, f(x_i))}{\partial f(x_i)}\right]_{f=f_{m-1}}.$$

   (b) Randomly select without replacement W cases from the data set, where W is less than the total number of observations. This is a simple random sample, not a bootstrap sample, which seems to improve performance. How large W should be is discussed shortly.
   (c) Using the randomly selected observations, each with their own r_{im}, fit a regression tree with J_m terminal nodes to the r_{im}, giving regions R_{jm} for each terminal node $j = 1, 2, \ldots, J_m$.
   (d) For $j = 1, 2, \ldots, J_m$, compute the optimal terminal node prediction as

   $$\gamma_{jm} = \arg\min_\gamma \sum_{x_i \in R_{jm}} L(y_i, f_{m-1}(x_i) + \gamma),$$

   where region R_{jm} denotes the set of x-values that define the terminal node j for iteration m.
   (e) Drop all of the cases down the tree grown from the sample and, update $f_m(x)$ as

   $$f_m(x) = f_{m-1}(x) + \nu \cdot \sum_{j=1}^{J_m} \gamma_{jm} I(x \in R_{jm}).$$

   where ν is a "shrinkage" parameter that determines the learning rate. The importance of ν is discussed shortly.

3. Output $\hat{f}(x) = f_M(x)$.

Ridgeway (1999) has shown that using this algorithmic structure, all of the procedures within the generalized linear model, plus several extensions of it, can properly be boosted by the stochastic gradient method. Stochastic gradient boosting relies on an empirical approximation of the true gradient (Hastie et al. 2001: Sect. 10.10). The trick is determining the right r_i for each special case; the "residuals" need to be defined. Among the current definitions of r_{im} are the following, each associated with a particular kind of regression mean function: linear regression, logistic regression, robust regression, Poisson regression, quantile regression, and others.

---

[4]Other initializations such as least squares regression could be used, depending on loss function (e.g., for a quantitative response variable).

1. Gaussian: $y_i - f(x_i)$: the usual regression residual.
2. Bernoulli: $y_i - \frac{1}{1+e^{-f(x_i)}}$: the difference between the binary outcome coded 1 or 0 and the fitted ("predicted") proportion for the conventional logit link function for logistic regression.
3. Poisson: $y_i - e^{f(x_i)}$: the difference between the observed count and the fitted count for the conventional log link function as in Poisson regression
4. Laplace: $\text{sign}[y_i - f(x_i)]$: the sign of the difference between the values of the response variable and the fitted medians, a form of robust regression.
5. Adaboost: $-(2y_i - 1)e^{-(2y_i-1)f(x_i)}$: based on exponential loss and closely related to logistic regression.
6. Quantile: $\alpha(I(y > f(x_i)) - (1 - \alpha)I(y_i \le f(x_i))$: for quantile regression the weighted difference between two indicator variables equal to 1 or 0 depending on whether residual is positive or negative with the weights α or $(1 - \alpha)$, and α as the percentile target.

There are several other options built into *gbm( )*. Hastie and his colleagues (2001: 321) derive the gradient for a Huber robust regression. Ridgeway (2012) offers boosted proportional hazard regression. Other less well-documented options include multinomial logistic regression, and regression based on a t-distribution. No doubt there will additional distributions added in the future.

Stochastic gradient boosting also can be linked to various kinds of penalized regression of the general form discussed in earlier chapters. One insight is that the sequence of results that is produced with each pass over the data can be seen as a regularization process akin to shrinkage (Bühlmann and Yu 2004; Friedman et al. 2004).

In short, with stochastic gradient boosting, each tree is constructed much as a conventional regression tree. The difference is how the "target" for the fitting is defined. Using disparities defined in particular ways, a wide range of fitting procedures can be boosted. It is with good reason that "gbm" stands for "generalized boosted regression models."

6.3.1 Tuning Parameters

Stochastic gradient boosting has a substantial number of tuning parameters, many of which affect the results in similar ways. There is no analytical way to arrive at an optimal tuning parameter values in part because how they perform is so dependent on the data (Buja et al. 2008). An algorithmic search over values might be helpful in principle, but would be computationally demanding, and there would likely be many sets of tuning parameter values leading to nearly the same performance. Fortunately, the results from stochastic gradient boosting are often relatively robust with respect to sensible variation in the tuning parameters, and common defaults usually work quite well.

The most important tuning parameters provided by *gbm( )* are as follows:

1. Number of Iterations — The number of passes through the data is typically the most important tuning parameter and is in practice empirically determined. Because there is no convergence and no clear stopping rule, the usual procedure is to run a large number of iterations and inspect a graph of the fitting error (e.g., residual deviance) plotted against the number of iterations. The error should decline rapidly at first and then level off. If after leveling, there is an inflection point at which the fitting error begins to increase, the number of iterations can be stopped shortly before that point. If there is no inflection point, the number of iterations can be determined by when reductions in the error effectively cease. There is a relatively large margin for error because plus or minus 50–100 iterations rarely lead to meaningful performance differences.

2. Subsample Size — A page is taken from bagging with the use of random sampling in step 2b to help control overfitting. The sampling is done without replacement, but as noted earlier, there can be an effective equivalence between sampling with and without replacement, at least for conventional bagging (Buja and Stuetzle 2006). When sampling without replacement, the sample size is a tuning parameter, and the issues are rather like those that arise when one works with split samples. How large should the training sample, evaluation sample, and test sample be? There seems to be no formal or general answer. Practice seems to favor a sample size of $N/2$. But it can make sense for any given data analysis to try sample sizes that also are about 25 % smaller and larger.

3. Learning Rate — A slow rate at which the updating occurs can be very useful. Setting the tuning parameter ν to be less than 1.0 is standard practice. A value of .001 often seems to work reasonably well, but values larger and smaller by up to a factor of 10 are sometimes worth trying as well. By slowing down the rate at which the algorithm "learns," a larger number of basis functions can be computed. Flexibility in the fitting process is increased, and the small steps increase shrinkage, which improves stability. A cost is a larger number of passes through the data. Fortunately, one can usually slow the learning process down substantially without a prohibitive increase in computing.

4. Interaction Depth — Another tuning parameter that affects the flexibility of the fitting function is the "depth" of the interaction. This name is a little misleading because it does not directly control the order of the interactions allowed. Rather it controls the number of splits allowed. If the interaction depth is 1, there is only a split of the root node data. If the interaction depth is 2, the two resulting data partitions of the root node data are split. If the interaction depth is 3, the four resulting partitions are split. And on it goes. Interaction depth is a way to limit the size of the regression trees, and values from 1 to 10 are used in practice. As such, the interaction depth determines the *maximum* order of any interactions, but the order of the interactions can be less than the interaction depth. For example, an interaction depth of 2 may result in four partitions defined

by a single predictor at different break points. There are no interactions effects because interaction effects are commonly defined as the product of two or more predictors. If interaction depth is set to 2, the largest possible interaction effect is 2 (i.e., a two-way interaction involving two predictors).

5. Terminal Node Size — Yet another tuning parameter that affects fitting function flexibility is the minimum number of observations in each tree's terminal node. For a given sample size, smaller node sizes imply larger trees and a more flexible fitting function. But smaller nodes also lead to less stability for whatever is computed in each terminal node. Minimum terminal node sizes of between 5 and 15 seem to work reasonably well in many settings, but a lot depends on the loss function that is being used.

In practice, the tuning parameters can interact. For example, terminal node size may be set too high for the interaction depth specified to be fully implemented. Also, more than one tuning parameter can be set in service of the same goal. The growth of larger trees, for instance, can be encouraged by small terminal node sizes and by greater interaction depth. In short, sometimes tuning parameters compete with one another and sometimes tuning parameters complement one another.

How one tunes depends heavily on the kind of stochastic gradient boosting being undertaken. The advice available typically depends on craft lore, but the interpolation perspective discussed earlier has more formal implications for classification. It can be useful to set tuning parameters to better approximate an interpolation of the data. Perhaps most important, a minimum size of 1 for terminal nodes is often very effective, at least for classification. In the same spirit, deep trees and a very large number of iterations should be considered. Examples will be provided later.

A major obstacle to effective tuning is the need for test data. Even with the sampling built into stochastic gradient boosting, there is no provision for retaining the unsampled data for performance evaluation. The out-of-bag data may be used only to help determine the number of iterations.[5] Common tuning advice, therefore, is limited to in-sample performance. But recall that for classification, one can have a perfect fit to the data and still reduce generalization error with more iterations. For classification and regression, using the test data for performance evaluation seems like a good idea.

6.3.2 Output

The key output from stochastic gradient boosting is much the same as the key output from random forests. However, unlike random forests, there are not the usual out-of-bag observations that can be used as test data. Consequently, confusion tables depend on resubstituted data; the data used to grow the trees are also used to evaluate their

---

[5]For gbm(), the data not selected for each tree are called "out-of-bag" data although that is not fully consistent with the usual definition because in *gbm()*, the sampling is without replacement.

performance. The same applies to fitted values for numerical response variables. Consequently, overfitting can be a complication although the updating over lots of trees helps a lot. Ideally, this problem should be addressed with real test data.

Just as for random forests, the use of multiple trees means that it is impractical to examine tree diagrams to learn how individual predictors perform. The solutions currently available are much like those implemented for random forests. There are variable importance measures and partial dependence plots that are similar to those used in random forests.

The partial dependence plots must be treated cautiously when the outcome variable is binary. Recall that in an effort to classify well, boosting can push the fitted probabilities away from .50 toward 0.0 and 1.0. For *gbm()*, partial dependence plots with binary response variables use either a probability or logit scale (i.e., $p_i/(1-p_i)$) on the vertical axis. Both are vulnerable if measures of classification performance are being used to tune. If tuning is done through measures of fit such as the deviance, one has no more than the usual concerns about overfitting. But, in that case, classification accuracy (should one care) will perhaps be sacrificed.

The exact form taken by the variable importance measures depends on options in the software. One common choice is reductions of the loss function that can be attributed to each predictor. The software sums for each tree how much the loss decreases when any predictor defines a data partition. For example, if for a given tree a particular predictor is chosen 3 times to define data partitions, the three reductions in the loss function are summed as a measure of that predictor's contribution to the fit for that tree. Such sums are averaged over trees to provide the contribution that each predictor makes to the overall fit. The contributions can be reported in raw form or as percentages of the overall reduction in loss. In gbm(), there is on a somewhat experimental basis a random shuffling approach to importance based on predictive accuracy. To date, however, out-of-bag observations are not used so that true forecasting accuracy is not represented. Recall that for random forests, importance is defined by contributions to prediction accuracy in the out-of-bag data.

6.4 Asymmetric Costs

All of the available loss functions for categorical outcomes use symmetric costs. False positives count the same as false negatives. For stochastic gradient boosting, there are two ways to easily introduce asymmetric costs. The first is to place a threshold on the fitted values that differs from .5 (or on the logit scale that differs from 0.0). This option was discussed earlier for several other procedures. For example, if a positive is coded 1 and a negative is coded 0, placing the threshold at .25 means false negatives are 3 times most costly than false positives. The problems with this approach were also discussed. All other boosting output is still based on symmetric costs. Moreover, there can be complications if the distribution of the fitted values is either very dense or very sparse in the neighborhood of the threshold. If very dense, small changes in the threshold that make no material difference can alter classification performance dramatically. If very sparse, it can be difficult set the threshold so that the desired cost ratio in a confusion tables is produced.

The second alternative is to use weights. This is much like altering the prior for CART. And like with CART, some trial and error is involved before the classification table with the desired cost ratio is produced. But the intent is to upweight the outcome for which classifications errors are more costly relative to the outcome for which classification error is less costly. An example is provided below.

For numerical response variables, the options are more limited. The only loss function for which asymmetric costs are naturally available is the quantile regression loss function. By choosing the appropriate quantile, underestimates can be given different costs from overestimates. For example, if one estimates the 75th percentile, underestimates are 3 times more costly than overestimates. Looking back at the quantile regression residual expression shown earlier when the algorithm for stochastic gradient boosting was introduced, the value of α is set to the target percentile and is the weight given to all positive residuals. The value of $(1 - \alpha)$ is the weight given to all negative residuals. Positive residuals are underestimates, and negative residuals are overestimates.

Figure 6.2 shows the shape of the loss function when the quantile is greater than .50. As illustrated by the red line, the loss grows more rapidly for underestimates (i.e., positive residuals) than overestimates (i.e., negative residuals). For quantiles less than .50, the reverse is true. For a quantile of .50, the red and blue line have the same rate of growth.

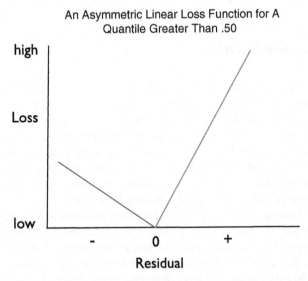

Fig. 6.2 Asymmetric loss function for the quantile loss function with the quantile set at .75

6.5   Boosting, Estimation, and Consistency

The most important output from boosting is the fitted values. For a level I analysis, these are just statistics computed for the data on hand. But, often there is an interest in using the values as estimates of the fitted values in the joint probability distribution responsible for the data. This is a level II analysis. Just as for random forests, no claims are made that boosting will provide accurate estimates of the true response surface. At best, one can get a consistent estimate of generalization error for a given sample size,[6] boosting specification and set of tuning parameters values (Jiang, 2004, Zhang and Yu 2005, Bartlett and Traskin 2007). But existing proofs either impose artificial conditions or are limited to a few of the "easier" loss functions such as exponential loss and quadratic loss. And even then, the implications for practice are not clear. There can be a Goldilocks stopping strategy for a given number of observations at which the number of iterations is neither too few nor too many. But how to find that sweet spot for a given analysis is not explained.

The best one can do in practice is apply some empirical heuristic and hope for the best. As already noted, that heuristic can be the point at which the decrease in the loss function levels off. Some measure of fit between the observed response values and the fitted values can then be used as a rough proxy for generalization error for that sample size, stopping decision, specification, and associated tuning parameter settings. Conventionally, this is an in-sample estimate. A more honest estimate of generalization error can be obtained from a test sample and as described earlier, one can use the nonparametric bootstrap to approximate the variance in that estimate.

6.6   A Binomial Example

We return to the Titanic data for some applications of stochastic boosting as implemented in *gbm( )*. Recall that the response is whether or not a passenger survived. The predictors we use are gender ("sex"), age, class of cabin ("pclass"), number of siblings/spouses aboard("sibsp"), and the number of parents/children aboard ("parch"). The code used for the analysis with Bernoulli loss is provided in Fig.6.3. At the top, the data are loaded, and a new data set is constructed. A weighting variable is constructed for later use. All NA entries removed. Removing NAs in advance is required when a procedure does not discard them automatically.

Consistent with our earlier discussion, the minimum terminal node size is set to 1, and the interaction depth set to 3. Setting interaction depth to a larger value (e.g., 8) led to fewer iterations but essentially the same results. Setting it to a smaller value (e.g., 1) led to more iterations, but also essentially same results. The number of iterations was set to 4000 anticipating that 4000 should be plenty. If not, the number could be

---

[6]Even with the minimum number of observations allowed in terminal nodes specified, with more observations there can be larger trees. There can be more splits before the minimum is reached.

```
# Load and Clean Up Data
library(PASWR)
data("titanic3")
attach(titanic3)
wts<-ifelse(survived==1,1,3) # for asymmetric costs
Titanic3<-na.omit(data.frame(fare,survived,pclass,
                             sex,age,sibsp,parch,wts))

# Boosted Binomial Regression
library(gbm)
out2<-gbm(survived~pclass+sex+age+sibsp+parch,
          data=Titanic3,n.trees=4000,interaction.depth=3,
          n.minobsinnode = 1,shrinkage=.001,bag.fraction=0.5,
          n.cores=1,distribution = "bernoulli")

# Output
gbm.perf(out2,oobag.curve=T,method="OOB",overlay=F) # 3245
summary(out2,n.trees=3245,method=permutation.test.gbm,
        normalize=T)
plot(out2,"sex",3245,type="response")
plot(out2,"pclass",3245,type="response")
plot(out2,"age",3245,type="response")
plot(out2,"sibsp",3245,type="response")
plot(out2,"parch",3245,type="response")
plot(out2,c("subsp","parch"),3245,type="response") # Interaction

# Fitted Values
preds2<-predict(out2,newdata=Titanic3,n.trees=3245,
                type="response")
table(Titanic3$survived,preds2>.5)
```

Fig. 6.3 R code for Bernoulli regression boosting

increased. All else were the defaults, except that the number of cores available was one. Even with only one core, the fitting took about a second in real time.[7]

Figure 6.4 shows standard *gbm()* performance output. On the horizontal axis is the number of iterations. On the vertical axis is the change in the Bernoulli deviance based on the OOB observations. The OOB observations provide a more honest assessment than could be obtained in-sample. However, they introduce sampling error so that the changes in the loss bounce around a bit. The reductions in the deviance decline as the number of iterations grows and become effectively 0.0 shortly after the 3000th pass through the data. Any of the iterations between 3000 and 4000 lead to about

---

[7] For these analyses, the work was done on an iMac with a single core. The processor was a 3.4 Ghz Intel Core i7.

Fig. 6.4 Changes in
Bernoulli deviance in OOB
data with iteration 3245 as
the stopping point
(N = 1045)

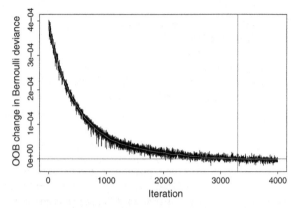

Fig. 6.5 Titanic data
variable importance plot for
survival using binomial
regression boosting
(N = 1045)

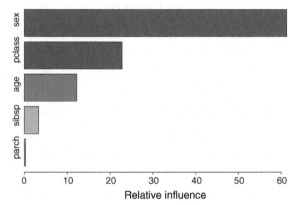

the same fit of the data, but the software selects iteration 3245 as the stopping point.
Consequently, the first 3245 trees are used in all subsequent calculations.[8]

Figure 6.5 is a variable importance plot shown in the standard *gbm( )* format for
the predictor shuffling approach. Recall that unlike in random forests, the reductions
are for predictions into the full dataset, not the subset of OOB observations. Also the
contribution of each input is standardized differently. All contributions are given as
percentages of the summed contributions. For example, gender is the most important
predictor with a relative performance of 60 (i.e., 60 %). The class of passage is the next
most important input with a score of about 25, followed by age with a score of about
12. If you believe the accounts of the Titanic's sinking, these contributions make
sense. But just as with random forests, each contribution includes any interaction
effects with other variables unless the tree depth is equal to 1 (i.e., *interaction.depth*
= 1). So, the contributions in Fig. 6.5 cannot be attributed to each input by itself.
Equally important, contributions to the fit are not regression coefficients and or

---

[8] If forecasting were on the table, it might have been useful to try a much larger number of iterations
to reduce generalization error.

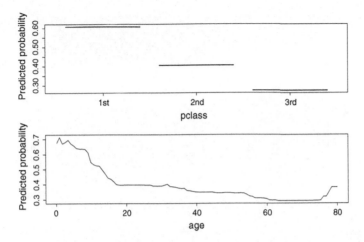

Fig. 6.6 Titanic data partial dependence plots showing survival proportions for class of passage and age using binomial regression boosting (N = 1045)

contributions to forecasting accuracy. It may not be clear, therefore, how to use them when real decisions have to be made.

Figure 6.6 presents two partial dependence plots with the fitted probability/proportion on the vertical axis. One has the option of reporting the results as probabilities/proportions or logits. One can see that class of passage really matters. The probability of survival drops from a little over 60 to a little under .30 from first class to second class to third class. Survival is also strongly related to age. The probability of survival drops from about .70 to about .40 as age increases from about 1 year to about 18. There is another substantial drop around age 55 and an increase around age 75. But there are very few passengers older than 65, so the apparent increase could be the result of instability.[9]

Figure 6.7 is a partial plot designed to show two-way interaction effects. The two inputs are the number of siblings/spouses aboard and the number of parents/children aboard, which are displayed as a generalization of a mosaic plot. The inputs are shown on the vertical and horizontal axes. The color scale is shown on the far right. A combination of sibsp >5 and parch >4 has the smallest chances survival; about a quarter survived. A combination of sibsp <2 and parch <3 has the largest chance of survival; a little less than half survived.[10] In this instance, there does not seem to be important interaction effects. The differences in the colors from top to bottom are about the same regardless of the value for sibsp. For example, when sibsp is 6, the proportion surviving changes top to bottom from about .25 to about .30. The

---

[9] The plots are shown just as *gbm()* builds them, and there are very few options provided. But just as with random forests, the underling data can be stored and then used to construct new plots more responsive to the preferences of data analysts.

[10] Because both inputs are integers, the transition from one value to the next is the midpoint between the two.

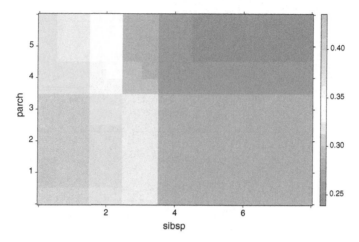

Fig. 6.7 Interaction partial dependence plot: survival proportions for the number of siblings/spouses aboard and the number of parents/children aboard using binomial regression boosting (N = 1045)

Table 6.1 Confusion table for Titanic survivors with default 1 to 1 weights (N = 1045)

	Forecast perished	Forecast survived	Model error
Perished	561	57	.09
Survived	126	301	.29
Use error	.18	.16	Overall error = .18

difference is −.05. When sibsp is 1, the proportion surviving changes from top to bottom from about .35 to about .40. The difference is again around −.05. Hence, the association between sibsp and survival is approximately the same for both values of sibsp.

It is difficult to read the color scale for Fig. 6.7 at the necessary level of precision. One might reach different conclusions if numerical values are examined. But the principle just illustrated is valid for how interaction effects are represented. And it is still true for these two predictors that a combination of many siblings/spouses and many parents/children is the worst combination of these two predictors whether or not their effects are only additive.

Table 6.1 is the confusion table that results when each case is given the same weight. In effect, this is the default. The empirical cost ratio that results is about 2.2 to 1 with misclassification errors for those who perished about twice as costly as misclassification errors for those who survived. Whether that is acceptable depends on how the results would be used. In this instance, there are probably no decisions to be made based on the classes assigned, so the cost ratio is probably of not much interest.

Stochastic gradient boosting does a good job distinguishing those who perished from those who survived. Only 9 % of those who perished were misclassified, and

Table 6.2 Confusion table for Titanic survivors with 3–1 weights (N = 1045)

	Forecast perished	Forecast survived	Model error
Perished	601	17	.03
Survived	195	232	.46
Use error	.24	.08	Overall error = .21

only 29 % of those who survived were misclassified. The forecasting errors of 18 % and 16 % are also quite good although it is hard to imagine how these results would be used for forecasting.

Table 6.2 repeats the prior analysis but with survivor observations weighted as 3 times more than the observations for those who perished. Because there are no decisions to be made based on the analysis, there is no grounded way to set the weights. The point is just to illustrate that weighting can make a big difference in the results that, in turn, affect the empirical cost ratio in a confusion table. That cost ratio is now 11.5 so that misclassifications of those who perished are now over 11 times more costly than misclassifications of those who survived. Consequently, the proportion misclassified for those who perished drops to 3 %, and the proportion misclassified for those who survived increases to 46 %. Whether these are more useful results than the results shown in Table 6.1 depend on how the results would be used.[11]

Should one report the results in proportions or probabilities? For these data, proportions seem more appropriate. As already noted, the Titanic sinking is probably best viewed as a one-time event that has already happened, which implies there may be no good answer to the question "probability of what?" Passengers either perished or survived, and treating such an historically specific event as one of many identical, independent trials seems a stretch. This is best seen as a level I analysis.

6.7 A Quantile Regression Example

For the Titanic data, the fare paid in dollars becomes the response variable, and the other predictors just as before. Because there are a few very large fares, there might be concerns about how well boosted normal regression would perform. Recall that boosted quantile regression is robust with respect to response variable outliers or a highly skewed distribution and also provides a way to build in relative costs for fitting errors. Figure 6.8 shows the code for a boosted quantile regression fitting the conditional 75th percentile.

There are two significant changes in the tuning parameters. First, the distribution is now "quantile" with alpha as the conditional quantile to be estimated. We

---

[11] It is not appropriate to compare the overall error rate in the two tables (.18–.21) because the errors are not weighted by costs. In Table 6.2, classification errors for those who perished are about 5 times more costly.

```
# Load Data and Clean Up Data
library(PASWR)
data("titanic3")
attach(titanic3)
Titanic3<-na.omit(data.frame(fare,pclass,
                             sex,age,sibsp,parch))

# Boosted Quantile Regression
library(gbm)
out1<-gbm(fare~pclass+sex+age+sibsp+parch,data=Titanic3,
          n.trees=12000,interaction.depth=3,
          n.minobsinnode = 10,shrinkage=.001,bag.fraction=0.5,
          n.cores=1, distribution = list(name="quantile",
          alpha=0.75))

#Output
gbm.perf(out1,oobag.curve=T) # 4387
summary(out1,n.trees=4387,method=relative.influence)
par(mfrow=c(2,1))
plot(out1,"sex",4387,type="link")
plot(out1,"age",4387,type="link")
plot(out1,"sibsp",4387,type="link")
plot(out1,"parch",4387,type="link")
plot(out1,c("pclass","age"),4448,type="link") # Interaction

# Fitted Values
preds1<-predict(out1,newdata=Titanic3,n.trees=4387,type="link")
plot(preds1,Titanic3$fare,col="blue",pch=19,
     xlab="Predicted Fare", ylab="Actual Fare",
     main="Results from Boosted Quantile Regression
     with 1 to 1 line Overlaid: (alpha=.75)")
     abline(0,1,col="red",lwd=2)
```

Fig. 6.8 R code for quantile regression boosting

begin by estimating the conditional 75th percentile. Underestimates are taken to be 3 times more costly than overestimates. Second, a much larger number of iterations is specified than for boosted binomial regression. For the conditional 75th percentile, only a little over 4000 iterations are needed. But we will see shortly that for other conditional percentiles, at least 12,000 iterations are needed. There is a very small computational penalty for 12,000 iterations for these data (Fig. 6.9).

Figure 6.10 is the same kind of importance plot as earlier except that importance is now represented by the average improvement over trees in fit for the quantile loss

Fig. 6.9 Changes in the
quantile loss function for the
fare paid with OOB Titanic
data and with iteration 4387
as the stopping point
(N = 1045)

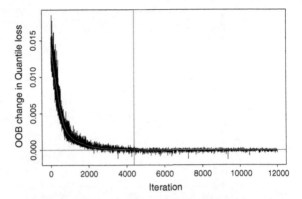

Fig. 6.10 Variable
importance plot for the fare
paid using quantile
regression boosting with the
75th percentile (N = 1045)

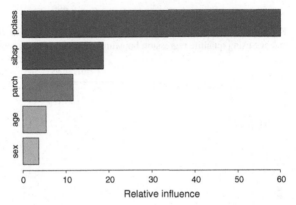

function as each tree is grown. This is an in-sample measure.[12] Nevertheless, the plot
is interpreted essentially in the same fashion. Fare is substantially associated with
the class of passage, just as one would expect. The number of siblings/spouses is the
second most important predictor, which also makes sense. With so few predictors,
and such clear differences in their contributions, the OOB approach and the in-sample
approach will lead to about the same relative contributions.

Figure 6.11 shows for illustrative purposes two partial response plots. The upper
plot reveals that the fitted 75th percentile is about $46 for females and a little less
than $36 for males with the other predictors held constant. It is difficult to know what
this means, because class of passage is being held constant and performs just as one
would expect (graph not shown). One possible explanation is that there is variation
in amenities within class of passage, and females are prepared to pay more for them.
The lower plot shows that variation in fare with respect to age is at most around $3
and is probably mostly noise, given all else that is being held constant.

Figure 6.12 is another example of an interaction partial plot. The format now
shows a categorical predictor (i.e., class of passage) and a numerical predictor

---

[12]The out-of-bag approach was not available in *gbm()* for boosted quantile regression.

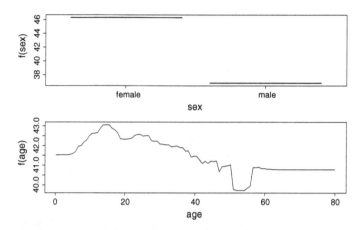

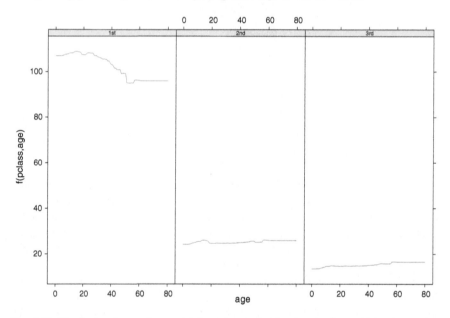

Fig. 6.11 Partial dependence plot for the Titanic data showing the fare paid for class of passage and age using quantile regression boosting fitting the 75th percentile (N = 1045)

Fig. 6.12 Titanic data interaction partial dependence plot showing the fare paid for the number of siblings/spouses aboard and the number of parents/children aboard using quantile regression boosting fitting the 75th percentile (N = 1045)

(i.e., age). There are apparently interaction effects. Fare declines with age for a first class passage but not for a second or third class passage. Perhaps older first class passengers are better able to pay for additional amenities. Perhaps, there is only one fare available for second and third class passage.

Fig. 6.13 Actual fare
against fitted fare for a
boosted quantile regression
analysis of the Titanic data
with a 1-to-1 line overlaid
(alpha = .75, N = 1045)

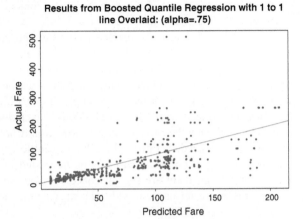

Fig. 6.14 Actual fare
against fitted fare for a
boosted quantile regression
analysis of the Titanic data
with a 1-to-1 line overlaid
(alpha = .25, N = 1045)

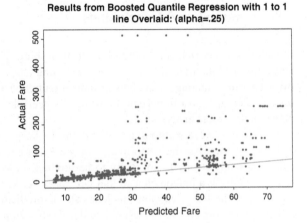

Figure 6.13 is a plot of the actual fare against the fitted fare for the 75th percentile.
Underestimates are 3 times more costly than overestimates. Overlaid is a 1-to-1
line that provides a point of reference. Most of the fitted values fall below the 1-
to-1 line, as they should. Still, four very large fares are grossly underestimated.
They are few and even with the expanded basis functions used in stochastic gradient
boosting, could not be fit well. The fitted values range from near $0 to over $200, and
roughly speaking, the fitted 75th percentile increases linearly with the actual fares.
The correlation between the two is over .70.

Figure 6.14 is a plot of the actual fare against the fitted fare for the 25th percentile.
Overestimates now are taken to be 3 times more costly than underestimates. Overlaid
again is a 1-to-1 line that provides a point of reference. Most of the actual fares fall
above the 1-to-1 line. This too is just as it should be. The fitted values range from

a little over \$0 to about \$75. Overall the fit still looks to be roughly linear, and the correlation is little changed.[13]

Without knowing how the results from a boosted quantile regression are to be used, it is difficult to decide which quantiles should be fitted. If robustness is the major concern, using the 50th percentile is a sensible default. But there are many applications where for subject-matter or policy reasons, other percentiles can be desirable. As discussed earlier, for example, if one were estimating the number of homeless in a census tract (Berk et al. 2008), stakeholders might be very unhappy with underestimates because social services would not be made available where they were most needed. Fitting the 90th percentile could be a better choice. Or, stakeholders might on policy grounds be interested in the 10th percentile if in a classroom setting, there are special concerns about students who are performing poorly. It is the performance of kids who struggle that needs to be anticipated.

6.8 Summary and Conclusions

Boosting is a very rich approach to statistical learning. The underlying concepts are interesting and their use to date creative. Boosting has also stimulated very productive interactions among researchers in statistics, applied mathematics, and computer science. Perhaps most important, boosting has been shown to be very effective for many kinds of data analysis.

However, there are important limitations to keep in mind. First, boosting is designed to improve the performance of weak learners. Trying to boost learners that are already strong is not likely to be productive. Whether a set of learners is weak or strong is a judgement call that will vary over academic disciplines and policy areas. If the list of variables includes all the predictors known to be important, if these predictors are well measured, and if the functional forms with the response variables are largely understood, conventional regression will then perform well and provide output that is much easier to interpret.

Second, if the goal is to fit conditional probabilities, boosting can be a risky way to go. There is an inherent tension between reasonable estimates of conditional probabilities and classification accuracy. Classification with the greatest margins is likely to be coupled with estimated conditional probabilities that are pushed toward the bounds of 0 or 1.

Third, boosting is not alchemy. Boosting can improve the performance of many weak learners, but the improvements may fall far short of the performance needed. Boosting cannot overcome variables that are measured poorly or important predictors that have been overlooked. The moral is that (even) boosting cannot overcome seriously flawed measurement and badly executed data collection. The same applies to all of the statistical learning procedures discussed in this book.

---

[13]The size of the correlation is being substantially determined by actual fares over \$200. They are still being fit badly, but not a great deal worse.

Finally, when compared to other statistical learning procedures, especially random forests, boosting will include a much wider range of applications, and for the same kinds of applications, perform competitively. In addition, its clear links to common and well-understood statistical procedures can help make boosting understandable.

Exercises

Problem Set 1

Generate the following data. The systematic component of the response variable is quadratic.

```
x1=rnorm(1000)
x12=x1^2 ysys=1+(-5*x12)
y=ysys+(5*rnorm(1000))
dta=data.frame(y,x1,x12)
```

1. Plot the systematic part of y against the predictor $x1$. Smooth it using *scatter.smooth()*. The smooth can be a useful approximation of the $f(x)$ you are trying to recover. Plot y against $x1$. This represents the data to be analyzed. Why do they look different?

2. Apply *gbm()* to the data. There are a lot of tuning parameters and parameters that need to be set for later output so here is some bare-bones code to get you started. But feel free to experiment. For example,

```
out<-gbm(y~x1,distribution="gaussian",n.trees=10000,
    data=dta)
gbm.perf(out,method="OOB")
```

Construct the partial dependence plot using

```
plot(out,n.trees=???),
```

where the ??? is the number of trees, which is the same as the number of iterations. Make five plots, one each of the following number of iterations: 100, 500, 1000, 5000, 10000 and the number recommended by the out-of-bag method in the second step above. Study the sequence of plots and compare them to the plot of the true $f(X)$. What happens to the plots as the number of iterations approaches the recommended number and beyond? Why does this happen?

3. Repeat the analysis with the interaction.depth = 3 (or larger). What in the performance of the procedure has changed? What has not changed (or at least not changed much)? Explain what you think is going on. (Along with n.trees, interaction.depth can make an important difference in performance. Otherwise, the defaults usually seem adequate.)

Problem Set 2

From the *car* library load the data "Leinhardt." Analyze the data using gbm(). The response variable is infant mortality.

1. Plot the performance of gbm(). What is the recommended number of iterations?

2. Construct a graph of the importance of the predictors. Which variables seem to affect the fit substantially and which do not? Make sure your interpretations take the units of importance into account.

3. Construct the partial dependence plot for each predictor. Interpret each plot.

4. Construct all of the two-variable plots. Interpret each plot. Look for interaction effects. (There are examples in the gbm documentation that can be accessed with *help().*)

5. Construct the three-variable plot. (There are examples in the *gbm()* documentation that can be accessed with *help().*) Interpret the plot.

6. Consider the quality of the fit. How large is the improvement compared to when no predictors are used? You will need to compute measures of fit. There are none in *gbm.object.*

7. Write a paragraph or so on what the analysis of these data has revealed about correlates of infant mortality at a national level.

8. Repeat the analysis using random forests. How do the results compare to the results from stochastic gradient boosting? Would you have arrived at substantially different conclusions depending on whether you used random forests or stochastic gradient boosting?

9. Repeat the analysis using the quantile loss function. Try values for α of .25, .50, and .75, which represent different relative costs for underestimates compared to overestimates. How do the results differ in the number of iterations, variable importance, partial dependence plots, and fit? How do the results compare to your early analysis using stochastic gradient boosting?

Problem Set 3

The point of this problem set is to compare the performance of several different procedures when the outcome is binary and decide which work better and which work worse for the data being analyzed. You also need to think about why the performance can differ and what general lessons there may be.

From the *MASS* library, analyze the dataset called Pima.tr. The outcome is binary: diabetes or not (coded as "Yes" and "No" for the variable "type."). Assume that the costs of failing to identify someone who has diabetes are 3 times higher than the costs of falsely identifying someone who has diabetes. The predictors are all of the other variables in the dataset.

The statistical procedures to compare are logistic regression, the generalized additive model, random forests, and stochastic gradient boosting. For each, you will need to determine how to introduce asymmetric costs. (Hint: for some you will need to weight the data by outcome class.) You will also need to take into account the data format each procedure is expecting (e.g., can missing data be tolerated?). Also feel free to try several different versions of each procedure (e.g., "Adaboost" v. "bernoulli" for stochastic gradient boosting). The intent is to work across material from several earlier chapters.

1. Construct confusion tables for each model. Be alert to whether the fitted values are for "resubstituted" data or not. Do some procedures fit the data better than others? Why or why not?

2. Cross-tabulate the fitted values for each model against the fitted values for each other model. How do the sets of fitted values compare?

3. Compare the "importance" assigned to each predictor. This is tricky. The units and computational methods differ. For example, how can sensible comparisons be made between the output of a logistic regression and the output of random forests?

4. Compare partial response functions. This too is tricky. For example, what can you do with logistic regression?

5. If you had to make a choice to use one of these procedures, which would you select? Why?

Chapter 7
Support Vector Machines

Support vector machines (SVM) was developed as a type of classifiers, largely in computer science, with its own set of research questions, conceptual frameworks, technical language, and culture. A substantial amount of the initial interest in support vector machines stemmed from the important theoretical work surrounding it (Vapnick 1996). For many, that remains very attractive.

The early applications of SVM were not especially compelling. But, over the past decade, the applications to which support vector machines have been applied have broadened (Christianini and Shawe-Taylor 2000; Moguerza and Munõz 2006; Ma and Gao 2014), available software has responded (Joachims 1998; Chen et al. 2004; Hsu et al. 2010; Karatzoglou et al. 2015), and relationships between support vector machines and other forms of machine learning have become better understood (Bishop 2006: Chaps. 6 and 7; Hastie et al. 2009: 417–437). SVM has joined a mainstream of many machine/statistical learning procedures. It incorporates some unique features to be sure, but many familiar features as well. In practice, SVM can be seen as a worthy competitor to random forests and boosting.

This chapter will draw heavily on material covered in earlier chapters. In particular, regression kernels, discussed in Chap. 2, will make an important encore appearance. Much of the earlier material addressing why boosting works so well also will carry over, at least in broad brush strokes. Support vector machines can be understood in part as a special kind of margin maximizer and in part as a loss function optimizer with an unusual loss function.

Different expositions of support vector machines often use rather different notation. In particular, the notational practices of computer science and statistics will rarely correspond. For example, the excellent treatment of support vector machines by Bishop (2006: Chap. 7) and the equally excellent treatment of support vector machines by Hastie and his colleagues (2009: Chap. 12) are difficult to compare without first being able to map one notional scheme on to the other. In this chapter,

The original version of this chapter was revised: See the "Chapter Note" section at the end of this chapter for details. The erratum to this chapter is available at https://doi.org/10.1007/978-3-319-44048-4_10.

the notation of Hastie and colleagues will be used by and large because it corresponds better to the notation used in earlier chapters.

7.1 Support Vector Machines in Pictures

Support vector machines has more demanding mathematical underpinnings than boosting or random forests. In some ways, it is another form of penalized regression. But before we get to a technical discussion, let's take a look at several figures that will make the key ideas accessible.

7.1.1 The Support Vector Classifier

Suppose there is a binary response variable coded, as is often done in boosting, as 1 and -1. There is also a $f(x)$, where x is a vector of one or more predictors. The function can be written in a familiar linear manner as

$$f(x) = \beta_0 + x^T \beta. \tag{7.1}$$

Equation 7.1 is essentially a linear regression with a binary outcome of 1 or -1 and no restrictions in practice on what numeric values the function yields. The $f(x)$ might be .6 for one observation, -1.2 for another observations, 2.1 for another observation, and so on. More is needed for classification. If $f(x)$ is a positive number, the label 1 is assigned to an observation. If $f(x)$ is a negative number, the label -1 is assigned to an observation. One can then compare the 1s and -1s from the function to the 1s and -1s of the response variable. The problem to be tackled in the pages ahead is how to make the two sets of 1s and -1s correspond as much as possible, not just in the data on hand, but in new realizations of the data. The task is to produce accurate classifications, which has been a major theme of past chapters. But the way SVM goes about this is novel. We begin with the support vector classifier.[1]

Figure 7.1 shows a three-dimensional scatter plot much like those used in earlier chapters. As before, there are two predictors (X and Z) and a binary response Y, that can take on values of red or blue. Red might represent dropping out of school, and blue might represent graduating. (Blue could be coded as 1, and red could be coded as -1.) The two predictors might be reading grade level and the number of truancies per semester. In this figure, the blue circles and red circles are each located in quite different areas of the two-dimensional space defined by the predictors. In fact, there is lots of daylight between the two groups, and a linear decision boundary easily could be drawn to produce perfect homogeneity. In SVM language, a linear

---

[1]In the SVM literature, the response variable is often called the "target variable," and the intercept in Eq. 7.1 is often called the "bias." Each observation is sometimes called an "example."

Fig. 7.1 A support vector classifier with two predictors X and Z and two linearly separable classes shown as *Red* or *Blue*

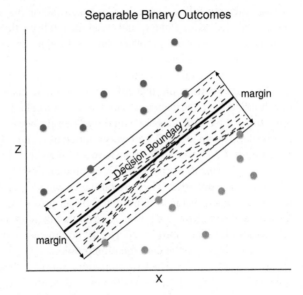

Separable Binary Outcomes

separating hyperplane could be drawn to produce separation between the two classes. More such SVM language will be introduced as we proceed.

In Fig. 7.1, there is a limitless number of linear decision boundaries producing separation. These are represented by the dashed lines in Fig. 7.1. Ideally, there is a way to find the best linear decision boundary.

Enter the support vector classifier. When there is separation, the support vector classifier solves the problem of which line to overlay by constructing two parallel lines on either side of, and the same distance from, the decision boundary. The two lines are placed as far apart as possible without including any observations within the space between them. One can think of the two lines as fences defining a buffer zone. In other words, the support vector classifier seeks two parallel fences that maximize their perpendicular distance from the decision boundary. There can be only one straight line parallel to the fences and midway between them. That decision boundary is shown with the solid black line.

Observations can fall right on either fence but not on their wrong sides. Here, there are no blue circles below the upper fence and no red circles above the lower fence. Observations that fall on top of the fences are called "support vectors" because they directly determine where the fences will be located and hence, the optimal decision boundary. In Fig. 7.1, there are two blue support vectors and three red support vectors.

In Fig. 7.1, the total width of the buffer zone is shown with the two double-headed arrows. The distance between the decision boundary and either fence is called the "margin," although some define the margin as the distance between the two fences (which amounts to the same thing). The wider the margin, the greater the separation between the two classes. Although formally the margin for a support vector classifier differs from the margins used by boosting and random forests, larger margins remain desirable because generalization error will usually be smaller.

Classification follows directly. Cases that fall on one side of the decision boundary are labeled as one class, and cases that fall on the other side of the decision boundary are labeled as the other class. Subsequently, any new cases for which the outcome class is not known will be assigned the class determined by the side of the decision boundary on which they fall. And that location will be a function of X and Z. The classification rule that follows from the decision boundary is called "hard thresholding," and the decision boundary is often called the "separating hyperplane." Sometimes the two fences are called the "margin boundary."

The data shown in Fig. 7.1 are very cooperative, and such cooperation is in practice rare. Figure 7.2 shows a plot that is much like Fig. 7.1, but the two sets of values are no longer linearly separable. Three blue circles and the two red circles violate their margin boundaries. They are on the wrong side of their respective buffer zone fences with each distance represented by an arrow. Moreover, there is no way to relocate and/or narrow the buffer zone so that there is a separating hyperplane able to partition the space into two perfectly homogeneous regions. There is no longer any linear solution to the classification problem.

One possible response is to permit violations of the buffer zone. One can specify some number of the observations that would be allowed to fall on the wrong side of their margin boundary. These are called "slack variables." One can try to live with a result that looks a lot like Fig. 7.2. The idea might be to maximize the width of the buffer zone conditional on the slack variables.

But that is not quite enough. Some slack variables fall just across their margin boundary, and some fall far away. In response, the distance between the relevant fence and the location of the slack variable can be taken into account. The sum of such distances can be viewed as a measure of how permissive one has been when

Fig. 7.2 A support vector classifier with predictors X and Z when there are two classes that are not linearly separable

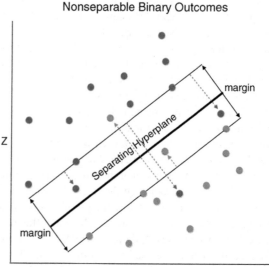

the margin is maximized. If one is more permissive by allowing for a larger sum, it may be possible to locate a separating hyperplane within a larger margin. Again, larger margins are good. More stable classifications can follow. But more permissive solutions imply more bias because misclassifications will be introduced. A form of the bias-variance tradeoff reappears. It follows that the sum of the distances can be a tuning parameter when a support vector classifier is applied to data. Fitting the support vector classifier with slack variables is sometimes called "soft thresholding."

7.1.2 Support Vector Machines

There is a complementary solution to classification problems when the classes are not linearly separable. One can allow for a nonlinear decision boundary in the existing predictor space by fitting a separating hyperplane in higher dimensions. We introduced this idea in Chap. 1 when linear basis expansions were discussed, and we elaborated on it in Chap. 2 when regression kernels were considered in some depth. Support vector classifiers become support vector machines when a kernel replaces a conventional set of predictors. However, the use of kernels is not straightforward. As already noted, there can be several kernel candidates with no formal guidance on which one to choose. In addition, kernels come with tuning parameters whose values usually have to be determined empirically. Finally, recall that kernel results are scale dependent (and normalizing papers over the problem) with categorical predictors a major complication.

In summary, support vector machines estimate the coefficients in Eq. 7.1 by finding a separating hyperplane producing the maximum margin, subject to a constraint on the sum of the slack variable distances. With those estimates in hand, fitted values are produced. Positive fitted values are assigned a class of 1, and negative fitted values are assigned a class of -1.

7.2 Support Vector Machines More Formally

With the main conceptual foundations of support vector machines addressed, we turn briefly to a somewhat more formal approach. To read the literature about support vector machines, some familiarity for the underlying mathematics and notation is essential. What follows draws heavily on Hastie and his colleagues (2009: 417–438) and on Bishop (2007: Chaps. 6 and 7).

7.2.1 The Support Vector Classifier Again: The Separable Case

There are N observations in the training data. Each observation has a value for each of p predictors and a value for the response. A response is coded 1 or -1. The separating hyperplane is defined by a conventional linear combination of predictors as

$$f(x) = \beta_0 + x^T \beta = 0. \tag{7.2}$$

Notice that the value of 0 is half way between -1 and 1. If you know the sign of $f(x)$, you know the class assigned. That is, classification is then undertaken by the following rule,

$$G(x) = \text{sign}(\beta_0 + x^T \beta). \tag{7.3}$$

A lot of information can be extracted from the two equations. One can determine for any i whether $y_i f(x_i) > 0$ and, therefore, whether it is correctly classified.[2] $\beta_0 + x^T \beta$ can be used to compute the signed distance of any fitted point in the predictor space from the separating hyperplane. Hence, one can determine whether a fitted point is on the wrong side of its fence and if so, how far.

Putting all this information together, we are ready to take on the margin maximization task. For the separable case, the trick is to find values β and β_0, to maximize the margin.

Let M be the distance from the separating hyperplane to the margin boundary. Then the goal is

$$\max_{\beta, \beta_0, \|\beta\|=1} M, \tag{7.4}$$

subject to

$$y_i(\beta_0 + x_i^T \beta) \geq M, \quad i = 1, \dots, N, \tag{7.5}$$

where for mathematical convenience the regression coefficients are standardized to have a unit length.[3] In words, our job is to find values for β and β_0 so that M is as large as possible for observations that are correctly classified. Notice that $2M$ is the margin.

The left-hand side of Eq. 7.5 in parentheses is the distance between the separating hyperplane and a fitted point. Because M is a distance centered on the separating hyperplane, Eq. 7.5 identifies correctly classified observations on or beyond their margin boundary. No cases are inside their fences. Thus, M is sometimes characterized as producing a "hard boundary" because it is statistically impermeable. That is basically the whole story for the support vector classifier when the outcomes are linearly separable.

---

[2]Because y is coded as 1 and -1, products that are positive represent correctly classified cases.

[3]Because there is no intention to interpret the regression coefficients, nothing important is lost.

It can be mathematically easier, if less intuitive, to work with an equivalent formulation:[4]

$$\min_{\beta,\beta_0} \|\beta\| \qquad (7.6)$$

subject to

$$y_i(\beta_0 + x_i^T \beta) \geq 1, \quad i = 1, \ldots, N. \qquad (7.7)$$

Because $M = 1/\|\beta\|$, Eq. 7.6 now seeks to *minimize the norm* of the coefficients through a proper choice of the coefficient values. (Hastie et al. 2009: Sect. 4.5.2). Equation 7.7 defines a linear constraint and requires that the points closest to the separating hyperplane are at a distance of 1.0, and that all other observations are farther away (i.e., distance > 1). Equations 7.6 and 7.7 do not change the underlying optimization problem and lead to a more direct, easily understood solution (Bishop 2007: 327–328).

7.2.2 The Nonseparable Case

We return for the moment to Eqs. 7.4 and 7.5, but for the nonseparable case, some encroachments of the buffer zone have to be tolerated. Suppose one defines a set of "slack" variables $\xi = (\xi_1, \xi_2, \ldots, \xi_N)$, $\xi_i \geq 0$, that measure how far observations are on the wrong side of their fence. We let $\xi_i = 0$ for observations that are on the proper side of their fence or right on top of it; they are correctly classified and not in the buffer zone. The farther an observation moves across its fence into or through the buffer zone, the larger is the value of the slack variable.

The slack variables lead to a revision of Eq. 7.5 so that

$$y_i(\beta_0 + x_i^T \beta) \geq M(1 - \xi_i) \qquad (7.8)$$

for all $\xi_i \geq 0$, and $\sum_{i=1}^{N} \xi_i \leq W$, with W as some constant quantifying how tolerant of misclassifications one is prepared to be.

The right-hand side of Eq. 7.8 equals M when an observation falls on top of its margin. For observations that fall on the wrong side of their margin, ξ_i is positive. As the value of ξ_i becomes larger, the margin-based threshold becomes smaller and more lenient as long as the sum of the ξ_i is less than W (Bishop 2007: 331–332). Equation 7.8, changes a hard thresholding as a function M into a soft thresholding as a function of $M(1 - \xi_i)$. The fence is no longer statistically impermeable.

There is again an equivalent and more mathematically convenient formulation, much like the one provided earlier as Eqs. 7.6 and 7.7 (Hastie et al. 2001: 373):

---

[4]The mathematics behind this is not deep, but there are several steps that require familiarity with vector algebra. Interested readers should be able to find excellent treatments on the web. See, for example, lectures on support vector machines by Patrick H. Winston of MIT or by Yaser Abu-Mostafa of Caltech.

$$\min_{\beta, \beta_0} \|\beta\| \tag{7.9}$$

subject to

$$y_i(\beta_0 + x_i^T \beta) \geq 1 - \xi_i, \quad i = 1, \ldots, N, \tag{7.10}$$

for all $\xi_i \geq 0$, and $\sum_{i=1}^{N} \xi_i \leq W$, with W as some constant. As before the goal is to minimize the norm of the coefficients but with special allowances for slack variables. For larger ξ_i's, the linear constraint is more lenient. Once again, there is soft thresholding. In expositions coming from computer science traditions, Eqs. 7.9 and 7.10 are considered "canonical."

Figure 7.3 is a small revision of Fig. 7.2 showing some important mathematical expressions. Observations for which $\xi_i > 1$ lie on the wrong side of the separating hyperplane and are misclassified. Observations for which $0 < \xi_i \leq 1$ lie in the buffer zone but on the correct side of the separating hyperplane. Observations for which $\xi_i = 0$ are correctly classified and on the margin boundary. The circles with borders are support vectors that will be discussed momentarily.

Equations 7.9 and 7.10 constitute a quadratic function with linear constraints whose quadratic programming solution can be found using Lagrange multipliers (Hastie et al. 2009: Sect. 12.2.1). Figure 7.4 shows a toy example in which there is single variable (i.e., x), a quadratic function of that variable in blue, and a linear constraint in red. The minimum when the constraint is imposed is larger than the minimum when the linear constraint is not imposed. The quadratic programming challenge presented by the support vector classifier is that the single x is replaced by the coefficients in Eq. 7.9, and the simple linear constraint is replaced by the N linear constraints in Eq. 7.10.

In the notation of Hastie et al. (2009: 421), the solution has

Fig. 7.3 A support vector classifier with some important mathematical expressions for predictors X and Z when there are two classes that are not separable (Support vectors are *circled*.)

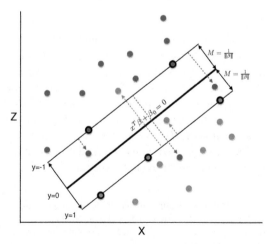

Nonseparable Binary Outcomes

Fig. 7.4 Finding the minimum of a quadratic function with a linear constraint

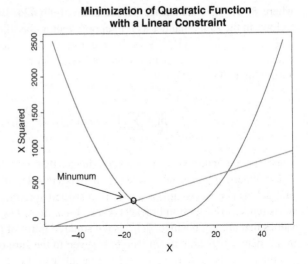

$$\hat{\beta} = \sum_{i=1}^{N} \hat{\alpha}_i y_i x_i, \qquad (7.11)$$

where $\hat{\alpha}_i$ represents a new coefficient for each i whose value needs to be estimated from the data. All of the N values for $\hat{\alpha}_i$ are equal to 0 except for the support vectors that locate the separating hyperplane. The value of $\hat{\beta}_0$ is estimated separately. With all of the coefficients in hand, classification is undertaken with Eq. 7.3: $\hat{G}(x) = \text{sign}(\hat{\beta}_0 + x^T \hat{\beta})$.

7.2.3 Support Vector Machines

We now turn from the support vector classifier to the support vector machine. The transition is relatively simple because support vector machines are essentially support vector classifiers that use kernels as predictors. Kernels were considered at some length in Chap. 2 and will not be reconsidered here. But as we proceed, it is important to recall that (1) the choice of kernel is largely a matter of craft lore and can make a big difference, (2) factors are formally not appropriate when kernels are constructed, and (3) there can be several important tuning parameters.

The Lagrangian is defined as before except that in place of the predictors contained in $\mathbf{X}$, support vector machines work with their linear basis expansions $\Phi(\mathbf{X})$ contained in $\mathbf{K}$. The result is

$$\hat{f}(x) = \hat{\beta}_0 + \sum_{i=1}^{N} \hat{\alpha}_i y_i K(x, x_i), \qquad (7.12)$$

where $K(x, x_i)$ is the kernel (Hastie et al. 2009: 424; Bishop 2007: 329). All else follows in the same manner as for support vector classifiers.

For $f(x) = h(x)^T \beta + \beta_0$, the optimization undertaken for support vector machines can be written in regularized regression-like form (Hastie et al. 2009: 426; Bishop 2007: 293):

$$\min_{\beta_0, \beta} \sum_{i=1}^{N} [1 - y_i f(x_i)]_+ + \frac{\lambda}{2} \|\beta\|^2, \tag{7.13}$$

where the $+$ next to the right bracket indicates that only the positive values are used. The product $y_i f(x_i)$ is negative when there is a misclassification. Therefore, the term in brackets is positive unless a case is classified correctly and is on the correct side of its fence.[5] The term in brackets is also linear in $y_i f(x_i)$ before becoming 0.0 for values that are not positive. $\|\beta\|^2$ is the squared norm of the regression coefficients, and λ determines how much weight is given to the sum of the slack variables. This is much like the way ridge regression penalizes a fit. A smaller value of λ makes the sum of slack variables less important and moves the optimization closer to the separable case. There will be a smaller margin, but the separating hyperplane can be more complex (Bishop 2007: 332).[6]

Equation 7.13 naturally raises questions about the loss function for support vector machines (Hastie et al. 2001: Sect. 12.3.2; Bishop 2007: 337–338). Figure 7.5 shows with a blue line the "hinge" SVM loss function. The broken magenta line is a binomial deviance loss of the sort used for logistic regression. The binomial deviance has been rescaled to facilitate a comparison.

Some refer to the support vector loss function as a "hockey stick." The thick vertical line in red represents the separating hyperplane. Values of $yf(x)$ to the left indicate observations that are misclassified. Values of $yf(x)$ to the right indicate observations that are properly classified. The product of y and $f(x)$ will be ≥ 1 if a correctly classified observation is on the proper side of its fence.

Consider the region defined by $yf(x) < 1$. Moving from left to right, both loss functions decline. At $yf(x) = 0$, the hinge loss is equal to 1.0, and an observation is a support vector. Moving toward $yf(x) = 1$, both loss functions continue to decline. The hinge loss is equal to 0 at $yf(x) = 1$. The binomial deviance is greater than 0. For $yf(x) > 1$, the hinge loss remains 0, but the binomial deviance continues to decline, with values greater than 0.

One can argue that the two loss functions are not dramatically different. Both can be seen as an approximation of misclassification error. The misclassification loss function would be a step function equal to 1.0 to the left $yf(x) = 0$ and equal to 0.0 at or to the right of $yf(x) = 0$. It is not clear in general when the hinge loss or the

---

[5] An example of a correct classification on the wrong side of its fence: $1 - (.9) = .1$. An example of a correct classification on the right side of its fence: $1 - (1.1) = -.1$. For a case that is a support vector: $1 - (1) = 0$.

[6] λ is equal to the reciprocal of the weight given to the sum of the slack variables in the usual Lagrange expression (Hastie et al. 2009: 420, 426).

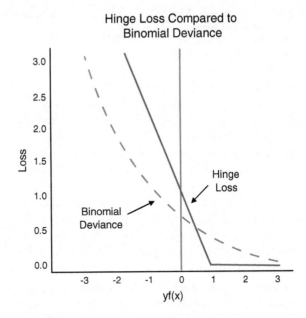

Fig. 7.5 Binomial and hinge loss as a function of the product of the true values and the fitted values

binomial deviance should be preferred although it would seem that the hinge loss would be somewhat less affected by outliers.

7.2.4 SVM for Regression

Support vector machines can be altered to apply to quantitative response variables. One common approach is to ignore in the fitting process residuals smaller in absolute value than some constant (called ϵ-insensitive regression). For the other residuals, a linear loss function is applied. Figure 7.6 provides an illustration.

The result is a robustified kind of regression. Any relative advantage in practice from support vector machine regression compared to any of several forms of robust regression is not clear, especially with what we have called kernelized regression in the mix. But readers interested in regression applications will find what they need in the *kernlab* or *e1071* libraries. For example, *kernlab* has a form of kernelized quantile regression.

7.2.5 Statistical Inference for Support Vector Machines

To this point, the discussion of support vector machines has been presented as a level I problem. But a level II analysis can be on the table. Equation 7.13 makes

Fig. 7.6 An example of an
ϵ-insensitive loss function
that ignores small residuals
and applies symmetric linear
loss to the rest

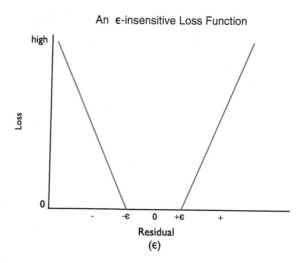

clear that support vector machines is a form of penalized regression. In particular, it is essentially kernelized ridge regression with a hinge loss function. Therefore, the discussion of statistical inference undertaken in Chap. 2 applies. A clear and credible account of an appropriate data generation process is essential. A proper estimation target must be articulated. And then, having legitimate test data can be very important, or at least an ability to construct sufficiently large split samples. As before, however, the results of support vector machines are sample size dependent because a kernel matrix is $N \times N$. This affects how the estimation target is defined. For example, kernels from split samples will necessarily be smaller than $N \times N$, which alters the estimation target. The estimation target is now a support vector machine for a kernel matrix based on fewer than N observations. In effect, the number of predictors in **K** is reduced.

7.3 A Classification Example

Support vector machines perform much like random forests and stochastic gradient boosting. However, there can be much more to tune. We undertake here a relatively simple analysis using the Mroz dataset from the *car* library in R. Getting fitted values with a more extensive set of inputs is not a problem. The problem is linking the inputs to outputs with graphical methods, as we will see soon.

The data come from a sample survey of 753 husband-wife households. The response variable is whether the wife is in the labor force. None of the categorical predictors can be used, which leaves household income exclusive of the wife's income, the age of the wife, and the log of the wife's expected wage. For now, two predictors are selected: age and the log of expected wage. About 60% of the wives are employed, so the response variable is reasonably well balanced, and there seems to be nothing else in the data to make an analysis of labor force participation problematic.

Figure 7.7 shows the code to be used. The recoding is undertaken to allow for more understandable variables and to code the response as a factor with values of

```
#### SVM With Mroz Employment Data ####
library(car)
data(Mroz)
attach(Mroz)

# Recodes
Participate<-as.factor(ifelse(lfp=="yes",1,-1)) # For clarity
Age<-age
LogWage<-lwg
Income<-inc
mroz<-data.frame(Participate,Age,LogWage,Income)

### Radial kernel with defaults: kpar="automatic",type="C-svc"
library(kernlab)
svm1<-ksvm(Participate~Age+LogWage,data=mroz,kernel="rbfdot",
           cross=5)
preds1<-predict(svm1,newdata=mroz) # Fitted values
summary(preds1) # Standard output
table(mroz$Participate,preds1) # Confusion table
prop.table(table(mroz$Participate,preds1),1) # Percentage
plot(svm1,data=mroz) # Plot separating hyperplane

### ANOVA kernel
#Define Weights
wts<-table(Participate) #Connects levels to Counts
wts[1]=.47 # Replace count for -1 class
wts[2]=.53 # Replace count for 1 class

library(kernlab)
svm2<-ksvm(Participate~Age+LogWage+Income,data=mroz,
           kernel="anovadot",kpar=list(sigma=1,degree=1),
           C=5,cross=3,type="C-svc",class.weights=wts)
svm2 # Standard output
preds2<-predict(svm2,newdata=mroz) # Fitted classes
table(mroz$Participate,preds2) # Confusion table
prop.table(table(mroz$Participate,preds2),1) # Percentage
plot(svm2,data=mroz,slice=list(Income=17)) # At median income
```

Fig. 7.7 R code for support vector machine analyses of labor force participation

1 and -1. The numerical values make the graphical output examined later easier to interpret.

The first analysis is undertaken with a radial kernel, which has a reputation of working well in a variety of settings. There are two tuning parameters. C is the penalty parameter determining the importance of the sum of the slack variables in the Lagrangian formulation. A larger value forces the fit toward the separable solution. We use the default value of 1. The other tuning parameter is σ, which sits in the denominator of the radial kernel. We let its value be determined by an empirical procedure that "estimates the range of values for the sigma parameter which would return good results when used with a Support Vector Machine (ksvm()). The estimation is based upon the 0.1 and 0.9 quantile of $\|x - x'\|^2$. Basically any value in between those two bounds will produce good results" (online documentation for ksvm() in the library kernlab). A single measure of spread is being provided for the entire set of predictors. The squared norm is larger when cases are more dissimilar over the full set of predictors. Finally, a cross-validation measure of classification error is included to get a more honest measure of performance.

Table 7.1 shows an in-sample confusion table. There are no out-of-bag observations or test data; the table is constructed in-sample. But C was set before the analysis began, and σ was determined with very little data snooping. The proportion misclassified in the training data was .28, and the fivefold cross-validation figure was .29.[7] Because the two proportions are very similar, overfitting apparently is not an important problem for this analysis.

Table 7.1 is interpreted like all of the earlier confusion tables, although the sign of the fitted values determines the class assigned. The empirical cost ratio is little less than two (i.e., 139/72). Incorrectly classifying a wife as in the labor force is about two times more costly than incorrectly classifying a wife as not in the labor force. That cost ratio would need to be adjusted should it be inconsistent with the preferences of stakeholders.

The results look quite good. Overall, the proportion misclassified is .28, although it should be cost weighted to be used properly as a performance measure. When a logistic regression was run on the same data with the same predictors, the proportion misclassified was .45. The large gap is an excellent example of the power of support vector machines compared to more conventional regression approaches. Model error

Table 7.1 SVM confusion table for forecasting labor force participation (radial kernel, default settings)

	Predict not labor force	Predict labor force	Model error
Not labor force	253	72	.22
Labor force	139	289	.32
Use error	.35	.20	Overall error = .28

[7] Both are included as part of the regular ksvm() output.

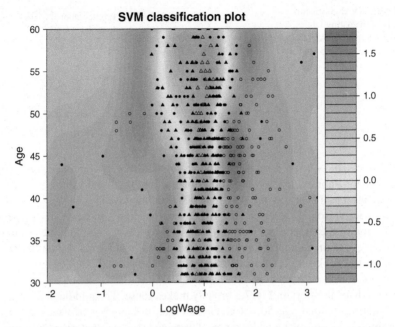

Fig. 7.8 Contour plot of SVM fitted values for labor force participation showing the separating hyperplane, observed values of the response, and support vectors (The *circles* are wives in the labor force. The *triangles* are wives not in the labor force. *Filled circles* or *triangles* are support vectors. A radial kernel with default settings was used.)

and use error also look good. For example, when a wife is predicted to be in the labor force, that classification is correct about 80 % of the time.

There are no variable importance plots or partial dependence plots available in *kernlab( )*.[8] However, one can plot the separating hyperplane for two predictors in the units of those predictors. Figure 7.8 is a contour plot showing the separating hyperplane for labor force participation in units of the fitted values. Positive fitted values in shades of blue mean that a wife was classified as in the labor force. Negative fitted values in shades of red mean that a wife was not classified as in the labor force. Age in years is on the vertical axis, and the log of expected wage is on the horizontal axis. Individuals in the labor force are shown with circles. Individuals not in the labor force are shown with triangles. Filled circles or triangles are support vectors.

The colors gradually shift from red to blue as the fitted values gradually shift from less than −1.0 to more than 1.5. The deeper the blue, the larger the positive fitted values. The deeper the red, the smaller the negative (i.e., more negative) fitted values. Deeper blues and deeper reds mean that an observation is farther from the separating hyperplane and more definitively classified. Consequently, the fitted values play a

---

[8]The other popular support vector machines library in R is *e1071*. It works well, but has fewer kernel options than *kernlab* and many fewer features for working with kernels. It also lacks variable importance plots and partial dependence plots.

Table 7.2 SVM confusion
table for forecasting labor
force participation (ANOVA
kernel, cost weighted, $\sigma = 1$,
degree $= 1$, C $= 5$)

	Predict not labor force	Predict labor force	Model error
Not labor force	225	100	.30
Labor force	113	315	.26
Use error	.33	.24	Overall error $= .29$

similar role to the vote proportions in random forests. Bigger is better because bigger
implies more stability. If one were doing forecasting, the fitted value for each case
could be used as a measure of the assigned class reliability.

The margin around the separating hyperplane is shown in white. Its shape and
the location of the support vectors may seem strange. But recall that the separating
hyperplane is estimated in a predictor space defined by a kernel. When the results
are projected back into a space defined by the predictors, complicated nonlinear
transformations have been applied.

But perhaps the story in Fig. 7.8 broadly makes sense. The middle pink area gets
wider starting around age 50. At about that age, the number of wives not in the
labor force increases over a wider range of expected wages. The larger blue areas on
either side indicate that either a low expected or a high expected wage is associated
with greater labor force participation. The former may be an indicator of economic
need. The latter may be an indicator of good job prospects. There is little evidence of
interaction effects because the pink area is effectively perpendicular to the horizontal
axis.

For illustrative purposes, the same data can be reanalyzed changing the kernel
and empirical cost ratio. An ANOVA kernel is used because in practice, it is often
recommended for regression applications. Also, just as in stochastic gradient boosting, one can apply case weights to alter the empirical cost ratio. Here, a weight of
.53 is applied to the 1s and a weight of .47 is applied to the -1s so that cases with
wives in the labor force are given more relative weight. Finally, a third predictor is
added to the mean function to illustrate later an interesting graphics option.

Table 7.2 shows the confusion table that results with the value for σ set to 1.0, the
value for degree set to 1, the value for C set to 5.0, and household income as a third
predictor. All three tuning values were determined after some trial and error using
performance in confusion tables to judge.

The empirical cost ratio is now about 1 to 1 (i.e., 113/100), and classification error
for being in the labor force has declined from .32 to .26. In trade, classification error
for not being in the labor force has increased from .22 to .30. The overall proportion
misclassified when *not weighted* by costs is effectively unchanged (i.e., .28) With so
many alterations compared to the previous analysis, it is difficult to isolate the impact
of each new feature of the analysis. However, it seems that including household
income does not make a large difference.

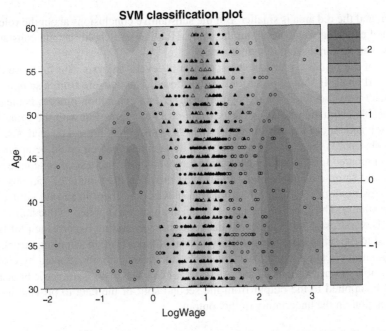

Fig. 7.9 Contour plot of SVM fitted values for labor force participation showing the separating hyperplane, observed values of the response, and support vectors (The circles are wives in the labor force. The triangles are wives not in the labor force. Filled circles or triangles are support vectors. An ANOVA kernel was used, cost weighted, with $\sigma = 1$, Degree $= 1$, $C = 5$, and household income values set to its median.)

Figure 7.9 shows the corresponding plot for the separating hyperplane. The layout is the same, but the content is different. Plots with two predictor dimensions means that the roles of only two predictors can be displayed. Here, there are three predictors. In response, the plotting function (*ksvm.plot()*) requires the predictors not displayed in the plot be set to some value. They are, in effect, held constant at that value. If any such predictors are not explicitly fixed at some value, the default has them fixed at 0.0. One can see from the last line of Fig. 7.7 that for all observations, the median of $17,000 is the assigned, fixed value.

This approach is less than ideal. It assumes that there are no interaction effects with the predictors whose values are fixed. An absence of interaction effects seems unlikely, so the issue is whether those interaction effects are large enough to matter. Perhaps the only practical way to get some sense is to examine a substantial number of plots like Fig. 7.9 with fixed values at other than the median. But even an exhaustive set of two-variable plots cannot be definitive unless there are only three predictors overall. That way, there are no interaction effects involving two or more of the fixed predictors.

The substantive message in Fig. 7.9 has not changed much. Because the 1s have been given more weight, more of them are forecast. As a result, the blue area is larger, and the red area is smaller. But the substantive conclusions about the roles of age and expected wage are about the same. Holding household income constant at its median does not seem to matter much.

All of the results so far have been a form of level I analysis. But for these data, a level II analysis should be seriously considered. The data are from a sample survey with a well-defined, finite population. The data generation process is clear. A reasonable estimation target is the population SVM regression with the same loss function and values for the tuning parameters as specified in the data analysis. The main obstacle is the lack of test data. A split sample approach could be applied if one is prepared to redefine the estimation target so that it has a smaller sample size.

A split sample reanalysis was undertaken in which the sample of 753 observations was randomly split into nearly equal halves (i.e., there is an odd number of observations). The code for the radial kernel analysis was applied to one half of the data. The confusion table code and the code for a separating hyperplane plot were applied to the other half. The results were very similar (within sampling error). An important implication is that in this instance, the results are not affected by cutting the number of observations in half. As in earlier chapters, a nonparametric bootstrap could be applied to the output from the second split of the data to provide useful information on the uncertainty of that output.

7.4 Summary and Conclusions

Support vector machines have some real strengths. SVM was developed initially for classification problems and performs well in a variety of real classification applications. As a form of robust regression, it may also prove to be useful when less weight needs to be given to more extreme residuals. And, the underlying fundamentals of support vector machines rest on well-considered and sensible principles.

Among academics, the adjective "interesting" is to damn with faint praise. But the recent applications discussed in Ma and Guo (2014) are genuinely interesting. They illustrate the rich set of data analysis problems to which support vector machines are being applied. They also document that a large number of talented researchers are working with and extending support vector machines. Its future looks bright.

In general, however, the comparative advantage of support vector machines compared to random forests and stochastic gradient boosting is not apparent. To begin, there is no evidence that it typically leads to smaller generalization error. Problems working with indicator predictor variables will often be a serious constraint. And choosing an appropriate kernel coupled with the required tuning can be a challenge. Finally, SVM may be overmatched by "big data."

Where support vector machines seem to shine is when the number of predictors and number of observations are modest. Then, kernels can have genuine assets that other machine learning procedures may not be able to match. The analysis immediately above is perhaps an example.

Exercises

Problem Set 1

Support vector machines begin with kernels. Review the section on kernels in Chap. 2 looking especially at the material on radial kernels. Load the R dataset *trees* and have a look at the three variables in the file. The code below will allow you to explore how the matrix derived from the radial kernel changes depending on the values assigned to σ. Try values of .01, .05, .1, and 1. Consider how the standard deviation changes, excluding matrix elements equal to 1.0. Also have a look at the three-dimensional histograms depending on the value of σ. Describe what you see. How do the changes you see affect the complexity of the function that can be estimated?

```
library(kernlab) # you may need to install this
library(plot3D) # you may need to install this
X<-as.matrix(trees)
rfb<-rbfdot(sigma=.01) # radial kernel
K<-kernelMatrix(rfb,X)
sd(K[K<1]) # standard deviation with 1's excluded.
hist3D(z=K,ltheta=45,lphi=50,alpha=0.5,opaque.top=T,scale=F)
```

Problem Set 2

Construct a dataset as follows.

```
w<-rnorm(500)
z<-rnorm(500)
w2<-w^2 x<-(-1+3*w2-1*z)
p<-exp(x)/(1 + exp(x))
y<-as.factor(rbinom(500,1,p))
```

1. Regress y on w and z using logistic regression and construct a confusion table with the resubstituted data. You know that the model has been misspecified. Examine the regression output and the confusion table. Now regress y on $w2$ and z using logistic regression and construct a confusion table with the resubstituted data. You know that the model is correct. Compare the two sets of regression coefficients, their hypothesis tests, and two confusion tables. How does the output from the two models differ? Why?
2. Can you do as well with SVM using w and z as when logistic regression is applied to the correct model? With w and z as predictors (not $w2$), use an ANOVA kernel in *ksvm()* from the library *kernlab*. You will need to tune the ANOVA kernel using some trial and error. (Have a look at the material on the ANOVA kernel in Chap. 2.) Start with $sigma = .01$ and $degree = 1$. Increase both in several steps until $sigma = 10$ and $degree = 3$. Chose the values that give you the fewest classification errors. How does this confusion table from the well-tuned SVM

compare to the confusion tables from the correct logistic regression? What is the general lesson?

3. Construct and interpret the SVM classification plot for the best SVM confusion table.

4. Repeat the SVM analysis, but with class weights. To construct the nominal weights with a ratio of, say 3 to 1, use

```
wts<-c(3,1) # specify weights
names(wts)<-c("0","1") #assign weights to classes
```

Insert these two lines of code before the call to *ksvm()* and then include the argument *class.weights=wts* in *ksvm()*. Try several different pairs of nominal weights until you get a cost ratio in the confusion table such that the 1s are three times as costly as the 0s. How do the results differ?

Problem Set 3

1. From the *MASS* library, load the Pima.tr dataset. The variable "type" is the response. All other variables are predictors. Apply *ksvm()* from the *kernlab* library and again use the ANOVA kernel and weights to address asymmetric costs. The doctor wants to be able to start treatment before the test results are in and thinks it is twice as costly to withhold treatment from a patient who needs it compared to giving treatment to a patient who does not need it. Apply SVM to the data so that the confusion table has a good approximation of the desired cost ratio and about as good performance as can be produced with these data. This will take some tuning of the ANOVA kernel and the tuning parameter C, which determines the weight given to the penalty in the penalized fit. (In Problem Set 2, C was fixed at the default value of 1.0.) A good strategy is to first set $C = 1$ and tune the ANOVA kernel. Then, see if you can do better altering the value of C.

2. Choose two predictors in which you think the doctor might be particularly interested and construct an SVM classification plot. Fix all other predictors at their means. Interpret the plot. Do you think there is any useful information in the plot to aid the physician. Why?

Chapter 8
Some Other Procedures Briefly

There are statistical learning procedures not discussed earlier that can be framed as regression analysis and deserve at least conceptual overviews. Perhaps the most widely known is neural networks. Although neural networks was the poster child for early work in machine learning, it is now an important niche player, primarily within some forms of "deep learning." Neural networks will be discussed briefly to give a general sense of its structure, associated concepts, and performance in practice.

A second procedure, squarely in statistical learning traditions, is Bayesian additive regression trees (BART). It has some of the look and feel of random forests, but tuning is done by placing prior distributions on decision tree parameters. Perhaps its primary strength is that uncertainty is explicitly and defensibly addressed within Bayesian perspectives. But so far at least, it too is a niche player. Nevertheless, there is a lot of interest in BART. It is certainly worth a brief overview.

A third approach is reinforcement learning, which some view as the conceptual paradigm for artificial intelligence. We will use genetic algorithms as an illustration. Reinforcement learning shares many features with boosting, but it is less a stand-alone procedure and more a key component in some forms of deep learning or in guidance and control systems used in robotics. Reinforcement learning is briefly discussed because it is considered by many to be a form of machine learning.

8.1 Neural Networks

Neural networks, neural nets for short, was an early attempt within computer science to develop software that approximated the way collections of neurons function. We now know that the neural network algorithms are a vastly oversimplified rendering of

The original version of this chapter was revised: See the "Chapter Note" section at the end of this chapter for details. The erratum to this chapter is available at https://doi.org/10.1007/978-3-319-44048-4_10.

© Springer International Publishing Switzerland 2016   311
R.A. Berk, *Statistical Learning from a Regression Perspective*,
Springer Texts in Statistics, DOI 10.1007/978-3-319-44048-4_8

Fig. 8.1 A neural net with one response, one hidden layer, and no feedback

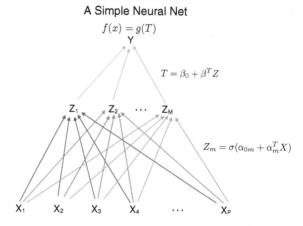

A Simple Neural Net

$$f(x) = g(T)$$

$$T = \beta_0 + \beta^T Z$$

$$Z_m = \sigma(\alpha_{0m} + \alpha_m^T X)$$

neural activity, but viewed as another machine learning procedure, they can perform well.[1] From a statistical learning perspective, neural nets are a way to combine inputs in a nonlinear manner to arrive at outputs. Put another way, a complicated $f(X)$ is approximated by a composition of many, far more simple functions. By now, this should have a familiar ring.

For notational consistency, we build on Hastie et al. (2009: Sect. 11.3). Figure 8.1 is a schematic of a very simple neural network. The inputs are represented by $x_1, x_2, \ldots, x_p$. These are just the usual set of predictors. There is a single output, Y, although more complicated networks can have several different outputs. Y can be numerical or categorical and is just the usual response variable. There is also a single "hidden layer" $z_1, z_2, \ldots, z_M$ that can be seen as a set of M unobserved, latent variables. All three components (i.e., inputs, output, and latent variables) are linked by associations that would be causal if one were trying to represent the actions of a collection of neurons (with no feedback).

It all starts with the inputs that are combined in a linear fashion for each latent variable. That is, each latent variable is a function of its own linear combination of the predictors. For the mth latent variable, one has

$$Z_m = \sigma(\alpha_{0m} + \alpha_m^T X), \tag{8.1}$$

where αs are coefficients (also called "weights") that vary over the M latent variables, X is the set of p inputs, and σ is commonly a sigmoid "activation function." A key idea behind the S-shape is that a linear combination of inputs will be more likely to trigger an impulse as that linear combination of the inputs increases in value, but

---

[1]An excellent introductory lecture on neural nets by Patrick Winston of MIT can be found at http://teachingexcellence.mit.edu/inspiring-teachers/patrick-winston-6-034-lecture-12-learning-neural-nets-back-propagation. If one is willing to learn a somewhat different notational scheme, Christopher Bishop's treatment is superb (2006: Chap. 5).

variation in the linear combination towards the middle of its range alters Z_m the most.[2]

In the next step, a linear combination of the latent variable values is constructed as

$$T = \beta_0 + \beta^T Z, \tag{8.2}$$

where now the βs are the coefficients (also called "weights") and Z is the set of latent variables. One has a linear combination of the M latent variables. Finally, the linear combination can be subject to a transformation

$$f(x) = g(T), \tag{8.3}$$

where g is the transformation function. When Y is numerical, the transformation simply may be an identity. When Y is categorical, the transformation may be logistic, much as in logistic regression.

There is no explicit representation of any disturbances, either for Z or Y, which is consistent with early machine learning traditions. The need to fit data with a neural net implies the existence of residuals, but they are not imbued with any formal statistical properties. It is not apparent, therefore, how to get from a level I analysis to a level II analysis. There is also no generative model, let alone a causal model. Despite its name, a neural network is algorithmic (Breiman 2001b).

If one substituted the M versions of Eq. 8.1 into 8.2, each version of Eq. 8.1 would be multiplied by its corresponding value of β. Consequently, the impact of the inputs would be re-weighted as a product of its β_m; a nonlinear, multiplicative transformation has been applied to the inputs. When those results are inserted into Eq. 8.3, there is the option of applying another nonlinear transformation. In short, one has built a set of sequential, nonlinear transformations of the inputs to arrive at the output; a series of simple nonlinear transformations are used to approximate a complicated $f(X)$. In the process, there is a new blackbox algorithm from which the associations between inputs and outputs are no longer apparent. Neural nets succeeds or fails by how well its fitted values for Y correspond to the actual values of Y.

Estimating the values of both sets of weights would be relatively straightforward if Z were observable. One would have something much like a conventional structural equation model in econometrics. But with Z unobservable, estimation is undertaken in a more complicated fashion that capitalizes on the sequential structure of the neural net: from X to Z to Y.

As usual, a loss function associated with the response must be specified. For example, if the response is quantitative, quadratic loss would be a likely choice. Then, because of the sequential nature of Eqs. 8.1–8.3, the inputs are used to construct the values of the latent variables that in turn are combined to arrive at $\hat{Y}$. But one still needs values for both sets of the weights. Consistent with many statistical leaning

---

[2]The color coding of the arrows in Fig. 8.1 is meant to indicate that each hidden layer has its own set of weights. These weights will typically differ from one another; the set of α_m will typically differ. Their common color is not meant to convey that the weights are the same.

algorithms discussed in earlier chapters, these first need to be initialized. Values randomly chosen close to 0.0 are often a good choice because one starts out with something very close to a linear model; products of the weights do not matter much.

Given the known values of X and an initialized weight for each α, fitted values for each Z_m follow directly. The set of initialized weights for the βs then determine the fitted values for Y. From these, the loss is computed.

One hopes that by revising the weights, it is possible to reduce the loss overall. Recall from the earlier discussion of stochastic gradient boosting, that a gradient is a partial derivative. Consider first the βs. The gradient expression for each β is the partial derivative of the loss with respect to that β. Things are little more complicated for the αs because their impact on the loss is altered by the βs. But by the chain rule in calculus, one can arrive at the gradient expression for each α, which is the partial derivative of the loss with respect to that α (Hastie et al. 2009: Sect. 11.4).

The expressions for the gradients are evaluated using the fitting disparities employed as arguments in the loss function. One proceeds by working backwards from the disparities to arrive the gradients' numerical values for the βs and then, the αs. This process is called backpropagation. With these values in hand, one can apply gradient descent to update the weights. At that point, the fitting and backpropagations begin again and repeat until the loss cannot be further reduced.

The backpropagation approach comes with several complications. First, start values can really matter because the loss functions are not convex. One can get stuck in a local minimum. A common approach is to repeat the estimation several times with different sets of start values and then choose the result with the smallest value of the loss. Also, there is some reason to think that for very high dimensional data, the local minimums will not be all that different from the global minimum. Second, with so many weights, overfitting can be a serious problem. Some form of regularization can help. Penalizing the fit in the spirit of ridge regression is one option. Test data can also be very important. Third, the different units in which the inputs are measured can make a big difference. Standardizing the inputs is usually helpful. Fourth, in Fig. 8.1, each input is connected to each latent variable, and each latent variable is connected to the response. The network is saturated. No inputs are directly linked to the response, although that can be an option. In short, there can be a large number of different network structures, which implies that inductively some weights can be set to 0.0. A form of model selection has been introduced. Finally, the number of latent variables and hidden layers are tuning parameters typically arrived at through some combination of subject-matter knowledge and performance in cross-validation. In effect, they are tuning parameters. Sometimes as many as 100 latent variables will be required.

There have been some recent enhancements in neural networks that are beyond the scope of this discussion, but two examples are worth brief mention. First, with so many parameters, a form of regularization can be introduced by imposing a prior distributions on each. The result is "Bayesian neural nets" that for estimation relies on extensive preprocessing of the data and very sophisticated Markov Chain Monte Carlo (MCMC) methods (Neal and Zhang 2006). In practice, Bayesian neural nets seems to perform very well and can be competitive with the other statistical learning procedures discussed earlier.

Second, one of the problems with traditional neural networks is that by today's standards, its fitting procedure is insufficiently adaptive and flexible. Deep learning can be seen as an effort to overcome these liabilities. It is common in deep learning to employ a very large number of latent variables and latent variable ("hidden") layers that are used to fit highly complex and highly nonlinear relationships (Deng and Yu 2014). This has led to considerable success in pattern recognition with very high dimensional image or speech datasets. One example is identifying small tumors on x-rays of lung tissue. In addition, one can introduce feedback loops and ensembles of neural networks, both of which can make deep learning deeper (Schmidthuber 2014).

It is also possible to deploy a neural network in a manner that reduces computational burdens apparently with no appreciable decline in accuracy. For example, one can fit the network by moving through hidden layers in a stagewise fashion. That is, the weights for the latent variables within one hidden layer are determined over many iterations before moving on to the weights for latent variables within the next hidden layer. Another strategy is to partition the x-values into subsets that can be learned separately before being combined. For example, different parts of an image can be learned separately. An important variant of this idea is to capitalize on spatial autocorrelation in an image and treat contiguous pixels that are much alike as a single observational unit by applying a transformation called "convolution". For example, 36 pixels can be treated as a single spatial neighborhood. The set of such spatial neighborhoods can comprise an image of reduced dimensionality that is further processed. In the end, one has a "convolution neural network" (Bishop 2006: Sect. 5.5.6). Much more is going on than can be considered here, and there are excellent treatments on the web (e.g., https://ujjwalkarn.me/2016/08/11/intuitive-explanation-convnets/).

Deep learning seems to dominate when extremely precise fits are required, and very small improvements can make a large practical difference. For example, a reduction in a loss function of 1 % can be a big deal. There are, however, at least three significant obstacles to widespread use. First, the computational burdens are enormous and growing. Despite innovations in hardware and software, the appetite for more computing power will not soon (or ever) be satisfied. Second, time consuming and complicated tuning is required. There is virtually no formal guidance, and the available craft lore is too rarely definitive. It can take weeks to tune a single application. Finally, there are now many flavors of deep learning with the number expanding rapidly. New claims of superior performance are routinely made even when the improvements seem to be data dependent. It will take a while for the field of deep learning to become better consolidated.

Formally, deep learning seems to be solely a level I enterprise. The data are treated as a very large finite population. There is no scaffolding on which to build inferences beyond the data. But in practice, inferences are often drawn to realizations that have not yet materialized. One might argue that with so many observations, there is no sampling error to worry about. This view only addresses the variance in fitted values.

Should the new realizations come from a different joint probability distribution, there can be substantial bias. One can get very reliable estimates of values that are systematically wrong. In response, some might claim that because very large neural networks can fit complicated functions, bias must be very small. Yet, this overlooks that complex neural networks can only fit the data they have. If the new realizations come from a different joint probability distribution, it is possible that fitting the data on hand better can make generalization error worse. In short, deep learning has the same inferential problems that all machine learning procedures share.

Deep learning procedures in R currently are a bit behind the curve, but they are catching up rapidly. For example, the library *h20()* (Candel et al. 2016) is a platform for a wide variety of machine learning procedures including random forests, gradient boosting, and "deep" neural nets as well as several unsupervised machine learning procedures such as principal components. There are claims that *h20()* can handle billions of observations in memory. An essential requirement for such impressive overall performance is that the data analyst has access to multiple cores, usually in a computer cluster. Other promising implementations of deep learning in R include the packages *mxnet, darch, deeplearning,* and *deepnet.*

8.2 Bayesian Additive Regression Trees (BART)

Bayesian additive regression trees (Chipman et al. 2010) is a procedure that capitalizes on an ensemble of classification or regression trees in the spirit of random forests and stochastic gradient boosting. Random forests generates an ensemble of random trees by treating the tree parameters as fixed while sampling the training data and predictors. Stochastic gradient boosting also capitalizes on sampling. Both operate with frequentist statistical traditions. Parameters such as the terminal node proportions are treated as fixed, and the data are treated as a collection of random realizations from a joint probability distribution of random variables. Bayesian additive regression trees turn this upside-down. Just as in Bayesian traditions more generally, the data are treated as fixed, and parameters characterizing the ensemble of trees are treated as random.

Each tree in the BART ensemble is realized at random in a manner that is determined by three kinds of hyperparameters:

1. Two hyperparameters for determining the probability that a node will to be split;
2. A hyperparameter determining the probability that any given predictor will be selected for the split; and
3. A hyperparameter determining the probability that a particular split value for the selected predictor will be used.

From the first two hyperparameters, the probability of a split is determined by

$$p(\text{split}) = \alpha(1 + d)^{-\beta},\tag{8.4}$$

where d is the tree "depth", defined as the number of stages beyond the root node; 0 for the root node (i.e., $d = 0$), 1 for the first split (i.e., $d = 1$), 2 for two splits beyond the root node (i.e., $d = 2$), and so on. The values of α and β affect how large a given tree will be. For a given value of β, smaller values for α make a split less likely. For a given value of α, smaller values of β make the penalty for tree depth more binding so that a split for a given value of d is less likely. The probability of a split also declines as the value of d increases. Possible values of α range from 0 to 1 with .95 a common choice. Possible values for β are nonnegative, but small values such 2 often work well and can be treated as sensible defaults (Kapelner and Bleich 2014).

If there is to be a split, a predictor is chosen at random by the value of the second hyperparameter. For example, if there are p predictors, each predictor can have a probability of $1/p$ of being selected. In a similar manner for the third hyperparameter, the split value for the selected predictor can be chosen with equal probability. It is possible to alter either random selection strategy if the situation warrants it. For example, if on subject-matter grounds some predictors are thought to be more important than others, they may be chosen with a higher probability than the rest. The relevant hyperparameter value would be altered accordingly.

The hyperparameters define very large Bayesian forests composed of potential trees that can be realized at random. Each tree is grown as usual with indicator variables for linear basis expansions of the predictors. Over trees, one has a very rich menu of possible expansions, a subset of which is realized for any given data analysis. In other words, the role of the hyperparameters is to produce a rich dictionary of linear basis expansions.

Figure 8.2 is meant to provide a sense of how this works in practice. Imagine a ball rolling down an inclined plane. In Fig. 8.2, the ball is shown in red at the top. The ball hits the first nail, and its path is displaced to the left or to the right in a manner that cannot be predicted in advance. The first nail is analogous to the first

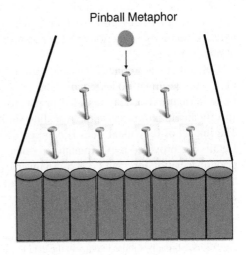

Fig. 8.2 Cartoon illustration of a pinball process (The ball is at the top, the nails are the splits, and the cups at the bottom are the terminal nodes.)

Pinball Metaphor

random split. Each subsequent nail is a subsequent potential split that can shift the path of the ball to the left or to the right in the same unpredictable fashion. After the third set of nails, the ball drops into the closest canister. The canisters at the bottom represent terminal nodes.

Imagine now that 25 balls are sequentially rolled down the plane. The 25 balls represent the cases constituting a dataset. Some of the balls are red and some are blue. The balls will follow a variety of paths to the canisters, and the proportions of red and blue balls in each canister will likely vary. The exercise can be repeated over and over with the same 25 balls. With each replication, the proportion of red balls and blue balls in each canister will likely change.

In Fig. 8.2, there are two sets of nails after the first nail at the top. To be more consistent with BART, the number of nail rows can vary with each replication. In addition, the rows can vary in the number nails and where they are placed. For example, the two left most nails in the bottom row of Fig. 8.2 might not be included. The result is a large number of inclined planes, with varying numbers of nail rows, nail placements and proportions of red and blue balls in each canister. One has a fixed collection of red and blue balls that does not change from replication to replication, but what happens to it does.[3]

Unlike random forests, the realized trees are not designed to be independent, and the trees are used in a linear model (Chipman et al. 2010):

$$Y = \sum_{j=1}^{m} g(x; T_j, M_j) + \varepsilon, \tag{8.5}$$

and as usual,

$$\varepsilon \sim N(0, \sigma^2). \tag{8.6}$$

Y is numerical, and there are m trees. Each tree is defined by the predictors x, T_j, which represents the splits made at each interior node, and M_j, which represents the set of means over terminal nodes. The trees are combined in a manner something like conventional backfitting such that each tree's set of conditional means is related to the response by a function that has been adjusted for the sets of conditional means of all other trees.

But, we are not done. First, we need a prior for the distribution of the means of Y over terminal nodes conditional on a given tree. That distribution is taken to be normal. Also, Y is rescaled in part to make the prior's parameters easier to specify and in part because the rescaling shrinks the conditional means toward 0.0. The impact of individual trees is damped down, which slows the learning process. Details are provided by Chipman and colleagues (2010: 271). Second, we need a prior distribution for σ^2 in Eq. 8.6. An inverse χ^2 distribution is imposed that has two hyperparameters. Here too, details are provided by Chipman and colleagues (2010: 272).

---

[3]Wu, Tjelmeland and West (2007) define a "pinball prior" for tree generation. The pinball prior and Fig. 8.2 have broadly similar intent, but the details are vastly different.

The algorithms used for estimation involve a complicated combination of Gibbs sampling and Markov Chain Monte Carlo methods that can vary somewhat depending on the software (Kapelner and Bleich 2014). In R, there is *bartMachine* written by Adam Kapelner and Justin Bleich, and *BayesTree* written by Hugh Chipman and Robert McCulloch. Currently, *bartMachine* is the faster in part because it is parallelized, and it also has a richer set of options and outputs. For example, there is a very clever way to handle missing data.

A discussion of the estimation machinery is beyond the scope of this short overview and requires considerable background in Bayesian estimation. Fortunately, both procedures can be run effectively without that background and are actually quite easy to use. In the end, one obtains the posterior distributions for the conditional means from which one can construct fitted values. These represent the primary output of interest. One also gets "credibility intervals" for the fitted values.

BART is readily applied when the response is binary. Formally,

$$p(Y = 1|x) = \Phi[G(x)], \tag{8.7}$$

where

$$G(x) \equiv \sum_{j=1}^{m} g(x; T_j, M_j), \tag{8.8}$$

and $\Phi[G(x)]$ is the probit link function used in probit regression. When used as a classifier, the classes are assigned in much the same way they are for probit regression. A threshold is applied to the fitted values (Chipman et al. 2010: 278). Otherwise, very little changes compared to BART applications with a numerical response.

It is difficult to compare the performance of BART to the performance of random forests, stochastic gradient boosting, and support vector machines. The first three procedures have frequentist roots and make generalization error and expected prediction error the performance gold standard. Because within a Bayesian perspective the data are fixed, it is not clear what sense out-of-sample performance makes. If the data are fixed, where do test data come from? If the test data are seen as random realizations of some data generation process, uncertainty in the data should be taken into account, and one is back to a frequentist point of view. Nevertheless, if one slides over these and other conceptual difficulties, BART seems to perform about as well as random forests, stochastic gradient boosting, and support vector machines. Broadly conceived, this makes sense. BART is "just" another way to construct a rich menu of linear basis expansions to be combined in a linear fashion.

BART's main advantage is that statistical inference is an inherent feature of the output; a level II analysis falls out automatically. But one has to believe the model. Are there omitted variables, for example? Does one really want to commit to a linear combination of trees with an additive error term? One also has to make peace with the priors. Most important, one has to be comfortable with Bayesian inference. But, even for skeptics, Bayesian inference might be considered a reasonable option given all of the problems discussed earlier when frequentist inference is applied to statistical learning procedures. It is also possible to use BART legitimately as a level I tool. The hyperparameters and priors distributions can be seen as tuning parameters and given no Bayesian interpretations. BART becomes solely a data fitting exercise.

BART has some limitations in practice. At the moment, only binary categorical response variables can be used. There is also no way to build in asymmetric costs of classification or fitting errors. And if one wants to explore the consequences of changing the hyperparameters (e.g., α and β), it not clear that conventional resampling procedures such as cross-validation make sense with fixed data.

In summary, BART is a legitimate competitor to the random forests, stochastic gradient boosting, and support vector machines. If one wants to do a level II analysis within a Bayesian perspective, BART is the only choice. Otherwise, it is difficult to see why one would pick BART over the alternatives. On the other hand, BART is rich in interesting ideas and for the more academically inclined, can be great fun.

8.3   Reinforcement Learning and Genetic Algorithms

Recall how boosting algorithms work. Observations that are fit less well in one pass through the data are given more weight in the next pass through the data. The algorithm learns with each pass how to better target problematic observations and is rewarded with an improved set of fitted values. One can say that the reweighting strategy is reinforced with each iteration, and the algorithm alters how it proceeds in a manner that responds to its performance. A fitting task can be more challenging when the training data are sampled because the data to be fit change with each iteration. But the same reinforcement process applies. In the end, the sets of fitted values are linearly combined.

Reinforcement learning can be seen as variants on, and extensions of, the foundations of boosting. Sutton and Barto (2016) provide an excellent introduction. For reinforcement learning, there are rules by which algorithms operate and an environment in which the algorithm is applied. The algorithm receives feedback on its performance in that environment and alters its actions in response. The environment may or may not change as well. Then, the process is repeated. The entire process is repeated many times until some satisfactory outcome is achieved. And like boosting, it never looks back; there are no do-overs.

Reinforcement learning is sometimes included within the tent of machine learning. Of late, it has gotten lots of attention as a component of deep learning. To provide a grounded sense of reinforcement learning, we briefly consider genetic algorithms (Mitchell 1998: 95–96).

8.3.1   Genetic Algorithms

Sometimes computer code written to simulate some natural phenomenon turns out to be a potential data analysis tool. Neural networks seems to have morphed in this fashion. Genetic algorithms appear to be experiencing a similar transformation. Whereas neural networks were initially grounded in how neurons interact, genetic algorithms share the common framework of natural selection. When used to study evolution, they are not tasked with data analysis, either as a data summary tool or as a data generation model. Applied to optimization problems, they can proceed in the same spirit as gradient descent or Newton-Raphson when as a practical matter, the loss function cannot be optimized. This came up earlier in a different context when for CART, a greedy algorithm was employed because evaluating all possible trees was untenable.

Here's the basic idea. There is an optimization problem and an initial population of candidate solutions, each evaluated for their fitness. Based on that fitness, an initial culling of the population follows. The survivors "reproduce," but in the process, the algorithm introduces "genetic" mutations, crossovers and sometimes other alterations to some of the progeny. Crossovers, for example, produce offspring whose makeup is a combination of the features of two members of the population. Fitness is again evaluated, and the population is culled a second time. The process continues until population fitness attains a target level of fitness (Affenseller 2009: Sect. 1.2). Thus, genetic algorithms are not "algorithmic" in Breiman's sense. They do not link inputs to outputs but can be a key components of how the linking gets done.

To illustrate how this can work, we revisit neural nets and the problem of which links should be included between inputs, latent variables and outputs. In a somewhat artificial fashion, we lift out one part of the fitting challenge: what should be the structure of the neural network? The discussion that follows draws heavily from Mitchell's introductory application of genetic algorithms to neural network architecture (1998: 70–71).

Fig. 8.3 A matrix representation of simple neural network (A 1 denotes a link, and a 0 denotes no link. The red entries can be varied between 1 and 0. The black entries are fixed. Two solution candidates are shown below the matrix.)

A Neural Network in Matrix Format

	X1	X2	X3	X4	X5	X6	Z1	Z2	Z3	Y
X1	—									
X2	0	—								
X3	0	0	—							
X4	0	0	0	—						
X5	0	0	0		—					
X6	0	0	0	0		—				
Z1	1	1	1	1	0	0	—			
Z2	1	0	0	1	0	0	0	—		
Z3	0	0	1	1	1	0	0	0	—	
Y	0	0	0	0	0	1	1	1	1	—

Network #1: 111100100100000111000000001111

Network #2: 110101100100000101100000100111

Figure 8.3 is a matrix representation of a simple neural network with 6 inputs $(X1 \ldots X6)$, 3 latent variables $(Z1 \ldots Z3)$, and 1 numerical response (Y). There is no feedback. The 1s denote links, and the 0s denote the absence of links. Consistent with usual practice, there are no links between inputs. But there are potential links between inputs, latent variables, and the response that need to be specified. For example, $X5$ is connected to $Z3$, but not to the other latent variables. $X6$ is connected to none of the latent variables but is connected directly to Y.

Network #1 is a vector of binary indicators consistent with the figure. The indicators are entered by row as one would read words in an English sentence. Network #2 is another vector of binary indicators that represents another structure for the 6 inputs, 3 latent variables, and 1 response. Both representations can be seen as candidate solutions for which fitness is measured by a loss function with Y and $\hat{Y}$ as arguments. The algorithm would begin with a substantial number of such candidate solutions. A neural network would be fit with each. The task is to find the neural net specification that minimizes the loss, and that loss will depend in part on the architecture of the network.

One might think that there is a brute-force solution. Just try all possible network specifications and find the one with the best fit. However, for all but relatively simple networks, the task may not be computationally feasible. Each possible network specification would require its own set of fitted values. We faced a similar problem earlier when we considered all possible classification trees for a given dataset. Much as a greedy algorithm can provide a method to arrive at a good tree, a genetic algorithm can provide a method to arrive at a good network specification. "Good" should not be read as "best."

One might proceed as follows (Mitchell 1998: 10–11).

1. Generate a random population of N network specifications, two of which are illustrated by network #1 and network #2 in Fig. 8.3. There would be some constraints such as not allowing links between inputs and requiring at least one path from an input to the response. The population of specifications would not be exhaustive.
2. Suppose Y is numeric. Compute the mean squared error for each candidate specification as a measure of fitness. This means fitting a neural net for each.
3. Sample with replacement a pair of candidate specifications with the probability proportional to fitness.
4. With a specified probability (a tuning parameter) cross the pair of candidate specifications at a randomly chosen point. That point would be selected with equal probability. For example, suppose for network #1 and #2, the equivalent of a coin flip comes up heads. A crossover is required. There are 28 possible break points, and suppose the 5th possible break point (going left to right) is selected at random. The values of 1, 1, 0, 0, 1 from the network solution #1 would be swapped with values 1, 1, 0, 1, 0 from the network #2 solution.
5. Mutate locations in each pair with some small probability (another tuning parameter). This means on occasion changing a 0 to a 1 and a 1 to a 0 where such changes are allowed (e.g., not between inputs).
6. Compute the mean squared error for each of the two progeny.

7. Repeat steps 3–6 until N offspring have been produced and replace the old population with the new population.
8. Repeat steps 2–7 and repeat until there have been a sufficient number of generations (e.g., 100).
9. Select the network structure from the population of network structures that is most fit (i.e., has the smallest mean squared error).[4]

One can now see why genetic algorithms are said to "learn", and why they can be a form of reinforcement learning. The algorithms discover what works. With steps that have parallels to natural selection, solutions that are more fit survive. In contrast, to conventional optimization methods like gradient descent, there is no overall loss function being minimized. Still, a solution is likely to be good in part because of built-in random components that help prevent a genetic algorithm from getting mired in less desirable, local results. For these and other more technical reasons, genetic algorithms can be folded into discussions of machine learning. They can also be a key feature of recent developments in deep learning when conventional numerical methods may be overmatched, and local solutions can be a serious pitfall.

---

[4]Readers interested in running genetic algorithms in R should consider using the library *GA* written by Luca Scrucca (Scrucca 2013).

Chapter 9
Broader Implications and a Bit of Craft Lore

9.1 Some Integrating Themes

Over the past decade, the number of statistical learning procedures that can be viewed as a form of regression has grown. By and large, they are variants on, or extensions of, the procedures discussed in earlier chapters. The major advances are to be found in deeper understandings of the underlying mechanisms and increasingly, some common themes.

The major players, random forests, boosting, and support vector machines, share with niche players like neural networks and Bayesian additive regression trees the use of linear basis expansions to provide a rich collection of predictors. How this is done can vary. Random forests arrives at its basis expansions by building inductively over a large number of regression or classification trees, sampling the training data and predictors. Stochastic gradient boosting proceeds by sampling and reweighting the data with each iteration. Support vector machines get the job done by constructing rich predictor kernels in advance of the data analysis. Neural networks imposes nonlinear transformations of the predictors through its hidden layers. BART generates an ensemble of trees by stochastic decision rules while treating the data as fixed. It should not be surprising that when properly implemented, one can often get similar performance across these statistical learning methods.

The reliance on complicated linear basis expansions usually leads to blackbox procedures. One can get fitted values that perform very well, but the role of the predictors responsible is typically obscure. There have been recent efforts to develop auxiliary algorithms that can help, and more such advances are in the offing. But the blackbox problem underscores that statistical learning procedures depend on algorithms not models in which ends can justify means. If one's primary data analysis

The original version of this chapter was revised: See the "Chapter Note" section at the end of this chapter for details. The erratum to this chapter is available at https://doi.org/10.1007/978-3-319-44048-4_10.

© Springer International Publishing Switzerland 2016
R.A. Berk, *Statistical Learning from a Regression Perspective*,
Springer Texts in Statistics, DOI 10.1007/978-3-319-44048-4_9

goal is to explain, statistical learning is not likely to be helpful, and formal causal inference is typically off the table. When feasible, one is better off doing experiments.

Each of the procedures discussed can be represented as $Y = f(X) + \varepsilon$, where $\hat{f}(X)$ is arrived at by minimizing some loss function. The introduction of ε and loss function optimization can be seen as recasting machine learning as statistical learning. In practice, however, any of the procedures we have discussed properly can sail under either flag.

The formulation relying on $Y = f(X) + \varepsilon$ does not imply that $f(X)$ is the true response surface. It is called an approximation for good reason. When there is estimation, the target is an acknowledged approximation. The goal is to arrive at an effective approximation with the understanding that there will be bias and variance separating the estimate from the "truth." In the end, statistical learning earns its keep by explicitly constructing approximations of the true response surface that by several criteria are usually better than the unacknowledged approximations constructed by conventional models.

There remains hard work to be done understanding why statistical learning procedures work so well. Margin maximization, loss function optimization, and interpolation all play some role. But the accounts are at best incomplete. For example, there is somewhat limited understanding of why certain kernels work well in certain settings but not others.

All of the statistical learning procedures we have discussed are conceptually and operationally challenged by statistical inference, statistical tests, and confidence intervals. Bayesian additive regression trees tackles the problem head on, but in a manner that many find unsatisfactory. All of the other methods have their greatest success when the training data can be seen credibly as IID realizations from a joint probability distribution and when there are test data to provide honest performance assessments.

9.2   Some Practical Suggestions

Just as for any other set of statistical procedures, practice is guided significantly by craft lore. In that spirit, we turn to a bit of craft lore about the use of statistical learning. It is important to keep in mind, however, craft lore can change dramatically with experience, and the experience with statistical learning to date is somewhat spotty.

9.2.1   Choose the Right Procedure

Recall Breiman's distinction between two cultures: a "data modeling culture" and an "algorithmic modeling culture" (2001b). The data modeling culture favors the generalized linear model and its various extensions. A data analysis begins with a mathematical expression meant to represent the mechanisms by which nature works. Estimation serves to fill in the details. The algorithmic modeling culture is concerned solely with linking inputs to outputs. The subject-matter mechanisms connecting the two are not represented and there is, therefore, no a priori vehicle by which inputs are transformed into outputs. A data analysis is undertaken to invent such a vehicle so that a good fit results. There is no requirement whatsoever that the vehicle reveals nature's machinery.

But, there is in practice no clear distinction between procedures that belong in the data modeling culture and procedures that belong in the algorithmic modeling culture. In both cultures, information extracted from data is essential. Even for a correct regression model, parameter estimates are obtained from data. Rather, there is a continuum characterized by how much the results depend on substantively informed constraints imposed on the analysis. For conventional regression, at one extreme, there are extensive constraints meant to represent the machinery by which nature proceeds. At the other extreme, random forests and stochastic gradient boosting mine associations in the data with virtually no substantively informed restrictions. Many procedures, such as those within the generalized additive model, fall in between.

How then should a data analysis tool be selected? As a first cut, the importance of explicitly representing nature's machinery should be determined. If explanation is the dominant data analysis motive, procedures from the data modeling culture should be favored. If prediction is the dominant data analysis motive, procedures from the algorithmic modeling culture should be favored. If neither is dominant, procedures should be used that are a compromise between the two extremes.

If one is working within the data modeling culture, the choice of procedures is determined primarily by the correspondence between subjective-matter information available and features of a candidate modeling approach. The correspondence should be substantial. For example, if nature is known to proceed through a linear combination of causal variables, a form of conventional regression may well be appropriate.

Working within the algorithmic modeling culture, the choice of procedures ideally is primarily determined by out-of-sample performance. One might hope that through formal mathematics and forecasting contests, clear winners and losers could be identified. Unfortunately, the results are rarely definitive. One major problem is that forecasting performance is typically dataset specific; accuracy depends on particular features of data that can differ across datasets. A winner on one forecasting task will often be a loser on another forecasting task. Another major problem is how to tune the procedures so that each is performing as well as it can on a given dataset. Because the kinds and numbers of tuning parameters vary across algorithmic methods, there is usually no way to ensure that fair comparisons are being made. Still another problem is that a lot depends on exactly how forecasting performance is measured. For example, the area under an ROC curve will often pick different winners from those evaluated by cost-weighted classification error.

However, all of the algorithmic methods emphasized in earlier chapters can perform well in a wide range of applications. In practice, perhaps the best strategy is for a data analyst to select a method that he or she adequately understands, that has features responding best to the application at hand, and that has the most instruc-

tive output. For example, only some of the procedures discussed can easily adapt
to forecasting errors that have asymmetric costs, and some can handle very large
datasets better than others. The procedures can also differ by whether there are, for
example, partial dependence plots and how variable importance is measured. Forecasting accuracy is but one of several criteria by which algorithmic procedures can
be compared. Among these other criteria are:

1. *ease of use* — A combination of the procedure itself and the software with which
   it is implemented;
2. *readily available software* — R usually a good place to start in part because
   commercial packages are often several years behind;
3. *good documentation* — for both the procedure and the software (be wary of
   commercial products that hide the details for their procedures by calling them
   proprietary);
4. *adaptability* — the procedure and its software should be easily adapted to unanticipated circumstances such as the need for test data;
5. *processing speed* — a function of the nature of the procedure, the number of
   observations, the number of variables, and the quality of the code (e.g., paral-
   lelization);
6. *ease of dissemination* — some procedures and some kinds of output are easier to
   explain to users of the results;
7. *special features of the procedure* — examples include the ability to handle classification with more than two classes, ways to introduce asymmetric costs from
   fitting errors, and tools for peering into the blackbox; and
8. *cost* — some commercial products can be quite pricey.

If there is no clear winner, it can always be useful to apply more than one procedure
and report more than one set of results.

9.2.2 Get to Know Your Software

There is not yet, and not likely to be in the near future, a consensus on how any of
the various statistical learning procedures should be implemented in software. For
example, a recent check on software available for support vector machines found
working code for over a half dozen procedures. There is, as well, near anarchy in
naming conventions, and notation. Thus, the term "cost," for instance, can mean
several different things, and a symbol such as γ can be a tuning parameter in one
derivation and a key argument in another derivation.

One cannot assume that a description of a procedure in a textbook (including this
one) or journal article corresponds fully to software using the very same name, even
by the same authors. Consequently, it is very important to work with software for
which there is good technical documentation on the procedure and algorithms being
used. There also needs to be clear information on how to introduce inputs, obtain
outputs, and tune the procedure. Descriptions of two computer programs can use the

same name for different items, or use very different names for the same item. And in either case, the naming conventions may not correspond to the naming conventions in the technical literature.

Even when the documentation looks to be clear and complete, a healthy dose of skepticism is useful. There are sometimes errors in the documentation, or in the software, or in both. So, it is usually important to "shake down" any new software with data that have previously been analyzed properly to determine if the new results come out as expected. In addition, it is usually helpful to experiment with various tuning parameters to see if the results make sense. In short, *caveat emptor*.

It is also very important keep abreast of software updates, which can come as often as five or six times a year. As a routine matter, new features are added, existing features are deleted, bugs fixed, and documentation rewritten. These changes are often far more than cosmetic. Working with an older version of statistical learning software can lead to unnecessary problems.

Finally, a key software decision is whether to work primarily with shareware such as found in R or Python, or with commercial products. The tradeoffs have been discussed earlier at various points. Cost is certainly an issue, but perhaps more important is the tension between having the most current software and having the most stable software and documentation. Shareware is more likely to be on the leading edge, but often lacks the convenience and stability of commercial products. One possible strategy for individuals who are unfamiliar with a certain class of procedures is to begin with a good commercial product, and then once some hands-on skill has been developed, migrate to shareware.

9.2.3 Do Not Forget the Basics

It is very easy to get caught up in the razzle-dazzle of statistical learning and for any given data analysis, neglect simple fundamentals. All data analyses must start with an effort to get "close" to the data. This requires a careful inspection of elementary descriptive statistics: means, standard deviations, histograms, cross-tabulations, scatterplots, and the like. It also means understanding how the data were generated and how the variables were measured. Moving into a statistical learning procedure without this groundwork can lead to substantial grief. For example, sometimes numeric values are given to missing data. Treating these values as legitimate values can seriously distort any data analysis, including ones undertaken with statistical learning.

It will often be helpful to apply one or more forms of conventional regression analysis before moving to statistical learning. One then obtains an initial sense of how good the fit is likely to be, of the likely signs of key relationships between predictors and the response, and of problems that might be more difficult to spot later (e.g., does one really have a weak learner?). An important implication is that it will often be handy to undertake statistical learning within a software environment in which a variety of statistical tools can be applied to the same data. This can weigh against single-purpose, statistical learning software.

To take one simple example, a tuning parameter in random forests may require a distinct value for each response class. But the order in which those arguments are entered into the expression for the tuning parameter may be unclear. In the binary case, for example, which category comes first? Is it $\omega = c(1, 0)$ or $\omega = c(0, 1)$? A wrong choice is easily made. Random forests runs just the same and generates sensible-looking output. But the analysis has not been tuned as it should have been. It can be difficult to spot such an error unless one knows the marginal distribution of the response variable and the likely sign of relationships between each predictor and the response. A few cross-tabulations and a preliminary regression analysis can help enormously.

Finally, one must not forget that preliminary analyses of the data can introduce data snooping, especially if relationships between potential predictors and potential responses are examined. This does not mean that one should avoid these analyses. What it means is that often, test data are essential.

9.2.4 Getting Good Data

As noted many times, there is no substitute for good data. The fact that boosting, for example, can make weak classifiers stronger, does not mean that boosting can make weak data stronger. There are no surprises in what properties good data should have: a large number of observations, little measurement error, a rich set of predictors, and a reasonably well-balanced response variable distribution. The clear message is that it is very important to invest time and resources in data collection. One cannot count on statistical learning successfully coming to the rescue. Indeed, some forms of statistical learning can be quite fussy and easily pulled off course by noisy data, let alone data that have systematic measurement error.

The case for having legitimate test data can be quite strong. Statistical learning procedures that use out-of-bag data or the equivalent may not formally need a test dataset. The out-of-bag observations can serve that purpose. But most statistical learning procedures currently are not designed to work with random samples of the data, even when that might make a lot of sense. Therefore, having access to test data is usually very important.

Even for random forests, test data beyond the out-of-bag observations can come in handy. Comparisons between how random forests performs and how other approaches (including conventional regression) perform are often very instructive. For example, one might learn that the key relationships are linear and that it is not worth losing degrees of freedom fitting more complex functions. Yet such comparisons cannot be undertaken unless there are test data shared by all of the statistical procedures in play. Finally, having a true test dataset can help a great deal if random forests is applied repeatedly to the same training data after changes in the tuning parameters. At the very end of the tuning process, there is still the opportunity to get a more honest measure of performance from data that until that moment have not been used.

9.2.5 Match Your Goals to What You Can Credibly Do

Much of the literature on statistical modeling is formulated around some $f(X)$. There is a real mechanism by which the data were generated. An essential goal of a data analysis is to recover the data-generation function from a dataset. It can be very tempting, therefore, to frame all data analyses in a similar manner.

But, one of the themes of this book has been that in reality, more modest goals are likely to be appropriate. Perhaps most important, statistical learning is not built around a regression model of the data generation process. The data are realized from a joint probability distribution and analyzed by algorithmic methods. In addition, one will usually not have access to all of the requisite predictors, let alone predictors that are all well measured. Finally, various kinds of data snooping will often be impossible to avoid. For these and other reasons, a level I analysis will be the primary enterprise.

But there also will be circumstances when a level II analysis can be justified and properly undertaken. These circumstances are addressed in various sections of the book. Perhaps the major take-home message is that level II analyses are never routine. They require clear and careful thought. For example, the vote proportions produced by random forests are not probabilities and do not represent the chances that a given observation falls into a particular outcome class. They are a measure of the internal reliability of the random forest algorithm.

Although causal thinking can be important as the research task is being formulated and the data are being collected, statistical learning procedures are not designed for Level III analyses. It can be very tempting to use some forms of statistical learning output, such as variable importance plots, to make causal statements. But the various definitions of importance do not comport well with the canonical definition of a causal effect, and the output is not derived from a causal model.

An important implication is that using a statistical learning procedure to do variable selection can lead to a conceptual swamp. If the purpose is to screen for important causal variables, it is not apparent how the statistical learning output is properly used for that purpose. This does not preclude dimension reduction in service of other ends. For example, regularization is an essential tool when the intent is to improve the stability of statistical learning output.

9.3 Some Concluding Observations

Over the past decade, statistical learning has become one of the more important tools available to applied statisticians and data analysts. But, the hype in which some procedures are wrapped can obscure important limitations and lead to analyses undertaken without sufficient care.

Statistical learning properly done will often require a major attitude adjustment. One of most difficult obstacles to effective applications is letting go of premises from conventional modeling. This will be especially difficult for experienced data analysts trained in traditional methods. One of the most common errors is to overlay statistical learning on top of model-based conceptions. Statistical learning is not just more of the same.

Finally, users of results from statistical learning must proceed with care. There is lots of money to be made and professional reputations to be built with statistical razzle-dazzle that is actually voodoo statistics. It can be very important to have access to technical advice from knowledgeable individuals who have no skin in the game.

Erratum to: Statistical Learning from a Regression Perspective

Erratum to:
R.A. Berk, *Statistical Learning*
from a Regression Perspective, **Springer Texts in Statistics,**
https://doi.org/10.1007/978-3-319-44048-4

The book was incorrectly published with errors in Chapters 1 to 9. The erratum book has now been updated with the changes.

The updated original online version of this book can be found at
https://doi.org/10.1007/978-3-319-44048-4

© Springer International Publishing Switzerland 2017
R.A. Berk, *Statistical Learning from a Regression Perspective*,
Springer Texts in Statistics, https://doi.org/10.1007/978-3-319-44048-4_10

References

Affenseller, M., Winkler, S., Wagner, S., & Beham, A. (2009). *Genetic algorithms and genetic programming: Modern concepts and practical applications*. New York: Chapman & Hall.

Akaike, H. (1973). Information theory and an extension to the maximum likelihood principle. In B. N. Petrov & F. Casaki (Eds.), *International Symposium on Information Theory* (pp. 267–281). Budapest: Akademia Kiado.

Angrist, J. D., & Pischke, J. (2009). *Mostly harmless econometrics*. Princeton: Princeton University Press.

Baca-García, E., Perez-Rodriguez, M. M., Basurte-Villamor, I., Saiz-Ruiz, J., Leiva-Murillo, J. M., de Prado-Cumplido, M., et al. (2006). Using data mining to explore complex clinical decisions: A study of hospitalization after a suicide attempt. *Jounal of Clinical Psychiatry, 67*(7), 1124–1132.

Barber, D. (2012). *Bayesian reasoning and machine learning*. Cambridge: Cambridge University Press.

Bartlett, P. L., & Traskin, M. (2007). Adaboost is Consistent. *Journal of Machine Learning Research, 8*(2347–2368), 2007.

Beck, A. T., Ward, C. H., Mendelson, M., Mock, J., & Erbaugh, J. (1961). An inventory for measuring depression. *Archives of General Psychiatry, 4*(6), 561–571.

Berk, R. A. (2003). *Regression analysis: A constructive critique*. Newbury Park: Sage.

Berk, R. A. (2005). New claims about executions and general deterrence: Déjà vu all over again? *Journal of Empirical Legal Studies, 2*(2), 303–330.

Berk, R. A. (2012). *Criminal justice forecasts of risk: A machine learning approach*. New York: Springer.

Berk, R. A., & Freedman, D. A. (2003). Statistical assumptions as empirical commitments. In T. Blomberg & S. Cohen (Eds.), *Law, punishment, and social control: Essays in honor of Sheldon Messinger, Part V* (pp. 235–254). Berlin: Aldine de Gruyter (November 1995, revised in second edition).

Berk, R. A., & Rothenberg, S. (2004). Water Resource Dynamics in Asian Pacific Cities. Statistics Department Preprint Series, UCLA.

Berk, R. A., Kriegler, B., & Ylvisaker, D. (2008). Counting the Homeless in Los Angeles County. In D. Nolan & S. Speed (Eds.), *Probability and statistics: Essays in Honor of David A. Freedman* Monograph Series for the Institute of Mathematical Statistics.

Berk, R. A., Brown, L., & Zhao, L. (2010). Statistical inference after model selection. *Journal of Quantitative Criminology, 26*, 217–236.

Berk., R. A., Brown, L., Buja, A., Zhang, K., & Zhao, L. (2014). Valid post-selection inference. *Annals of Statistics, 41*(2), 802–837

© Springer International Publishing Switzerland 2016
R.A. Berk, *Statistical Learning from a Regression Perspective*,
Springer Texts in Statistics, DOI 10.1007/978-3-319-44048-4

Berk, R. A., Brown, L., Buja, A., George, E., Pitkin, E., Zhang, K., et al. (2014). Misspecified mean function regression: Making good use of regression models that are wrong. *Sociological Methods and Research, 43*, 422–451.

Berk, R. A., & Bleich, J. (2013). Statistical procedures for forecasting criminal behavior: A comparative assessment. *Journal of Criminology and Public Policy, 12*(3), 515–544.

Berk, R. A., & Bleich, J. (2014). Forecast violence to inform sentencing decisions. *Journal of Quantitative Criminology, 30*, 79–96.

Berk, R. A., & Hyatt, J. (2015). Machine learning forecasts of risk to inform sentencing decisions. *Federal Sentencing Reporter, 27*(4), 222–228.

Bhat, H. S., Kumer, N., & Vaz, G. (2011). Quantile regression trees. Working Paper, School of Natural Sciences, University of California, Merced.

Biau, G. (2012). Analysis of a random forests model. *Journal of Machine Learning Research, 13*, 1063–1095.

Biau, G., Devroye, L., & Lugosi, G. (2008). Consistency of random forests and other averaging classifiers. *Journal of Machine Learning Research, 9*, 2015–2033.

Biau, G., & Devroye, L. (2010). On the layered nearest neighbor estimate, the bagged nearest neighbour estimate and the random forest method in regression and classification. *Journal Multivariate Analysis, 101*, 2499–2518.

Bishop, C. M. (2006). *Pattern recognition and machine learning.* New York: Springer.

Box, G. E. P. (1976). Science and statistics. *Journal of the American Statistical Association, 71*(356), 791–799.

Bound, J., Jaeger, D. A., & Baker, R. M. (1995). Problems with instrumental variables estimation when the correlation between the instruments and the endogenous explanatory variable is weak. *Journal of the American Statistical Association, 90*(430), 443–450.

Breiman, L. (1996). Bagging predictors. *Machine Learning, 26*, 123–140.

Breiman, L. (2001a). Random forests. *Machine Learning, 45*, 5–32.

Breiman, L. (2001b). Statistical modeling: Two cultures (with discussion). *Statistical Science, 16*, 199–231.

Breiman, L., Friedman, J. H., Olshen, R. A., & Stone, C. J. (1984). *Classification and regression trees.* Monterey: Wadsworth Press.

Breiman, L., Meisel, W., & Purcell, E. (1977). Variable kernel estimates of multivariate densities. *Technometrics, 19*, 135–144.

Bring, J. (1994). How to standardize regression coefficients. *The American Statistician, 48*(3), 209–213.

Bühlmann, P. (2006). Boosting for high dimensional linear models. *The Annals of Statistics, 34*(2), 559–583.

Bühlmann, P., & Yu, B. (2002). Analyzing bagging. *The Annals of Statistics, 30*, 927–961.

Bühlmann, P., & Yu, B. (2004). Discussion. *The Annals of Statistics, 32*, 96–107.

Bühlmann, P., & Yu, B. (2006). Sparse boosting. *Journal of Machine Learning Research, 7*, 1001–1024.

Bühlmann, P., & van de Geer, S. (2011). *Statistics for high dimensional data.* New York: Springer.

Buja, A., & Rolke, W. (2007). Calibration for simultaneity: (Re) sampling methods for simultaneous inference with application to function estimation and functional data. Working Paper. https://www-stat.wharton.upenn.edu/~buja/.

Buja, A., & Stuetzle, W. (2000). Smoothing effects of bagging. Working Paper. http://www-stat.wharton.upenn.edu/~buja/.

Buja, A., & Stuetzle, W. (2006). Observations on bagging. *Statistica Sinica, 16*(2), 323–352.

Buja, A., Mease, D., & Wyner, A. J. (2008). Discussion of Bühlmann and Hothorn. *Statistical Science,* forthcoming.

Buja, A., Stuetzle, W., & Shen, Y. (2005). Loss functions for binary class probability estimation and classification: Structure and applications. Unpublished manuscript, Department of Statistics, The Wharton School, University of Pennsylvania.

Buja, A., Berk, R. A., Brown, L., George, E., Pitkin, E., Traskin, M. et al. (2015). Models as approximations — a conspiracy of random regressors and model violations against classical inference in regression. $imsart - stsver.2015/07/30 : Buja\_et\_al\_Conspiracy-v2.tex$ date: July 23, 2015.

Camacho, R., King, R., & Srinivasan, A. (2006). 14th International conference on inductive logic programming. *Machine Learning*, *64*, 145–287.

Candel, A., Parmar, V., LeDell, E., & Arora, A. (2016). Deep learning with H_2O. Mountain View: H_2O.ai Inc.

Candes, E., & Tao, T. (2007). The Dantzig selector: Statistical estimation when p is much larger than n (with discussion). *Annals of Statistics*, *35*(6), 2313–2351.

Chaudhuri, P., Lo, W.-D., Loh, W.-Y., & Yang, C.-C. (1995). Generalized regression trees. *Statistic Sinica*, *5*, 641–666.

Chaudhuri, P., & Loh, W.-Y. (2002). Nonparametric estimation of conditional quantiles using quantile regression trees. *Bernoulli*, *8*(5), 561–576.

Chen, P., Lin, C., & Schölkopf, B. (2004). A tutorial on v-support vector machines. Department of Computer Science and Information Engineering, National Taiwan University, Taipei, Taiwan.

Chen, T., & Guestrin, C. (2016). XGBoost: a scalable tree boosting system. arXiv:1603.02754v1 [cs.LG].

Chipman, H. A., George, E. I., & McCulloch, R. E. (1998). Bayesian CART model search. *Journal of the American Statistical Association*, *93*(443), 935–948.

Chipman, H. A., George, E. I., & McCulloch, R. E. (1999). Hierarchical priors for Bayesian CART shrinkage. *Statistics and Computing*, *10*(1), 17–24.

Chipman, H. A., George, E. I., & McCulloch, R. E. (2010). BART: Bayesian additive regression trees. *Annals for Applied Statistics*, *4*(1), 266–298.

Christianini, N., & Shawe-Taylor, J. (2000). *Support vector machines* (Vol. 93(443), pp. 935–948). Cambridge, UK: Cambridge University Press.

Choi, Y., Ahn, H., & Chen, J. J. (2005). Regression trees for analysis of count data with extra Poisson variation. *Computational Statistics & Data Analysis*, *49*, 893–915.

Clarke, B., Fokoué, E, & Zhang, H. H. (2009). *Principles and theory of data mining and machine learning* New York: Springer.

Cleveland, W. (1979). Robust locally weighted regression and smoothing scatterplots. *Journal of the American Statistical Association*, *78*, 829–836.

Cleveland, W. (1993). *Visualizing data*. Summit, New Jersey: Hobart Press.

Cochran, W. G. (1977). *Sampling techniques* (3rd ed.). New York: Wiley.

Cook, D. R., & Weisberg, S. (1999). *Applied regression including computing and graphics*. New York: Wiley.

Crawley, M. J. (2007). *The R book*. New York: Wiley.

Dalgaard, P. (2002). *Introductory statistics with R*. New York: Springer.

Dasu, T., & Johnson, T. (2003). *Exploratory data mining and data cleaning*. New York: Wiley.

de Boors, C. (2001). *A practical guide to splines* (revised ed.). New York: Springer.

Deng, L., & Yu, D. (2014). *Deep learning: Methods and applications*. Boston: Now Publishers Inc.

Dijkstra, T. K. (2011). Ridge regression and its degrees of freedom. Working Paper, Department Economics & Business, University of Gronigen, The Netherlands.

Duvenaud, D., Lloyd, J. R., Grosse, R., Tenenbaum, J. B., & Ghahramani, Z. (2013). Structure discovery in nonparametric regression through compositional kernel search. *Journal of Machine Learning Research W&CP*, *28*(3), 1166–1174.

Dwork, C., Hardt, M., Pitassi, T., Reingold, O., & Zemel, R. (2011). Fairness through awareness. Retrieved November 29, 2011, from arXiv:1104.3913v2 [cs.CC]

Dwork, C., Feldman, V., Hardt, M., Pitassi, T., Reingold, O., & Roth, A. (2015). The reusable holdout: Preserving validity in adaptive data analysis. *Science*, *349*(6248), 636–638.

Edgington, E. S., & Ongehena, P. (2007). *Randomization tests* (4th ed.). New York: Chapman & Hall.

Eicker, F. (1963). Asymptotic normality and consistency of the least squares estimators for families of linear regressions. *Annals of Mathematical Statistics, 34*, 447–456.

Eicker, F. (1967). Limit theorems for regressions with unequal and dependent errors. *Proceedings of the Fifth Berkeley Symposium on Mathematical Statistics and Probability, 1*, 59–82.

Efron, B. (1986). How biased is the apparent error rate of prediction rule? *Journal of the American Statistical Association, 81*(394), 461–470.

Efron, B., & Tibshirani, R. (1993). *Introduction to the bootstrap*. New York: Chapman & Hall.

Ericksen, E. P., Kadane, J. B., & Tukey, J. W. (1989). Adjusting the 1980 census of population and housing. *Journal of the American Statistical Association, 84*, 927–944.

Exterkate, P., Groenen, P. J. K., Heij, C., & Van Dijk, D. J. C. (2011). Nonlinear forecasting with many predictors using kernel ridge regression. Tinbergen Institute Discussion Paper 11-007/4.

Fan, J., & Gijbels, I. (1992). Variable bandwidth and local linear regression smoothers. *The Annals of Statistics, 20*(4), 2008–2036.

Fan, J., & Gijbels, I. (1996). *Local polynomial modeling and its applications*. New York: Chapman & Hall.

Fan, G., & Gray, B. (2005). Regression tree analysis using TARGET. *Journal of Computational and Graphical Statistics, 14*, 206–218.

Fan, J., & Li, R. (2006). Statistical challenges with dimensionality: Feature selection in knowledge discovery. In M. Sanz-Sole, J. Soria, J.L. Varona & J. Verdera (Eds.), *Proceedings of the International Congress of Mathematicians* (Vol. III, pp. 595–622).

Fan, J., & Lv, J. (2008). Sure independence screening for ultrahigh dimensional feature space (with discussion). *Journal of the Royal Statistical Society, B70*, 849–911.

Fan, J., & Gijbels, I. (1996). Variable bandwidth and local linear regression smoothers. *The Annals of Statistics, 20*(4), 2008–2036.

Faraway, J. (2004). Human animation using nonparametric regression. *Journal of Computational and Graphical Statistics, 13*, 537–553.

Faraway, J. J. (2014). Does data splitting improve prediction? *Statistics and computing*. Berlin: Springer

Finch, P. D. (1976). The poverty of statisticism. *Foundations of Probability Theory, Statistical Inference, and Statistical Theories of Science, 6b*, 1–46.

Freedman, D. A. (1981). Bootstrapping regression models. *Annals of Statistics, 9*(6), 1218–1228.

Freedman, D. A. (1987). As others see us: A case study in path analysis (with discussion). *Journal of Educational Statistics, 12*, 101–223.

Freedman, D. A. (2004). Graphical models for causation and the identification problem. *Evaluation Review, 28*, 267–293.

Freedman, D. A. (2009a). *Statistical models cambridge*. UK: Cambridge University Press.

Freedman, D. A. (2009b). Diagnostics cannot have much power against general alternatives. *International Journal of Forecasting, 25*, 833–839.

Freund, Y., & Schapire, R. (1996). Experiments with a new boosting algorithm. In *Macine Learning: Proceedings for the Thirteenth International Conference* (pp. 148–156). San Francisco: Morgan Kaufmann.

Freund, Y., & Schapire, R. E. (1997). A decision-theoretic generalization of online learning and an application to boosting. *Journal of Computer and System Sciences, 55*, 119–139.

Freund, Y., & Schapire, R. E. (1999). A short introduction to boosting. *Journal of the Japanese Society for Artificial Intelligence, 14*, 771–780.

Friedman, J. H. (1991). Multivariate adaptive regression splines (with discussion). *The Annals of Statistics, 19*, 1–82.

Friedman, J. H. (2001). Greedy function approximation: A gradient boosting machine. *The Annals of Statistics, 29*, 1189–1232.

Friedman, J. H. (2002). Computational statistics and data analysis. *Stochastic Gradient Boosting, 38*, 367–378.

Friedman, J. H., & Hall, P. (2000). On bagging and nonlinear estimation. Technical Report. Department of Statistics, Stanford University.

Friedman, J. H., Hastie, T., & Tibshirani, R. (2000). Additive logistic regression: A statistical view of boosting (with discussion). *Annals of Statistics, 28*, 337–407.

Friedman, J. H., Hastie, T., Rosset, S., Tibshirani, R., & Zhu, J. (2004). Discussion of boosting papers. *Annals of Statistics, 32*, 102–107.

Gareth, M., & Radchenko, P. (2007). Sparse generalized linear models. Working Paper, Department of Statistics, Marshall School of Business, University of California.

Gareth, M., & Zhu, J. (2007). Functional linear regression that's interpretable. Working Paper, Department of Statistics, Marshall School of Business, University of California.

Geurts, P., Ernst, D., & Wehenkel, L. (2006). Extremely randomized trees. *Machine Learning, 63*(1), 3–42.

Ghosh, M., Reid, N., & Fraser, D. A. S. (2010). Ancillary statistics: A review. *Statistica Sinica, 20*, 1309–1332.

Gifi, A. (1990). *Nonlinear multivariate analysis*. New York: Wiley.

Good, P. I. (2004). *Permutation, parametric and bootstrap tests of hypotheses*. New York: Springer.

Grandvalet, Y. (2004). Bagging equalizes influence. *Machine Learning, 55*, 251–270.

Granger, C. W. J., & Newbold, P. (1986). *Forecasting economic time series*. New York: Academic Press.

Green, P. J., & Silverman, B. W. (1994). *Nonparametric regression and generalized linear models*. New York: Chapman & Hall.

Grubinger, T., Zeileis, A., & Pfeiffer, K.-P. (2014). Evtree: Evolutionary learning of globally optimal classification and regression trees in R. *Journal of Statistical Software, 61*(1). http://www.jstatsoft.org/.

Hall, P. (1997). *The bootstrap and Edgeworth expansion* New York: Springer.

Hand, D., Manilla, H., & Smyth, P. (2001). *Principles of data mining*. Cambridge, MA: MIT Press.

Hastie, T., Tibshirani, R., & Friedman, J. (2009). *The elements of statistical learning* (2nd ed.). New York: Springer.

Hastie, T. J., & Tibshirani, R. J. (1990). *Generalized additive models*. New York: Chapman & Hall.

Hastie, T. J., & Tibshirani, R. J. (1996). Discriminant adaptive nearest neighbor classification. *IEEE Pattern Recognition and Machine Intelligence, 18*, 607–616.

He, Y. (2006). Missing data imputation for tree-based models. Ph.D. dissertation for the Department of Statistics, UCLA.

Hoeting, J., Madigan, D., Raftery, A., & Volinsky, C. (1999). Bayesian model averaging: A practical tutorial. *Statistical Science, 14*, 382–401.

Horváth, T., & Yamamoto, A. (2006). International conference on inductive logic programming. *Journal of Machine Learning, 64*, 3–144.

Hothorn, T., & Lausen, B. (2003). Double-bagging: Combining classifiers by bootstrap aggregation. *Pattern Recognition, 36*, 1303–1309.

Hothorn, T., Hornik, K., & Zeileis, A. (2006). Unbiased recursive partitioning: A conditional inference framework. *Journal of Computational and Graphical Statistics, 15*(3), 651–674.

Huber, P. J. (1967). The behavior of maximum likelihood estimates under nonstandard conditions. *Proceedings of the Fifth Symposium on Mathematical Statistics and Probability, I*, 221–233.

Hurvich, C. M., & Tsai, C. (1989). Regression and time series model selection in small samples. *Biometrika, 76*(2), 297–307.

Hsu, C., Chung, C., & Lin, C. (2010). A practical guide to support vector classification. Department of Computer Science and Information Engineering National Taiwan University, Taipei, Taiwan. http://www.csie.ntu.edu.tw/~cjlin/libsvm.

Ishwaran, H. (2015). The effect of splitting on random forests. *Machine Learning, 99*, 75–118.

Ishwaran, H., Kogalur, U. B., Blackstone, E. H., & Lauer, T. S. (2008). Random survival forests. *The Annals of Applied Statistics, 2*(3), 841–860.

Ishwaran, H., Gerds, T. A., Kogalur, U. B., Moore, R. D., Gange, S. J., & Lau, B. M. (2014). Random survival forests for competing risks. *Biostatistics, 15*(4), 757–773.

Janson, L., Fithian, W., & Hastie, T. (2015). Effective degrees of freedom: A flawed metaphor. *Biometrika, 102*(2), 479–485.

Jiang, W. (2004). Process consistency for adaboost. *Annals of Statistics, 32*, 13–29.

Jiu, J., Zhang, J., Jiang, X., & Liu, J. (2010). The group dantzig selector. *Journal of Machine Learning Research, 9*, 461–468.

Joachims, T. (1998). Making large-scale SVM learning practical. In B. Schölkopf, C. J. C. Burges, & A. J. Smola (Eds.), *Advances in kernel methods - support vector learning*. Cambridge, MA: MIT Press.

Jordan, M. I., & Mitchell, T. M. (2015). Machine learning: Trends, perspectives, and prospects. *Science, 349*(6234), 255–260.

Karatzoglou, A., Smola, A., & Hornik, K. (2015). kernlab – An S4 Package for Kernel Methods in R. https://cran.r-project.org/web/packages/kernlab/vignettes/kernlab.pdf.

Kass, G. V. (1980). An exploratory technique for investigating large quantities of categorical data. *Applied Statistics, 29*(2), 119–127.

Katatzoglou, A., Smola, A., Hornik, K., & Zeileis, A. (2004). Kernlab – An S4 package for Kernel methods in R. *Journal of Statistical Software, 11*(9). http://www.jstatsoft.org.

Kaufman, S., & Rosset, S. (2014). When does more regularization imply fewer degrees of freedom? Sufficient conditions and counter examples from the lasso and ridge regression. *Biometrica, 101*(4), 771–784.

Kapelner, A., & Bleich, J. (2014). BartMachine: Machine learning for bayesian additive regression trees. arXiv:1312.2171v3 [stat.ML].

Kessler, R. C., Warner, C. H., & Ursine, R. J. (2015). Predicting suicides after psychiatric hospitalization in US army soldiers: The army study to assess risk and resilience in service members (Army STARRS). *JAMA Psychiatry, 72*(1), 49–57.

Kuhn, M., & Johnson, K. (2013). *Applied predictive modeling*. New York: Springer.

Krieger, A., Long, C., & Wyner, A. (2001). Boosting noisy data. In *Proceedings of the International Conference on Machine Learning*. Amsterdam: Mogan Kauffman.

Kriegler, B. (2007) Boosting the quantile distribution: A cost-sensitive statistical learning procedure. Department of Statistics, UCLA, working paper.

Lafferty, J., & Wasserman, L. (2008). Rodeo: sparse greedy nonparametric regression. *Annals of Statistics, 36*(1), 28–63.

Lamiell, J. T. (2013). Statisticism in personality psychologists' use of trait constructs: What is it? How was it contracted? Is there a cure? *New Ideas in Psychology, 31*(1), 65–71.

Leamer, E. E. (1978). *Specification searches: Ad hoc inference with non-experimental data*. New York: Wiley.

LeBlanc, M., & Tibshirani, R. (1996). Combining estimates on regression and classification. *Journal of the American Statistical Association, 91*, 1641–1650.

Lee, S. K. (2005). On generalized multivariate decision tree by using GEE. *Computational Statistics & Data Analysis, 49*, 1105–1119.

Lee, S. K., & Jin, S. (2006). Decision tree approaches for zero-inflated cont data. *Journal of Applied Statistics, 33*, 853–865.

Leeb, H., & Pötscher, B. M. (2005). Model selection and inference: Facts and fiction. *Econometric Theory, 21*, 21–59.

Leeb, H., & Pötscher, B. M. (2006). Can one estimate the conditional distribution of post-model-selection estimators? *The Annals of Statistics, 34*(5), 2554–2591.

Leeb, H., & Pötscher, B. M. (2008). Model selection. In T. G. Anderson, R. A. Davis, J.-P. Kreib & T. Mikosch (Eds.), *The handbook of financial time series* (pp. 785–821). New York: Springer.

Lin, Y., & Jeon, Y. (2006). Random forests and adaptive nearest neighbors. *Journal of the American Statistical Association, 101*, 578–590.

Lipton, P. (2005). Testing hypotheses: Prediction and prejudice. *Science, 307*, 219–221.

Little, R., & Rubin, D. (2015). *Statistical analysis with missing data* (3rd ed.). New York: Wiley.

Liu, J., Wonka, P., & Ye, J. (2012). Multi-stage Dantzig selector. *Journal of Machine Learning Research, 13*, 1189–1219.

Loh, W.-L. (2014). Fifty years of classification and regression trees (with discussion). *International Statistical Review, 82*(3), 329–348.

Loader, C. (2004). Smoothing: Local regression techniques. In J. Gentle, W. Hardle, & Y. Mori (Eds.), *Handbook of computational statistics*. New York: Springer.

Lockhart, R., Taylor, J., Tibshirani, R. J., & Tibshirani, R. (2014). A significance test for the lasso (with discussion). *Annals of Statistics, 42*(2), 413–468.

Loh, W.-Y. (2002). Regression trees with unbiased variable selection and interaction detection. *Statistica Sinica, 12*, 361–386.

Ma, Y., & Gao, G. (2014). *Support vector machines applications*. New York: Springer.

Maindonald, J., & Braun, J. (2007). *Data analysis and graphics using R* (2nd ed.). Cambridge, UK: Cambridge University Press.

Madigan, D., Raftery, A. E., Volinsky, C., & Hoeting, J. (1996). Bayesian model averaging. In *AAA Workshop on Integrating Multiple Learned Models* (pp. 77–83). Portland: AAAI Press.

Mallows, C. L. (1973). Some comments on CP. *Technometrics, 15*(4), 661–675.

Manly, B. F. J. (1997). *Randomization, bootstrap and Monte Carlo methods in biology*. New York: Chapman & Hall.

Mammen, E., & van de Geer, S. (1997). Locally adaptive regression splines. *The Annals of Statistics, 25*(1), 387–413.

Mannor, S., Meir, R., & Zhang, T. (2002). The consistency of greedy algorithms for classification. In J. Kivensen & R. H. Sloan (Eds.), *COLT 2002*. LNAI (Vol. 2375, pp. 319–333).

Maronna, R., Martin, D., & Yohai, V. (2006). *Robust statistics: Theory and methods*. New York: Wiley.

Marsland, S. (2014). *Machine learning: An algorithmic perspective* (2nd ed.). New York: Chapman & Hall.

Mathlourthi, W., Fredette, M. & Larocque, D. (2015). Regression trees and forests for non-homogeneous poisson processes. *Statistics and Probability Letters, 96*, 204–211.

McCullagh, P., & Nelder, J. A. (1989). *Generalized linear models* (2nd ed.). New York: Chapman & Hall.

McGonagle, K. A., Schoeni, R. F., Sastry, N., & Freedman, V. A. (2012). The panel study of income dynamics: Overview, recent innovations, and potential for life course research. *Longitudinal and Life Course Studies, 3*(2), 268–284.

Mease, D., & Wyner, A. J. (2008). Evidence contrary to the statistical view of boosting (with discussion). *Journal of Machine Learning, 9*, 1–26.

Mease, D., Wyner, A. J., & Buja, A. (2007). Boosted classification trees and class probability/quantile estimation. *Journal of Machine Learning, 8*, 409–439.

Meinshausen, N. (2006). Quantile regression forests. *Journal of Machine Learning Research, 7*, 983–999.

Meinshausen, N., & Bühlmann, P. (2006). High dimensional graphs and variable selection with the lasso. *The Annals of Statistics, 34*(3), 1436–1462.

Mentch, L., & Hooker, G. (2015). Quantifying uncertainty in random forests via confidence intervals and hypothesis tests. Cornell University Library. arXiv:1404.6473v2 [stat.ML].

Meyer, D., Zeileis, A., & Hornik, K. (2007). The strucplot framework: Visualizing multiway contingency tables with vcd. *Journal of Statistical Software, 17*(3), 1–48.

Michelucci, P., & Dickinson, J. L. (2016). The power of crowds: Combining human and machines to help tackle increasingly hard problems. *Science, 351*(6268), 32–33.

Milborrow, S. (2001). rpart.plot: Plot rpart models. An enhanced version of plot.rpart. R Package.

Mitchell, M. (1998). *An introduction to genetic algorithms*. Cambridge: MIT Press.

Moguerza, J. M., & Munõz, A. (2006). Support vector machines with applications. *Statistical Science, 21*(3), 322–336.

Mojirsheibani, M. (1997). A consistent combined classification rule. *Statistics & Probability Letters, 36*, 411–419.

Mojirsheibani, M. (1999). Combining classifiers vis discretization. *Journal of the American Statistical Association, 94*, 600–609.

Mroz, T. A. (1987). The sensitivity of an empirical model of married women's hours of work to economic and statistical assumptions. *Econometrica, 55*, 765–799.

Murphy, K. P. (2012). *Machine learning: A probabilistic perspective*. Cambridge: MIT Press.

Murrell, P. (2006). *R graphics*. New York: Chapman & Hall/CRC.

Nagin, D. S., & Pepper, J. V. (2012). *Deterrence and the death penalty*. Washington, DC: National Research Council.

Neal, R., & Zhang, J. (2006). High dimensional classification with bayesian neural networks and dirichlet diffusion trees). In I. Guyon, S. Gunn, M. Nikravesh & L. Zadeh (Eds.), *Feature extraction, foundations and applications*. New York: Springer.

Peña, D. (2005). A new statistic for influence in linear regression. *Technometrics*, *47*, 1–12.

Quinlan, R. (1993). *Programs in machine learning*. San Mateo, CA: Morgan Kaufman.

Raftery, A. D. (1995). Bayesian model selection in social research. *Sociological Methodology*, *25*, 111–163.

Ridgeway, G. (1999). The state of boosting. *Computing Science and Statistics*, *31*, 172–181.

Ridgeway, G. (2012). Generalized boosted models: A guide to the gbm package. Available at from gbm() documentation in R.

Ripley, B. D. (1996). *Pattern recognition and neural networks*. Cambridge, UK: Cambridge University Press.

Rosset, S., & Zhu, J. (2007). Piecewise linear regularized solution paths. *The Annals of Statistics*, *35*(3), 1012–1030.

Rozeboom, W. W. (1960). The fallacy of null-hypothesis significance tests. *Psychological Bulletin*, *57*(5), 416–428.

Rubin, D. B. (1986). Which ifs have causal answers. *Journal of the American Statistical Association*, *81*, 961–962.

Rubin, D. B. (2008). For objective causal inference, design trumps analysis. *Annals of Applied Statistics*, *2*(3), 808–840.

Ruppert, D. (1997). Empirical-bias bandwidths for local polynomial nonparametric regression and density estimation. *Journal of the American Statistical Association*, *92*, 1049–1062.

Ruppert, D., & Wand, M. P. (1994). Multivariate locally weighted least squares regression. *Annals of Statistics*, *22*, 1346–1370.

Ruppert, D., Wand, M. P., & Carroll, R. J. (2003). *Semiparametric regression*. Cambridge, UK: Cambridge University Press.

Schwartz, G. (1978). Estimating the dimension of a model. *Annals of Statistics*, *6*, 461–464.

Shakhnarovich, G. (Ed.). (2006). *Nearest-neighbor methods in learning and vision: Theory and practice*. Cambridge, MA: MIT Press.

Schapire, R. E., Freund, Y., Bartlett, P., & Lee, W.-S. (1998). Boosting the margin: A new explanation for the effectiveness of voting methods. *The Annals of Statistics*, *26*(5), 1651–1686.

Schapire, R. E. (1999). A brief introduction to boosting. In *Proceedings of the Sixteenth International Joint Conference on Artificial Intelligence*.

Schapire, R. E., & Freund, Y. (2012). *Boosting* Cambridge: MIT Press.

Schmidhuber, J. (2014). Deep learning in neural networks: An overview. arXiv:1404.7828v4 [cs.NE].

Schwarz, D. F., König, I. R., & Ziegler, A. (2010). On safari to random jungle: A fast implementation of random forests for high-dimensional data. *Bioinformatics*, *26*(14), 1752–1758.

Scrucca, L. (2014). GA: A package for genetic algorithms in R. *Journal of Statistical Software*, *53*(4), 1–37.

Seligman, M. (2015). Rborist: Extensible, parallelizable implementation of the random forest algorithm. R package version 0.1-0. http://CRAN.R-project.org/package=Rborist.

Sill, M., Heilschher, T., Becker, N., & Zucknick, M. (2014). c060: Extended Inference with lasso and elastic-net regularized cox and generalized linear models. *Journal of Statistical Software*, *62*(5), 1–22

Sutton, R. S., & Barto, A. G. (2016). *Reinforcement learning* (2nd ed.). Cambridge, MA: MIT Press.

Therneau, T. M., & Atkinson, E. J. (2015). An introduction to recursive partitioning using the RPART routines. Technical Report, Mayo Foundation.

Thompson, S. K. (2002). *Sampling* (2nd ed.). New York: Wiley.

Tibshirani, R. J. (1996). Regression shrinkage and selection via the lasso. *Journal of the Royal Statistical Society, Series B, 25*, 267–288.

Tibshirani, R. J. (2015). Adaptive piecewise polynomial estimation via trend filtering. *Annals of Statistics, 42*(1), 285–323.

Vapnick, V. (1996). *The nature of statistical learning theory.* New York: Springer.

Wager, S. (2014). Asymptotic theory for random forests. Working Paper. arXiv:1405.0352v1.

Wager, E., Hastie, T., & Efron, B. (2014). Confidence intervals for random forests: The jackknife and infinitesimal jackknife. *Journal of Machine Learning Research, 15*, 1625–1651.

Wager, S., & Walther, G. (2015). Uniform convergence of random forests via adaptive concentration. Working Paper. arXiv:1503.06388v1.

Wahba, G. (2006). Comment. *Statistical Science, 21*(3), 347–351.

Wang, H., Li, G., & Jiang, F. (2007). Robust regression shrinkage and consistent variable selection through the LAD-lasso. *Journal of Business and Economic Statistics, 25*(3), 347–355.

White, H. (1980a). Using least squares to approximate unknown regression functions. *International Economic Review, 21*(1), 149–170.

White, H. (1980b). A heteroskedasticity-consistent covariance matix estimator and a direct test for heteroskedasticity. *Econometrica, 48*(4), 817–838.

Weisberg, S. (2014). *Applied linear regression* (4th ed.). New York: Wiley.

Winham, S. J., Freimuth, R. R., & Beirnacka, J. M. (2103) A weighted random forests approach to improve predictive performance. *Statitical Analysis and Data Mining, 6*(6), 496–505.

Witten, I. H., & Frank, E. (2000). *Data mining.* New York: Morgan and Kaufmann.

Wood, S. N. (2000). Modeling and smoothing parameter estimation with multiple quadratic penalties. *Journal of the Royal Statistical Society, B, 62*(2), 413–428.

Wood, S. N. (2003). Thin plate regression splines. *Journal of the Royal Statistical Society B, 65*(1), 95–114.

Wood, S. N. (2004). Stable and efficient multiple smoothing parameter estimation for generalized additive models. *Journal of the American Statistical Association, 99*, 673–686.

Wood, S. N. (2006). *Generalized additive models* New York: Chapman & Hall.

Wright, M. N. & Ziegler, A. (2015). Ranger: A fast implementation of random forests for high dimensional data in C++ and R. arXiv:1508.04409v1 [stat.ML].

Wu, Y., Tjelmeland, H., & West, M. (2007). Bayesian CART: Prior specification and posterior simulation. *Journal of Computational and Graphical Statistics, 16*(1), 44–66.

Wyner, A. J. (2003). Boosting and exponential loss. In C. M. Bishop & B. J. Frey (Eds.), *Proceedings of the Ninth Annual Conference on AI and Statistics Jan* (pp. 3–6). Florida: Key West.

Wyner, A. J., Olson, M., Bleich, J., & Mease, D. (2015). Explaining the success of adaboost and random forests as interpolating classifiers. Working Paper. University of Pennsylvania, Department of Statistics.

Xu, B., Huang, J. Z., Williams, G., Wang, Q., & Ye, Y. (2012). Classifying very high dimensional data with random forests build from small subspaces. *International Journal of Data Warehousing and Mining, 8*(2), 44–63.

Xu, M., & Golay, M. W. (2006). Data-guided model combination by decomposition and aggregation. *Machine Learning, 63*(1), 43–67.

Zeileis, A., Hothorn, T., & Hornik, K. (2008). Model-based recursive partitioning. *Journal of Computational and Graphical Statistics, 17*(2), 492–514.

Zelterman, D. (2014). A groaning demographic. *Significance, 11*(5), 38–43.

Zemel, R., Wu, Y., Swersky, K., Pitassi, T., & Dwork, C. (2013). Learning fair representations. *Journal of Machine Learning Research, W & CP, 28*(3), 325–333.

Zhang, C. (2005). General empirical bayes wavelet methods and exactly adaptive minimax estimation. *The Annals of Statistics, 33*(1), 54–100.

Zhang, H., & Singer, B. (1999). *Recursive partitioning in the health sciences.* New York: Springer.

Zhang, H., Wang, M., & Chen, X. (2009). Willows: A memory efficient tree and forest construction package. *BMC Bioinformatics, 10*(1), 130–136.

Ziegler, A., & König, I. R. (2014). Mining data with random forests: Current options for real world applications. *Wiley Interdisciplinary Reviews: Data Mining and Knowledge Discovery, 4*(1), 55–63.

Zhang, T., & Yu, B. (2005). Boosting with early stopping: Convergence and consistency. *Annals of Statistics, 33*(4), 1538–1579.

Zou, H. (2006). The adaptive lasso and its oracle properties. *The Journal of the American Statistical Association, 101*(467), 1418–1429.

Zou, H., & Hastie, T. (2005). Regularization and variable selection via elastic net. *Journal of the Royal Statistical Association, Series B, 67*(2), 301–320.

Zou, H., Hastie, T., & Tibshirani, R. (2005). Space principal component analysis. *Journal of Computational and Graphical Statistics, 15*, 265–286.

Index

© Springer International Publishing Switzerland 2016
R.A. Berk, *Statistical Learning from a Regression Perspective*,
Springer Texts in Statistics, DOI 10.1007/978-3-319-44048-4

CPSIA information can be obtained
at www.ICGtesting.com
Printed in the USA
BVOW07*0444300118
506592BV00013B/5/P

9 783319 440477